D0612812

Psychiatry, Ministry and Pastoral Counseling

PSYCHIATRY, MINISTRY & PASTORAL COUNSELING

*A.W. Richard Sipe
& Clarence J. Rowe · Editors*

Second Edition

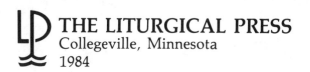

THE LITURGICAL PRESS
Collegeville, Minnesota
1984

First printing, January 1984
Second printing, October 1984

Printed in the United States of America.
Cover design by Don Bruno.

Library of Congress Cataloging in Publication Data

Main entry under title:

Psychiatry, ministry, and pastoral counseling.

Rev. ed. of: Psychiatry, the clergy, and pastoral counseling / Dana L. Farnsworth, Francis J. Braceland, editors.

Bibliography: p.

1. Pastoral counseling—Addresses, essays, lectures. 2. Pastoral psychology—Addresses, essays, lectures. 3. Psychiatry and religion—Addresses, essays, lectures. I. Sipe, A. W. Richard, 1932–   . II. Rowe, Clarence J. III. Psychiatry, the clergy, and pastoral counseling.

BV4012.2.P75 1983   253.5   83-18711

ISBN 0-8146-1324-1

Dedicated to
BALDWIN W. DWORSCHAK, O.S.B.
teacher, leader, pastor, counselor

Contents

7

Part Three — Common Pastoral Problems

The Authors

FRANCIS J. BRACELAND, M.D.: The Institute of Living, Hartford, Connecticut; former editor, *American Journal of Psychiatry;* past president, American Board of Psychiatry and Neurology

J. ALEXIS BURLAND, M.D.: Clinical professor of psychiatry and human behavior, Jefferson Medical College of Thomas Jefferson University, Philadelphia, Pennsylvania; training and supervising analyst, Philadelphia Psychoanalytic Institute

JOSEPH CIARROCCHI, PH.D.: Director of Addictions Services, Taylor Manor Hospital, Ellicott City, Maryland

BARRY K. ESTADT, O.F.M. CAP., PH.D.: Director, Pastoral Counseling Program, Loyola College, Baltimore, Maryland; diplomate, American Board of Examiners in Professional Psychology; fellow, American Associate of Pastoral Counselors

JAMES W. EWING, PH.D.: Executive director, American Association of Pastoral Counselors, Fairfax, Virginia; former professor of pastoral care, Eden Theological Seminary, St. Louis, Missouri

HERBERT S. GASKILL, M.D.: Director, Denver Institute for Psychoanalysis, Denver, Colorado; former president of the American Psychoanalytic Association

JUDD MARMOR, M.D.: Franz Alexander Professor Emeritus of Psychiatry, University of Southern California, Los Angeles, California; adjunct professor of psychiatry, UCLA School of Medicine; past president, American Psychiatric Association

ROBERT J. MCALLISTER, M.D., PH.D.: Adjunct associate professor, Gonzaga University, Spokane, Washington; seminary board, Mater Dei Institute of Priestly Formation, Spokane, Washington

CHARLES MCCAFFERTY, M.D.: Medical director, Adolescent Psychiatric Unit, United Hospitals, St. Paul, Minnesota; clinical associate professor of psychiatry, University of Minnesota Medical School, Minneapolis, Minnesota

9

WILLIAM W. MEISSNER, S.J., M.D.: Clinical professor of psychiatry, Harvard Medical School; training and supervising analyst, Boston Psychoanalytic Institute, Boston, Massachusetts

WALTER D. MINK, PH.D.: Professor and co-chair, department of psychology, Macalester College, St. Paul, Minnesota

PATRICK F. OWEN, M.A.: Licensed clinical psychologist, United Hospitals, St. Paul, Minnesota

MICHAEL R. PETERSON, M.D.: President and medical director, Saint Luke Institute, Inc., Suitland, Maryland; clinical assistant professor, department of psychiatry, Georgetown University Medical School, Washington, D.C.

PAUL W. PRUYSER, PH.D.: Henry March Pfeiffer Professor and Director, Interdisciplinary Studies Program, The Menninger Foundation, Topeka, Kansas

JOSEPH J. REIDY, M.D.: Associate professor, department of psychiatry, The Johns Hopkins University, Baltimore, Maryland; teaching analyst, Baltimore-District of Columbia Institute for Psychoanalysis

HOWARD P. ROME, M.D.: Professor of psychiatry emeritus, Mayo Graduate School of Medicine, Rochester, Minnesota; chairman, faculty of the Cook Institute, The Constance Bultman Wilson Center, Faribault, Minnesota

CLARENCE J. ROWE, M.D.: Medical director, adult psychiatric services, United Hospitals of St. Paul, Minnesota; psychiatric consultant, The Constance Bultman Wilson Center, Faribault, Minnesota; clinical professor of psychiatry, University of Minnesota Medical School, Minneapolis, Minnesota

NATHAN SCHNAPER, M.D.: Professor of psychiatry and oncology, School of Medicine, University of Maryland; distinguished physician, distinguished alumnus, Washington College, Chestertown, Maryland; Humanitarian of the Year (1983), Arlene R. Wyman Guild

A. W. RICHARD SIPE, M.S., C.C.M.H.C.: Board certified clinical mental health counselor, adjunct professor, pastoral counseling, St. Mary's Seminary and University, Baltimore, Maryland

NANCY BRITTON SOTH, M.A.: Librarian, The Constance Bultman Wilson Center, Faribault, Minnesota

M. ROBERT WILSON, M.D.: Psychiatrist-in-chief, The Constance Bultman Wilson Center, Faribault, Minnesota

Foreword

The restoration of health and maintenance of good health are not solely the responsibility of doctors, nurses, and other medical professionals. We all bear a responsibility in this regard, both as individuals and as members of larger social and religious institutions.

> —U.S. Roman Catholic Bishops,
> Pastoral Letter on Health and
> Health Care (1981)

In my reflection and reading of this second edition of *Psychiatry, Ministry, and Pastoral Counseling,* I found myself discovering that I am actually living within that dialogue between religion and psychiatry which has evolved so dramatically in the past thirty years and which is so well described in this book.

As a physician and psychiatrist *and* a Roman Catholic priest, I realize that this dialogue began within me many years ago and continues with each passing year. In practical terms the tension between psychiatry and religion unfolds in many ways. As a psychiatrist, someone ostensibly interested in human behavior and the human mind, I ask where do my counseling and diagnostic skills and interest stop and my Christian ministry begin? Do they end at the neck and disregard the heart? Where does my professional identity extend? Does the internist to whom I send my psychiatric patients feel that I am stepping on his professional toes if I treat the hypertension as well as the depressive symptoms and behaviors? Other questions come and go.

The "tension" between medical professionals, such as physicians and psychiatrists—and even within myself trained as a physician first and a psychiatrist second—will always exist. Very likely, with changes in our understanding of the pathophysiology of diseases and technological advances to deal with them, we shall likely see an increased number of specializations and an even greater blurring of professional borders. Each patient will be subjected to an increasing number of the specialists, who because of their skills see only part of the human person and seldom his or her wholeness. Yet the great upsurge and popularity of holistic approaches to patients and their life problems give the lie to a growing desire to see the person from a perspective of specialized multidisciplinary and multidimensional viewpoints—to restore the wholeness of the patient as a human being.

The Christian and Jewish ministers, who share a common tradition, have seen a dramatic change in the expectations heaped upon them by their people in the past thirty years. Not only are they expected to fulfill their traditional religious roles, but they are presumed to have those special skills of assessing the social, cultural, and family problems experienced in our highly complex society. Yet the minister cannot also be the social or psychiatric social worker, even though he or she unwittingly is thrust into such a position. So where does the role of minister end and where does the role of mental health professional begin? Do not the minister and mental health professional look at the same human being? Yet because of their own specializations either in religion or science, they tend to see human problems in fragmented and partial ways.

The recent development of pastoral counseling, with its own sophisticated and unique methodologies, seems to indicate a viable response to this problem of fragmentation, i.e., of treating only a part of a person without considering the whole. When I think of myself as a Christian minister within the Roman Catholic tradition, the same conflict arises: where does my role as psychiatrist end and my role as minister of the gospel begin? I have not found the answer. It is not so easy to define for and within myself the boundaries of psychiatry and ministry.

As a teacher in a superb professional school for pastoral psychology, I had my first lesson in humility with respect to Christian ministry and pastoral counseling. I found myself teaching psychiatric assessment skills to men and women who were far more experienced than I in dealing with human problems and misery and who had a greater enthusiasm for learning than I ever saw in my medical students. These were persons constantly asking *why* and whether our skills were being applied in the psychiatric profession with the proper understanding of the gospel.

I have learned that only in dialogue with such men and women—only in learning how other disciplines encounter human behavior and the total human person—will I be able to succeed in my own task of healing the troubled human being. I have learned that healing cannot be effected by a single source, but that there must be a variety of approaches from a variety of healing sources before a person can be touched at the many levels of experience and understanding. Each day in the rehabilitation program I direct, I grow more aware, professionally and personally, of my dependence upon a highly skilled and diverse professional staff.

Without each of these staff members' contributions to each patient in the treatment program, there could be no healing of the whole person.

To many readers my observations may seem quite simplistic. You may be thinking, "Where has this man been in the last few years?" I have been to the finest colleges, medical schools, graduate schools, and prestigious centers for medical research; yet I only vaguely remember hearing the word *holistic* or of the need to treat the whole person. I have had to live through this experience to understand it and now finally to contribute to its practice.

Psychiatry, Ministry, and Pastoral Counseling has managed to capture and elucidate these concerns, as expressed in the foregoing paragraphs. And I am sure they are the concerns of many others. The contributors to this volume are diverse in their professional education and experience and in their religious experiences and traditions. They embody the dialogue referred to in the preface, the dialogue between psychiatry and pastoral counseling. Together they offer a discussion that allows us to have a newer and richer perspective of our human problems, our human condition, and our human experiences.

Those in ministry and pastoral counseling can be proud of the contributions they are making in increasing the health of those they touch. This book can likewise be proud of its interdisciplinary approach, the breadth of topics included in the volume, and its sensitivity to the range of human needs and emotions.

Most impressive, and perhaps most important, is this book's underlying message that, with greater knowledge and understanding of how problems are assessed by the different professionals, the minister, who is on the "front line," can be more effective in the healing process. The Christian or Jewish minister touches more lives in a single lifetime through preaching and ministry than our whole medical profession could ever dream of. In order for them to be effective in their teaching and healing roles within their own traditions, they need more and more knowledge and education in the human sciences. This book, in my opinion, makes such a contribution to that educational process, and I would, therefore, recommend its reading to all who are interested in helping people.

— Rev. Michael R. Peterson, M.D.
St. Luke Institute,
archdiocese of Washington;
clinical assistant professor,
department of psychiatry,
Georgetown University Medical School

Preface

The old and the new

The first edition of this book was published in 1969 under the title *Psychiatry, the Clergy and Pastoral Counseling.* It was the by-product of the St. John's University Institute for Mental Health, which was organized in 1953. In 1976 the institute was reorganized as the Institute for Religion and Human Development. Comparing the two editions and the two institutes of which they are a part is like revisiting one's hometown after a period of years. The territory is the same but a great deal has changed. Landmarks can look different and indeed do take on new emphasis when the context around them shifts.

The spirit and intent of the Institute for Religion and Human Development as well as this volume are the same as that of their predecessors. Both book and institute are ecumenical religiously and professionally, but syncretism has been assiduously avoided. What was sought was an honest sharing of perspectives, and as Dr. Paul Pruyser points out in his chapter, " the perspectival model is more likely than any other model to promote mutual respect between disciplines and foster interdisciplinary collaboration."

Already in 1958 Dr. Hyman S. Lippman and Dr. David A. Boyd, Jr., members of the original board of directors, along with Dr. Francis J. Gerty, president of the American Psychiatric Association, read a report of the work of the institute at the 114th annual meeting of the association. They said the goal of the interdisciplinary exchange between religion and psychiatry at St. John's was practical—"improving the understanding and skills of the clergy, who were frequently the first to be consulted in times of trouble [and] engendering a deeper understanding of the human personality and the roots of human behavior."

Although the spirit of respectful collaboration and the goal of understanding human development remain intact, the focus on the clergy was broadened. In the 1950s "pastor" and "clergy" were synonymous with "clergy*man.*" Already in the 1960s the institute cooperated in sponsoring workshops for religious women, although these workshops remained separate but equal experiences. Only in the 1970s could the real burden of sexism be faced and thrown off. Also in the interim the concept of ministry broadened and divested itself of its exclusively clerical nature. Many functions, including pastoral counseling, are included in the gambit of religious ministrations, but not limited to either clerics or men. Women and laypersons have become more actively engaged in these helping professions. We felt that "ministry" even in the title of this edition reflects more accurately the present reality and the focus of the interchange in all of the chapters.

In some ways it is difficult to call this a second edition. Sixteen of its chapters are entirely new. They deal with the same issues, but naturally reflect shifts in emphasis and development of the past decade. Of the remaining five chapters only one remains in mint condition; that is Dr. H. Rome's treatment of crisis intervention, for the principles he outlines are likely to be just as valid in another decade. Dr. F. Braceland revised his three chapters, incorporating the wisdom and insights of his added years of experience. Dr. Herbert Gaskill's chapter on history-taking and diagnosis needed only minor revision to renew its usefulness.

Is there a need?

So much has been written in the past decade about religion and psychiatry generally and pastoral counseling specifically that most serious consideration had to be given to the usefulness of another book in the area, let alone a second edition. Did what the St. John's University Institute for Mental Health stand for, as reflected in its psychiatry and pastoral counseling, really merit a restatement? Our first reaction was cool, bordering on the negative; but the more knowledgeable people we consulted and the more specialists in the ministries and counseling we approached, the more astonished we were at the uniqueness of the original contribution and the soundness of the basic principles. Although outdated, the first edition had not been superseded. Thus, we have striven to abide by the basic principles of the first edition. Each discipline — medicine or theology — is respected. We are not trying to make therapists of ministers or ministers of physicians. At the same time we can acknowledge and respect the necessary struggle of the "bridge dwellers" whom J. Ewing describes. Confidence in one's discipline and an ecumenical openness mark both volumes.

Organization

The organization of this edition is essentially identical to the first edition, merely more explicit in its division into sections. (Two elements of the first edition — the section on sex, marriage, and the family and the section on related issues — have been planned for a coming volume.) Section 1 of this present volume is devoted to the dialogue between psychiatry and religion. The more distant and immediate practical history of this inter-action between religion and psychiatry, represented by the observations of R. McAllister and B. Estadt, are balanced by the ministerial application represented by the statements of H. Gaskill and P. Pruyser, erected on the solid basis of J. Marmor's seven basic principles. And J. Ewing struggles masterfully in the arena that reflects the dynamic tension of this dialogic focus.

Drs. F. Braceland and D. Farnsworth were pacesetters when they organized the core of the first edition around the developmental sequence. Now commonplace after the work of D. Levenson and perhaps almost too popular and glib since treatments like G. Sheehee's, for instance, the approach still has great merit. This volume neither uses the theme of developmental crisis nor seeks a unity of theory or outlook of authors. Instead, this book like its predecessor is not a closed structure of axioms but a blueprint for creative response. Individual differences and even contradictory viewpoints are willingly tolerated. This is the state — and the reality — of the art.

The real emphasis of this second section is on childhood observation and development, represented by the contributions of A. Burland and J. Reidy. Childhood reconstruction and observation after all have been the enduring and unquestionable gifts of psychiatry to the understanding of human development. Both students of religion and of human behavior have gained from the insight. Just as the observations of Spitz and Piaget are being mined continually for the gold of cognitive and moral development, the observations of Margaret Mahler have opened the way to a deeper understanding of the affective development of the person. What Mahler has uncovered, so well described by A. Burland, gives serious students of religious development the tools for a deeper understanding of the affective development of a sense of religion. In fact, this could be a worthy goal of the next decade for the institute: to truly understand the development and stress of the life cycle in terms of the personal journey from the primary other, with and through the significant other, to final union with the ultimate other. This edition only begins that journey, but it does have some clear roadmarks.

The third section of this edition is again devoted to common pastoral problems. The chapter on the affective disorders is the most paradigmatic of the dramatic shift in psychiatry in the past decade and predictive of its future direction. Psychiatry is medicine. No matter how respectful medicine becomes of the humanistic (i.e., the psycho-social), it must not lose its original base in the biophysical and biochemical phenomena. Nowhere have the biomedical discoveries of the past decade confronted psychiatry with its biological responsibilities and possibilities more forcefully than in the understanding of the biochemistry of mood. Instead of throwing psychiatry back to a mechanistic and reductionistic view of the human person as nothing but a machine, a chemical conglomerate, or a computer, it opens up, as C. Rowe says, a fertile avenue for cooperation between minister and physician, since support, insight, and understanding as well as chemical intervention are needed. What is recorded in the current chapter on the affective disorders will be compounded a hundredfold by the end of the century. The implications for all pastoral problems are staggering.

Readers

This edition is respectfully submitted to the new generation of ministers — people who care about people — that broad category of men and women who no longer see themselves hierarchically franchised by rather arbitrary trappings of sex or privilege or power structure. It is offered to the thoughtful and committed educator, preacher, cleric, counselor, and friend who believes in the value of understanding one's self and others, who artfully reveres human development as an awesome reality to be fostered, and who considers the reduction of human suffering and stress a worthy endeavor and a godsome vocation.

This edition is dedicated to Abbot Baldwin W. Dworschak, O.S.B., who served on the founding board of the Institute for Mental Health as well as the reorganized board of the Institute for Religion and Human Development. He is preeminently the modern minister. His pastoral wisdom infused each accomplishment because he chose to serve rather than rule over anyone. His example was a source of strength to those who wrote this book. We humbly hope that his spirit will inspire those who read it.

CLARENCE J. ROWE, M.D.
A. W. RICHARD SIPE, M.S.

St. Paul, Minnesota
Baltimore, Maryland

Acknowledgments

There is an element of presumption involved when two people assume the task of reediting a book that enjoyed originally the services of Dr. Francis J. Braceland, then editor of the *American Journal of Psychiatry,* and Dr. Dana L. Farnsworth, director of the Student Health Services of Harvard University. We presumed the solid basis on which the first edition was established and the goodwill that was engendered by the original production. We were not disappointed. And we were lucky to have the sage advice and active encouragement of Dr. Braceland throughout this project. We thank him for his help. We think his influence is clear in the final product, but reserve for ourselves any limitations or flaws this edition has over the first edition.

We are also indebted to the board of the St. John's University Institute for Religion and Human Development and especially its immediate past executive director, Fr. Timothy Kelly, O.S.B., for encouraging us to put our hand to the plow when Fr. Daniel Durken, O.S.B., director of The Liturgical Press proposed the task. Also Mr. John Dwyer, business manager of The Press, had a gentle persuasion in keeping our noses to the grindstone while he kept a practical eye to larger issues. This is a great service to the work that the Institute hopes to accomplish.

While no foundation funds were available to help with this book, several individuals were generous in their financial support. Dr. and Mrs. J. Alfred LeBlanc of Washington, D.C.; Dr. and Mrs. John Bunce of McLean, Virginia; and Dr. Marianne Benkert of Timonium, Maryland, demonstrated their continuing interest in all the projects of the Institute by generous financial investment in this edition.

Mr. Henry Tom of The Johns Hopkins University Press and a lay minister of Corpus Christi Church in Baltimore gave invaluable assistance during the editorial process. His influence more than any other individual is responsible for quality control.

Patricia M. Rowe, executive secretary of the Minnesota Psychiatric Society, offered warm hospitality and encouragement at several crucial junctures. Mrs. Beverly Brown typed and retyped manuscripts with a speed, accuracy, and good nature that at times improved even content.

To all these colleagues as well as to each author, new as well as old, we are indebted. We were impressed how the spirit that produced the first edition was demonstrated and rekindled anew. This is the spirit of St. John's, Collegeville, for which we are grateful.

PART ONE

Basic Issues: Dialogue

1

Psychiatry and Religion: Yesterday and Today

ROBERT J. MCALLISTER

The December 1980 issue of the *American Journal of Psychiatry* contained a special section on "Modern Religious Experiences and Psychiatry" and an editorial on "Charismatic Religious Experience and Large Group Psychology."[1] These articles published in the official journal of the American Psychiatric Association reflect a remarkable rapprochement between the disciplines of religion and psychiatry. Such was not always the case. Psychiatry's domain had been human emotions; religion's interest, that of values and morality. This was the traditional attitude. Yet recent years have witnessed an increasing awareness of religion's attention to the emotions. At the same time, psychiatry has taken an increasing interest in values and morality. These journal articles represented a behavioral science approach to religious topics such as the conversion experience, the nature of religiosity, cult leadership, and charismatic religious sects. They were an attempt to place values on some of the emotional components of religious experience and as such were examples of the many significant modifications that have occurred between psychiatry and religion.

Early twentieth-century psychiatry took as its subjects of research the behaviors, motivations, conflicts, and emotional and mental aberrations of persons. It approached these areas with a scientific stance that, for the most part, avoided transcendent topics of faith, spirit, and the supernatural. In the latter half of the twentieth century, psychiatry took quite a different attitude. *The Theory and Practice of Psychiatry* offered a clear statement of the reasons why psychiatry and religion share common ground. Their mutual interest

> stems from three needs: (1) a practical need of ministers to acquaint themselves with modern psychotherapeutic techniques; (2) the common interest of theologians and psychiatrists in the human "soul" and destiny; and (3) the needs of psychiatrists and psychologists to understand religious experience.[2]

One could expand this list of shared interests and values: both believe in the value and potential of life; both work toward self-regulation — they value human freedom; both defend values and rights of individuals; both recognize the healing effects of introspection. Religion and psychiatry see life as a process or journey — from primary other to ultimate other. They have a commitment to help persons organize their experiences and relationships in ways that make sense or have meaning and contribute to life. Although one discipline might primarily foster spiritual health and the other might look to eradicating physically related illness, both are involved with persons whom each discipline values. Religion is not reduced to humanism by acknowledging human values — but humanism is crucial to the development and progress of psychiatry, as Gregory Zilboorg said in the conclusion of his *History of Medical Psychology:*

> The whole course of the History of Medical Psychology is punctuated by the medical man's struggle to rise above the prejudices of all ages in order to identify himself with the psychological realities of his patients. Every time such an identification was achieved the medical man became a psychiatrist. The history of psychiatry is essentially the history of humanism. Everytime humanism has diminished or degenerated into mere philanthropic sentimentality, psychiatry has entered a new ebb. Every time the spirit of humanism has arisen, a new contribution to psychiatry has been made.[3]

In his 1980 presidential address to the American Psychiatric Association, Alan Stone called psychiatry "a noble profession because it is both a moral and a scientific enterprise."[4]

History of psychiatry

The history of psychiatry is interwoven with a thread of religion. Yet, it is impossible to recapture fully the shifting moods, the cautious contacts, and the precarious moments that have occurred even over the past eighty years in the uncharted border between religion and psychiatry. Whether considering the present century or earlier ones, it is important to remember that one focus of religion and the central focus of psychiatry have always been persons: developing, struggling, changing, anguished, and mentally afflicted individuals. Religion has always acknowledged the care of the sick as part of the broadly spiritual mission of churches. Medicine has as its *raison d'être* the care of the sick. Whatever interactions take place between the two or whatever understanding occurs, they are both profitable if in some way they help to bring comfort and peace to the mentally ill and the emotionally troubled.

When ministers and physicians explore their deepest origins, they find a common ancestor in the witch doctor — the medicine man. This fact as well as other shared values and traditions should not blur the distinct role each has in ministering to the sick and the afflicted. Conversely, awareness of one's heritage fosters true differentiation (identity, creativity, and cooperation) in three important ways. It establishes the development and continuity of thought in each profession. It clarifies the language that each profession has chosen to describe its observations, and it delineates the perspective from which each profession considers a particular segment of reality. Going to the well-springs of one's professional heritage makes one aware both how much has been accomplished and how much yet remains to be understood in one's field of study and service. It should also develop respect for diverse approaches to shared challenges.

Physicians and ministers will find dross as well as gold in their professional history. Vestiges of magic, materialism, mechanism, and rationalism coexist with objective observation and true spirituality. Early medicine had a great deal of ambiguity about the nature and causes of mental illness. At times it saw mental illness as moral turpitude; at other times, a manifestation of physical disease or a contagion. It equated illness with a fall from grace, a disorder of passion. Illness was weakness, a result of heredity. It attributed mental illness to demonic possession, incompatible body humors, environmental situations, and ancestral sins. Astrology still holds some popular appeal (although psychiatry has long abandoned it). These were some of the uncertainties and obscurities in the history of psychiatry. Through the centuries preceding our own, there were advances and retreats, clarifications and new complexities, and periods of improved understanding and improved care, and periods when gains were lost. From the earliest times through the Renaissance, western medicine struggled with a fragmented view of mental operations, and its medical interventions reflected its understanding. Some of its understanding was perceptive and truly prophetic.

In the fourth century B.C., Hippocrates, the Father of Medicine, wrote of four temperament types: sanguine, choleric, melancholic, and phlegmatic, each of which was thought to result from the interaction of the four bodily humors. Twenty-four centuries later, medicine, in the specialty of psychiatry, is discovering interrelationships between a person's neuroendocrine system (bodily humors) and his or her emotional states. In the Greek culture of Plato's time, one of the treatments of madness was incubation therapy. The patient went to sleep in underground corridors of the temple. During sleep the god Asklepios would appear in dreams and touch the patient's illness. On waking the patient would be healed and his or her dream would be decoded by an interpreter. These therapeutic maneuvers certainly bear a resemblance to modern sleep therapy and dream analysis.

In giving a detailed description of the passions, Cicero in the first century B.C. used the term *libido* to describe "violent desire." The Corpus Juris Civilis of Roman times described conditions of insanity and drunkenness and their effect in lessening criminal responsibility. St. Augustine, writing in the fifth century A.D., revealed insights into the psychology of children and into adult motivations, insights that correspond with those of modern dynamic psychiatry.

Thomas Aquinas in the thirteenth century expressed many ideas consonant with modern psychiatry. He acknowledged the importance of dreams and observed that dreams are often important to examining physicians because they indicate a patient's internal dispositions. He believed that feelings and passions could so affect thinking and judgment as to make people most unreasonable. He seemed to recognize "unconscious" motivations and intentions. He held that sensuality is an undifferentiated and chaotic force within the individual.[5] These ideas do not sound too dissimilar from Freud when he wrote: "The ego represents what we call reason and sanity, in contrast, to the id which is dominated by the passions."[6]

Modern psychiatry

Johann Weyer, who lived in the sixteenth century, is considered by some to be the Father of Modern Psychiatry. He wrote *De praestigiis daemonum,* a volume that contained a strong condemnation of those who believed in witchcraft as an explanation of mental illness. The break with former thinking represented by Weyer's thesis constituted a true revolution in medicine's understanding of mental illness. It acknowledged a biological base for the properties and functions of the mind and opened the door to modern medical psychology with its orientation to the physiological, descriptive, empirical, and experimental. Weyer's writings contain a particularly noteworthy concept, which seems to catapult us into the 1980s. He recommended that nuns in convents who displayed psychological symptoms be returned to their own families, because the needs of the individual took precedence over the rules of the institution. History indicates that Weyer's ideas aroused hostile reactions from theologians, philosophers, and physicians. His ideas were summarily and officially condemned, even though he demonstrated that he was a loyal and dedicated Christian scholar and gentleman. The ideas and spirit of the *Malleus maleficarum* (1487), which justified persecution of illness and provided a textbook for the Inquisition, prevailed for almost a century after Weyer's monumental contribution.

Paracelsus, a contemporary of Weyer, in his book *On the Diseases Which Deprive Man of Reason* (1567), made the first clear reference to the unconscious. He, like Weyer, rejected demonology but suggested the importance of sexual factors in the etiology of hysteria and neuroses. He advocated more humane treatment of mental patients. George Mora, in an historical review of Paracelsus's work, characterized this period as "a very unstable one, of transition from medieval to modern values and systems."[7] Although psychiatry was beginning to define its perspective more accurately with Paracelsus's publication, the word *psychiatry* did not yet appear. In fact, Francis Braceland pointed out that psychiatry was named only in the time of Phillipe Pinel (1801), whose humane approach to mental patients in the Bicêtre and Salpetrière in Paris was a logical extension of the understanding of Weyer and Paracelsus. The term *psychiatry* did not even receive general prominence until after 1918. But the growing interest in applying scientific methodology to the subject of mental disease continued throughout the seventeenth and eighteenth centuries. Paola Zacchia in the seventeenth century stated that only a physician was competent to judge the mental condition of a person (an early territorial claim that psychiatry continues to support).

Mental hospitals

Already in the fourteenth century several institutions had been established for the custody of the mentally ill. Although Bethlehem Hospital in London was founded in 1247, it did not receive lunatics until 1377. This is the same hospital later called Bedlam, where whipping and shackeling were common modes of treatment. Some monasteries and convents as well as certain homes and villages served as hospitable refuges for members of mentally troubled pilgrims in the Middle Ages and before. Some became famous shrines of mental healing, like Metz and Gheel.

The first mental hospital per se was founded in 1409 in Valencia. In 1632 the religious order of St. Vincent de Paul founded St. Lazare, a hospital for the care of the insane, and in 1668 the Brothers of Charity founded the Charité de Senlis for the same purpose. These institutions provided patients with isolation, reading, spiritual exercises, and interviews with the religious staff, and controlled contact with family members. It is by no means an exclusively twentieth-century phenomenon to have religious communities providing contemporary medical practices in the care of the mentally ill. It was in 1793 that Phillipe Pinel's symbolic act of freeing the mentally ill from their chains occurred at the Bicetre in Paris where mentally ill, mentally retarded, and criminals were housed together, and similarly abused. The spirit of decency and humanity prevailed outside revolution-torn France. The new spirit existed in York, England, where, in 1796, under the direction of William Tuke, the Retreat was opened. Here patients were treated as guests in a friendly, understanding atmosphere free from mechanical restraint.

American psychiatry profited from the reform spirit of mental hospitals in Europe and England. America had no history of institutions on its own shores, so when new institutions were established they were free of earlier punitive and restrictive treatment practices. Benjamin Franklin was influential in the establishment of the Pennsylvania Hospital in 1756, the first public mental institution in the United States. Another public hospital was opened in Williamsburg, Virginia, in 1773, and a number of private hospitals were founded in the early years of the nineteenth century, most of them with some religious affiliation.

So-called moral treatment was in vogue during this era. It involved the direct and personal care provided or supervised by the hospital superintendent. It emphasized kind attention and a supportive, accepting and protective milieu, providing adequate nourishment and healthy physical living conditions. The medications available were offered in concert with an emphasis on fostering the normal aspects of the psychotic patient's functioning.

Two champions of "good" psychiatric care were Benjamin Rush (1745–1813), considered the Father of American Psychiatry, and Dorothea Lynde Dix (1802–1887), who crusaded tirelessly in behalf of humane care for the mentally-ill indigent and persuaded lawmakers to establish state mental hospitals to provide health care. Rush's *Medical Inquiries and Observations upon the Disease of the Mind,* published in 1812, was the only American textbook on psychiatry until the end of the century. His ideas and ideals were influential in the establishment of ten state institutions and a number of smaller private mental hospitals founded during the early nineteenth century. The Association of Medical Superintendents of American Institutions for the Insane was founded in 1844 by thirteen directors of these hospitals. This represents the oldest medical society in the United States. *The American Journal of Insanity,* also established in 1844, was the original title of the present-day *American Journal of Psychiatry.*

In 1843, when Dorothea Lynde Dix, a former school teacher, became active in persuading fifteen state legislatures to construct large institutions for the care of the mentally ill, her intention was to extend and insure moral treatment for all who needed it. With the construction of large institutions, the more personal and direct care (what was called "moral treatment") gave way to treatment that was less personal and more physical and that provided limited interest in the familial ties and social needs of patients. Dorothea Dix sought quality patient care, but large institutions, the legislative response to her empassioned pleas, had ultimate difficulty in responding to individual needs, particularly when they separated patients geographically from their usual environment and were understaffed because of budgetary restrictions.

Dynamic psychiatry

The era of dynamic psychiatry began with the work of Sigmund Freud (1856–1939). Jean-Martin Charcot (1825–1893), Ambrose-August Liebeault (1823–1904), Hippolyte-Marie Bernheim (1837–1919), Pierre Janet (1859–1947) and Carl Gustav Jung (1876–1961) are among other names that must be linked with the beginning of this era. Teachers, students, or contemporaries of Freud, this group explored the unfamiliar coasts of the unconscious. Hypnosis was the ship which brought each to the new land. Freud and Jung established beachheads, each going in different directions to chart maps and move inland. It was a discovery that constituted a second revolution. Previously, fledgling psychiatry had been content to lay claim to charted territory – an understanding of mental illness. Psychiatry proclaimed itself the discipline most able to care for the mentally ill. That was no small task, however. It had to convince the courts that psychiatry afforded the mentally ill protection. It had to persuade the Church of the validity of this approach. And it had to teach society that the mentally ill should be treated rather than ridiculed. It can easily be understood why psychiatry took a long time to establish itself as the competent care-giver for the mentally ill.

In time, dynamic psychiatry reached beyond the care of the mentally ill and became interested in the motivating forces in all human behavior. It left the laboratory, the hospital, and the consulting room and entered the world outside these parameters. It became interested in the family, in the social environment, and in all those factors that influenced the individual's psychological development. Psychiatry reached beyond mental illness per se in an attempt to understand human behavior. It did so essentially to focus more acutely on treatment of mental illness. Just as the existence of physical diseases and attempts to treat them forced medicine to the scientific study of anatomy and physiology, so mental diseases pushed psychiatry in the twentieth century to become increasingly interested in patients' psychology, sociology, anthropology, and religion. These interests on the part of psychiatry have not developed without some "in-house" disagreements and turmoil. For the most part, psychiatry's interest and involvement in these other areas have been gradual.

Premature attempts to bridge the gap between psychiatry and religion — the area we are interested in — created some early antagonisms between the two disciplines. For example, Freud explained religion as a figment of man's dependency needs and God as an illusory counterpart of man's father image. Yet, Freud's position provoked many churchmen to look more carefully at this developing discipline called psychiatry. They were curious and suspicious; some were critical and some were hostile. They were made uneasy by the knowledge that a new discipline in the world also spoke of people's intellectual and emotional processes, not in the language of traditional philosophers but in strange dark terms.

These new psychiatrists talked about unconsious processes: id, ego, and superego. The "id" did not seem in any way related to the "passions" of Aquinas. The "ego" seemed at times to be synonymous with being "egocentric" and at other times to be a euphemism for a mechanistic, materialistic view of the person. The "superego" threatened to replace morality with a set of interdictions that were empty echoes of early parental prohibitions. New disciples of psychiatry spoke of sexual drives and sexual behavior without reference to a traditional norm for morality and often without consideration of social mores. They even spoke of sexuality in young children who had not yet reached the age of reason. With such misunderstanding about psychiatry, it is not surprising that those in the field of religion sounded an alarm. And rather typically of those who work in the fields of science, biological or social, these new scientists of human behavior and human maladjustment initially paid little heed to those in religion who began to talk to them, perhaps because so many of them seemed to be shouting.

The furor that Freud awakened in religion gradually abated as religious writers and philosophers distinguished between the acceptable and the unacceptable in emerging psychiatry. R. E. Brennan in *Thomistic Psychology* exemplified a new moderation: "The great merit of Sigmund Freud and his school is that of having shown the real importance of unconsious mental processes and their influence on conscious activities, particularly in the orientation of the individual toward a normal goal of life."[8] Brennan could accept the Freudian theory of instincts and psychoanalysis as a branch of psychiatric study as well as a method of probing the depths of the unconscious. What religion could not accept, according to Brennan, was a theory proposed as a philosophy of the grossest materialism.

In the late 1930s and during the 1940s, the conflict between psychiatry and religion reached its peak. Each side spoke and wrote *about,* rather than *to,* the other side. However, exceptional individuals searched for dialogue and rapprochement. Prominent among those who set the new direction were psychiatrists Thomas Verner Moore, Karl Stern, Gregory Zilboorg, psychologist Noël Mailloux, and theologian Seward Hiltner. Titles like Stern's "Religion and Psychiatry" in *Commonweal*[9] and Zilboorg's "Psychoanalysis and Religion" in the *Atlantic Monthly*[10] were clear signals of the change. American psychiatry was also regrouping its forces. In 1947 the Group for the Advancement of Psychiatry assembled and stated its belief in the dignity and integrity of the individual. It placed social responsibility as the major goal of treatment and emphasized that religion could play a major role in emotional, physical and moral well-being. The conflict between psychiatry and religion was evaporating in the shared sunshine of mutual openness. The most obvious meeting ground for religion and psychiatry was their common interest in the individual. Their mutual concern lay in the struggles, weakness, happiness, and fulfillment of the human being.

Social psychiatry

In the 1940s another trend developed in psychiatry which provided a second meeting place for these two disciplines. The neo-Freudians, led by Harry Stack Sullivan, Karen Horney, and Eric Fromm, were applying classical psychoanalytic concepts to broader social issues and cultural problems. Psychiatrists were becoming seriously concerned about poverty, urbanization, and automation, and their effects on families and individuals. They talked about "values," an area that would later become a "common territory" for psychiatry and religion. In many ways the 1940s set the stage for the improved relations of the 1950s and 1960s.

The 1950s brought psychiatry into close and direct contact with religion largely at the request of religious leaders. Religious leaders of the twentieth century have not been easily intimidated by science. After some initial "analysis" of their own, they found value in dynamic psychiatry: it was easy to accept psychiatry as the caretaker of the mentally ill. Yet, they went two or three steps further—and rather rapidly. They discovered that psychiatry had valid things to say about the development of the human personality and decided that psychiatry could help them in their work with individuals. They came to accept the idea that psychiatry could help them understand themselves better.

Defining the interface

It was principally in the 1950s that religious groups grew to appreciate and use the psychodynamic principles of modern psychiatry. This appreciation occurred in a number of ways. Religious communities sent increasing numbers of their members to institutes and universities for training in behavioral sciences. They were assisted by government subsidies for psychiatric social work, training in clinical psychology, and support of psychiatric residencies. In the 1950s there were but four or five clergy psychiatrists in the United States; in a decade or two that number increased ten times.

Seward Hiltner stated in 1965 that "the most conspicuous achievements in relating religion and psychiatry ten years ago were the programs of chaplaincy service and clinical pastoral training in mental hospitals." He pointed out that a "significant number" of Protestant theological schools appointed to their faculties clergymen from these clinical pastoral training programs and who thus had direct experience in working with psychiatrists. Hiltner maintained that these training programs contributed a great deal to establish early positive encounters between psychiatry and religion.[11]

Dialogue between the two disciplines increased in local psychiatric groups, medical schools, and theological schools. The Academy of Religion and Mental Health, founded in 1954, became a forum for the fruitful exchange of ideas. The American Foundation of Religion and Psychiatry served a similar purpose. More books and articles appeared addressing the issues.

A unique example of the growing cooperative spirit between religion and psychiatry was the St. John's University Institute for Mental Health in Collegeville, Minnesota. In 1953 Alexius Portz from St. John's Abbey and Joseph Quinlan, chaplain from the Hastings State Hospital (Minnesota), conceived the idea of getting together a knowledgeable group to discuss mental health problems and their implications for religion. The abbot and the bishop were supportive. The Hamm Foundation of St. Paul provided generous financial support. A board of directors was assembled, and by the summer of 1954 the first workshop in mental health for clergy of all faiths was held at Collegeville. Even the membership of the board was a sign of new directions: psychiatrists and ministers served together. The Catholic, Episcopalian, Lutheran, and Jewish faiths were represented.

Over the first twenty years of the institute's existence, eighty-two faculty members worked on the project. Nine have served as president of the American Psychiatric Association. The faculty represented clinical practice, university departments, and hospitals. They were chosen because of their high levels of competence in their profession and interest in the goals of the institute. The program brought six faculty members and forty clergy together for a five-day workshop. Three or four workshops of this kind were conducted each summer. Each day there were formal sessions, seminar discussions with groups of ten clergy and one faculty member, informal meetings and multiple opportunities for individual exchange between clergy and faculty. Over twenty-four hundred clergy participated in the workshops between 1954 and 1974. Participants came from all over the United States and Canada, Mexico, Italy, Belgium, Japan, and North Africa. Unquestionably, the St. John's University institute set an outstanding example of interaction between the fields of religion and psychiatry. Yet, this was only a secondary benefit. Its primary goal and primary benefit was to bring mental health training to twenty-four hundred clergy and make them better able to understand and serve others and to appreciate, enhance, and conserve their own gifts.

The spirit of cooperation was in the air. What happened at St. John's caught the mood and the melody. Others were not deaf. It was one among many who began to pick up the tune. Various religious denominations established mental health training in their seminaries, and other universities sponsored workshops on religion and psychiatry. And many psychiatrists who participated in the St. John's workshops served as faculty for other workshops throughout the United States. The Menninger Foundation set up a program for the training of pastoral counselors. Various religious communities organized annual mental health meetings to educate their members. As usual, communities of religious women lead the avant garde of this movement.

The trusting relationship between religion and psychiatry that was established during these years provided another indirect but important benefit. It made access to mental health care less of a stigma for devout

Church members. Certainly there had been an earlier period when many clergy questioned the "threats to faith" of psychiatric care. Indeed, a few may still question, but there is little or no support among their contemporaries for such a position. As psychiatric care became an acceptable treatment for parishioners, it also became an acceptable treatment for Catholic priests; Protestant pastors, their wives, and families; and the men and women of religious communities.

Not only did treatment of illness become acceptable, but so did evaluation of emotional health. Religious communities grew increasingly aware of emotional problems among their members and searched for understanding of these members and greater insight into the psychodynamics of illnesses. It followed quite naturally that these same religious communities asked for psychiatric testing and evaluation of candidates and persons in formation. The fact of mental illness in members of religious communities was accepted as a matter of frank appraisal, and articles appeared in professional journals discussing the subject.[12] [13] [14] For example, T. G. Esau and R. H. Cox[15] and M. K. Bowers[16] wrote on the mental health of Protestant ministers, their wives, and families.

There was still another encouraging involvement of psychiatry in the field of religion. The Second Vatican Council (1962–1965) brought about many changes in the Catholic Church, among them a theological atmosphere favorable to the influence of the behavioral sciences. These two factors, namely, a new theological atmosphere and the new dynamic concepts of the behavioral sciences, produced dramatic and far-reaching changes in religious life. Essays such as those in *Cross Currents of Psychiatry* and *Catholic Morality,* edited by W. Birmingham and J. E. Cunneen, brought together moral theology and psychodynamic principles in considering grace, psychic determinism, guilt, sanctity, and conscience.[17]

The development of conscience became a territory more open to exploration than it had previously been. Against this background, the morality of behavior took on new dimensions, and the validity of some moral decisions came under scrutiny. Clergy saw the importance of personality patterns and emotional states in determining the validity of religious and marriage vows. Psychodynamic insights and the cooperative efforts of the behavioral sciences contributed vital assistance in individual cases of dispensation or annulment. Of far greater importance, they provided theologians with tools to hammer out a much broader perspective in evaluating the questions of moral responsibility. It is clear that dynamic psychiatry has made an important contribution to the lives of thousands who benefited emotionally as well as spiritually from this awareness.

Religious feedback

During the past forty years improved understanding between religion and psychiatry has also led to subtle but no less important changes in psychiatry. The psychiatric literature reflects some of these changes. The fourth edition of E. A. Strecker's *Fundamentals of Psychiatry,* published in 1947, did not list religion in its index.[18] *Modern Clinical Psychiatry,* by A. P. Noyes and L. C. Kolb, followed suit.[19] By comparison, the *American Handbook of Psychiatry,* published little more than a decade later, devoted an entire chapter to religion and psychiatry, coauthored by Kenneth Appel, John Higgins, Mortimer Ostow, and Eilhard von Domarus.[20] *The Theory and Practice of Psychiatry,* by F. C. Redlich and D. X. Freedman, published in 1966, continued the new direction. It too had a section on the relationship between religion and psychiatry.[21]

A landmark volume, "Clinical Psychiatry and Religion," was edited by E. M. Pattison and published in the *International Psychiatric Clinics.*[22] It contains twenty-two articles dealing with the interrelationships between these two disciplines. In addition, it includes a contemporary bibliography on the subject listing over 120 books, twenty-six of which were published in the 1950s and eighty-seven in the 1960s. V. D. Sanua wrote in the *American Journal of Psychiatry* in 1969 that "psychiatry and religion share a common concern for the improvement of mental health. Yet, until a few years ago, there was little interaction or cooperation between these two areas in exchanging valuable information."[23] The remarkable changes in the relationship between psychiatry and religion that occurred during recent decades are a tribute to the many persons of goodwill in both disciplines who searched for dialogue, mutual respect, and understanding.

The moral dimension

Not only do religion and psychiatry share a common concern for mental health, they also have a common interest in moral issues, such as political oppression, social injustice, and family breakdown. Again, there is evidence of change in the position on the part of psychiatry. O. Diethelm, writing in *Treatment in Psychiatry,* published in 1950, stated: "Every physician must heed the patient's religious attitude and needs. However, this will always remain a side issue in the treatment . . . . The physician's own convictions cannot enter into the treatment. . . ."[24]

In the past many psychiatrists tried to keep their own moral convictions and values out of the treatment relationship. Yet, in his presidential address of the 133rd annual meeting of the American Psychiatric Association in 1980, Alan Stone observed:

Psychiatry does not stand outside history or morality, but how do we decide which history and which morality to accept? . . . Psychiatrists are taught to avoid value judgments in their dealing with patients, but I do not believe I make a radical claim when I assert that history and morality are a presence in the therapist's office.

Later he stated:

I am deeply suspicious of anyone who makes the contrary claim that history, morality and human values are all irrelevant to psychiatry . . . . I began to examine the scientific problem of prediction in psychiatry and the moral consequences of my professional activity.

In the same address he spoke of social psychiatry as "the fractious adolescent member of the psychiatric family, disrupting the serenity of the household by arguing about values, morality and social justice."[25] Dana Farnsworth, writing in *Hope: Psychiatry's Commitment,* also called for value systems in psychiatry: ". . . the therapeutic technique of complete tolerance does not represent the psychiatrist's actual belief; and psychiatrists must see that psychiatry as a profession can and should endorse responsible standards of behavior."[26] In the same volume Karl Menninger wrote: "The psychiatrist has the obligation to keep abreast of the moral and ethical implications of every significant development in his society."[27]

This century has indeed witnessed the metamorphosis of psychiatry. Although it clearly developed as a branch on the tree of medicine, there was a period in the 20s and 30s when it grew more detached from medicine. Psychiatrists, and psychoanalysts especially, seemed to be far removed from the laboratory, the general hospital, and the biological aspects of medicine. Psychiatric patients were generally separated from other patients in far off mental hospitals or in the remoteness of the psychiatrist's office. However, the picture began to change in the early 50s when new and effective psychotropic drugs became available for the treatment of mental illnesses. Psychiatrists renewed their acquaintance with physiology and pharmacology. In the past two decades research has intensified in the areas of neurophysiology, neurochemistry, and psychopharmacology, bringing psychiatry into ever closer alignment with its parent fields of medicine and basic sciences.

As psychiatrists moved back into the mainstream of medicine, their patients reentered the mainstream of society. The Community Mental Health Centers Act of 1963 provided a powerful instrument by which the treatment of the mentally ill could take place within their own communities. General hospitals set up psychiatric units or admitted psychiatric patients to medical units. As these changes occurred, more people became involved in the "team treatment" of the mentally ill, so that pastors could maintain contact with their mentally ill parishioners during the various stages of their treatment. Presently, the field of psychiatry represents a wide diversity of interests. The base of research into the biological foundations of human behavior is ever deepening at the same time that the breadth of interest and activity in social, political, and cultural issues is increasing. Yet the primary focus of psychiatry remains the treatment and prevention of mental illness. This focus keeps psychiatry always attendant upon the individual, for it is in the individual that the biological research and the social issues join. Psychiatry can thus meet religion primarily in the individual where the *person forms one basic unit of conviction and conversion.* Psychiatry and religion are both involved in helping and serving the individual whether one defines that service as healing or saving. Either discipline could have originated the comment made by Rimbaud: "It is through constant and confident appeal to responsibility, to moral judgment, and to the courage of being oneself that we will be able to rescue man from the mighty weight of a civilization of necessity and conformism."[28]

Theology and medicine are prepared and poised to wrestle with the conundrums of Job: the meaning as well as the alleviation of suffering and affliction; the preservation and the value of life in the face of limitations, reversals, and the inevitability of death. Their tasks are not identical nor are they in essential opposition. Each must remain true to its calling and at the same time respectful of other perspectives.

Theology and medicine have the commission to struggle deeply with the theory of life, its origin, nature, and destiny. Pastoral counseling needs to appreciate the explorations of both disciplines. Its particular task is to mediate the knowledge in ways that are consonant with human needs and consistent with one's essential identity. It is no small task. Psychiatry has not had an easy path through the history of medicine. Pastoral counseling can expect blind alleys and false starts and rocky terrain and steep grades in its journey toward self-definition. The value in forging a way is twofold: it makes it easier for others to follow, and it opens the way to greater service and productivity to one's fellow travelers.

NOTES

1. M. Galanter & J. Westermeyer. Special section: modern religious experience and psychiatry. *American Journal of Psychiatry* 137 (12), 1980.

2. F. C. Redlich & D. X. Freedman. *The Theory and Practice of Psychiatry.* New York: Basic Books, 1966, 836.

3. Gregory Zilboorg. *A History of Medical Psychology.* New York: W. W. Norton & Co., 1941.

4. A. Stone. A presidential address: conceptual ambiguity and morality in modern psychiatry. *American Journal of Psychiatry* 137 (8): 807–91, Aug. 1980.

5. M. Stock. Thomistic psychology and Freud's psycholanalysis. *The Thomist* 21 (2), 1958.

6. S. Freud. *The Ego and the Id* authorized translation by Joan Riviere. London: Hogarth, 1950, 30.

7. G. Mora. Paracelsus' psychiatry: On the 400th anniversary of his book, *Diseases That Deprive Man of His Reason* (1567): *American Journal of Psychiatry* 124 (6): 812, Dec. 1967.

8. R. E. Brennan. *Thomistic Psychology.* New York: Macmillan, 1941, 352–53.

9. K. Stern. Religion and psychiatry. *Commonweal* 49, 30–33, 1948.

10. G. Zilboorg. Psychoanalysis and religion. *Atlantic Monthly* 183 (47): 45–49, 1949.

11. S. Hiltner. An appraisal of religion and psychiatry since 1954. *Journal of Religion and Health* 4 (3): 217, 1965.

12. T. V. Moore. Insanity in priests and religious. *American Ecclesiastical Review* 95, 601, 1936.

13. M. W. Kelley. The incidence of hospitalized mental illness among religious sisters in the United States. *American Journal of Psychiatry* 115, 72, 1958.

14. R. J. McAllister & A. J. VanderVelt. Psychiatric illness in hospitalized Catholic religious. *American Journal of Psychiatry* 121, 881, 1965.

15. T. G. Esau & R. H. Cox. The mental health of ministers' wives and families. *International Psychiatric Clinics* 5 (4), 1969.

16. M. K. Bowers. *Conflicts of the Clergy.* New York: Thomas Nelson, 1963.

17. W. Birmingham & J. E. Cunneen, eds. *Cross Currents of Psychiatry and Catholic Morality.* New York: Random House, 1964.

18. E. A. Strecker. *Fundamentals of Psychiatry.* Philadelphia: J. B. Lippincott Co., 1947.

19. A. P. Noyes & L. C. Kolb. *Modern Clinical Psychiatry.* Philadelphia: W. B. Saunders Co., 1958.

20. S. Arieti, ed. *American Handbook of Psychiatry,* VL, II. New York: Basic Books, 1959.

21. F. C. Redlich & D. X. Freedman. *The Theory and Practice of Psychiatry.* New York: Basic Books, 1966.

22. E. M. Pattison, ed. Clinical psychiatry and religion. *International Psychiatric Clinics* 5 (4), 1969.

23. V. D. Sanua. Religion, mental health and personalities: a review of empirical studies. *American Journal of Psychiatry* 125 (9): 97, 1969.

24. O. Diethelm. *Treatment in Psychiatry.* Springfield: Charles Thomas, 1950, 43.

25. A. A. Stone. A presidential address: conceptual ambiguity and morality in modern psychiatry. *American Journal of Psychiatry* 137 (8): 888–90, Aug. 1980.

26. A. W. R. Sipe, ed. *Hope: Psychiatry's Commitment.* New York: Brunner/Mazel, 1970, 333.

27. Ibid. 377.

28. W. Birmingham & J. E. Cunneen. *Cross Currents of Psychiatry and Catholic Morality.* New York: Random House, 1970, 135.

2

Pastoral Counseling: Today and Tomorrow

BARRY K. ESTADT

A n article in the *Journal of Pastoral Care* (June 1981) called attention to the contemporary expectation that clergy be available for
counseling as part of their overall ministry:

> A national survey in 1969, in which 2,460 adults were interviewed, indicated
> that nearly one in four adult Americans felt sufficiently troubled to need help
> at some time; that one in seven sought help; that 42 percent of those seeking
> professional help had approached a clergyperson. Seven years later these
> figures were again affirmed in a study by Ronald Lee. These surveys con-
> firmed the continuing demand upon pastors to provide counseling.[1]

The response to this expectation over the past several decades by clergy,
religious, and lay ministers has given rise to the ministry of pastoral
counseling as we know it today.

In reflecting upon and seeking to conceptualize the role of counseling
within ministry, Henri Nouwen's simple schema presented in *Creative
Ministry* is helpful.[2] Nouwen ordered the many activities of ministry
under five headings: preaching, teaching, organizing, celebrating, and
individual pastoral care. In this chapter pastoral counseling will be
treated as a *specific form of individual pastoral care* in which ministers
utilize the knowledge and skills derived from the contemporary helping
professions within a theological and spiritual framework as they work to
meet the needs of individuals, couples, families, and groups who seek
their help.

Individual pastoral care has been a rich part of the tradition of Christian ministry from the earliest days. W. Clebsch and C. Jaekle, in *Pastoral Care in Historical Perspective,* developed the functions of pastoral care under the headings: healing, sustaining, guiding, and reconciling.[3] *Healing* entails helping a person to be restored to a condition of wholeness; *sustaining* consists of helping a hurting person to endure; *guiding* involves assisting perplexed persons to make confident choices; *reconciling* seeks to reestablish broken relationships with others and with God. The authors related these four functions to eight periods of Church history from "Primitive Christianity" to the present "Post-Christendom Era." While individual pastoral care has been part of Christian ministry for some twenty centuries, the effort to reach these goals through the process of pastoral counseling is a twentieth-century phenomenon.

Pastoral counseling, as a specific form of pastoral care, attempts to combine insights and techniques derived from the contemporary helping professions with the insights of theology and faith. The goal of training in pastoral counseling is to provide the minister with the opportunity to work towards a synthesis that includes: an incorporation of the body of knowledge common to the field of counseling theory and practice, the development of specific counseling skills and a general way of being which facilitates personal growth in clients, a formulation of one's personal theological understanding of ministry, and an understanding of one's personal spirituality. Succinctly, the goal of pastoral counseling training programs is to assist individuals in becoming knowledgeable and competent practitioners committed to the counseling ministry.

In the pages to follow emerging patterns in the developing field of pastoral counseling are addressed under six headings: (1) from Freud to growth-oriented eclecticism, (2) from mental health affiliates to ministers with holistic vision, (3) from the intrapsychic and interpersonal to the transpersonal, (4) from the pastoral practice to theological articulation, (5) from therapeutic isolation to denominational relatedness; and (6) from the therapy hour to counseling outreach. The article concludes with challenges facing the pastoral counseling movement.

From Freud to growth-oriented eclecticism

Counseling, as we know it today, grew out of the vocational-guidance movement pioneered by Frank Parsons (1909), the early mental health movement in the United States, the work of G. Stanley Hall in the child-study movement, and the introduction of psychoanalysis to this country in 1909 by Freud's lectures at Clark University. The impact of Freud's psychoanalytic theory predominated throughout the 20s and 30s, with many theorists (e.g., Adler, Fromm, Horney, Sullivan) developing, modifying, and refining the psychoanalytic concepts of Freud and, to some extent, Jung. The explosion of knowledge in American psychology in the 30s and 40s in terms of personality theory (e.g., Murray, Lowen, Allport, Sheldon; Trait and Factor Theory, Learning Theory) added to the sophistication of the contemporary helping professions. The development and popularization of client-centered therapy in the 40s and 50s contributed extensively to the development of contemporary counseling. This was followed by a host of developing theories in the 60s: behavioral counseling, existential counseling, transactional analysis, reality therapy, gestalt therapy, rational emotive therapy, and many more.

Ministers interested in incorporating counseling and psychotherapy into their ministry of pastoral care did so by drawing upon the prevailing theories of their day. The pioneers in pastoral counseling quite naturally sought to incorporate Freudian concepts into their understanding of human growth and development. Today, given the rich diversity of theory and technique in the field of counseling and psychotherapy, candidates preparing for the counseling ministry are encouraged to become familiar with a wide range of theorists in order to develop a personal style within the framework of a *growth-oriented eclecticism.* Underlying such a framework is the assumption that theoretical constructs and counseling techniques are the brushes and colors that the counseling artist uses in attempting to capture the richness of the human experience. Each school of thought offers a variety of constructs that are helpful in understanding the complexity of the human person. Each school has its unique techniques for facilitating the personal growth of the client. No school is complete in itself.

With a view towards facilitating the development of an integrated growth-oriented eclecticism, Howard Clinebell examined the concepts and techniques of each major theorist from the perspective of a "growth-hope" model, based on his assumption that the central task for the pastoral counselor was to awaken "realizable hopes for creative change" and to help people to actualize these hopes.[4] Clinebell highlighted, in each theory, the insights that illuminate the process of moving towards greater wholeness and identified methods that nourish such growth. The task for each individual pastoral counselor, and the goal of pastoral counseling training programs, is to work towards an integration of theory and practice in the person of the pastoral counselor—an integration that incorporates an understanding of the use of contemporary psychological theory and technique within the age-old ministry of pastoral care.

From mental health affiliates to ministers with holistic vision

During the 40s and 50s rapid developments within the field of counseling theory and technique left many clergy feeling inadequate in terms of their own pastoral care functions of healing, sustaining, guiding, and reconciling. Ministerial training in preparing for these traditional functions, though theologically thorough, typically lacked the richness of theory and therapeutic skills that had become part of the professionalism of the contemporary helper. At the same time, people sought out psychiatrists and psychologists, finding in them a new source of acceptance, support, direction, healing, and reconciliation. Psychiatrists and psychologists became for many people secular counterparts of the ministers. It is not surprising under such circumstances that many clergy began to feel like junior partners, even "mental health affiliates," as psychiatrists and psychologists took on an increasingly prominent role in providing many of the functions that were traditionally allotted to the minister.

The pastoral counseling movement had its origins in the interest of individual clergy and religious in utilizing the theoretical body of knowledge and clinical skills of the contemporary helping professions of psychiatry, psychology, and social work within the overall ministry of the Church. A large number of Protestant ministers who pursued this interest came from the ranks of the Association of Clinical Pastoral Education (ACPE), which gave birth in 1964 to the American Association of Pastoral Counselors (AAPC), an organization created to promote the ministry of pastoral counseling and the professional competence of pastoral counselors. Catholic clergy and religious with such interests gravitated toward universities for training in clinical and counseling psychology. In the 50s and 60s the psychology departments of Fordham University and The Catholic University of America, to mention only two institutions, had dozens of clergy and religious enrolled in doctoral programs. Many of these graduates were active in the American Catholic Psychological Association (ACPA), founded in 1947 as an ongoing forum for working towards an integration of psychological data and theories with religious thought and practice. ACPA's success in creating a climate for religious dialogue among psychologists is evidenced by the dissolution of the organization and the creation of a new division within the American Psychological Association, i.e., Division 36: Psychologists Interested in Religious Issues. Ecumenical in scope, Division 36 has grown to include 1,380 members, fellows, and associates.

Most candidates entering pastoral counseling programs today do so specifically because they wish to enhance their skills as ministers. They do not want to become psychiatrists, psychologists, or social workers but ministers able to utilize effectively the counseling process within the age-old ministry of individual pastoral care. They do not consider themselves as ancillary to mental health professionals; rather they view their counseling within the overall ministry of the Church. The primary goal of ministry is not to promote mental health, though frequently it does so. Rather the goal of ministry is to give witness to God's loving care as people search for meaning and purpose on life's journey. To the extent that the contemporary disciplines of psychiatry and psychology enrich the understanding of the human journey, and to the extent that they promote the well being of the human person, to that extent, psychology, psychiatry, and ministry are partners in a broad ministry of human caring.

From the intrapsychic and interpersonal to the transpersonal

In the 50s and 60s much of the focus in pastoral counseling was on the *clinical* and *scientific* method. Clergy manifested a keen interest in becoming truly "professional" in terms of acquiring a level of clinical and scientific expertise comparable to their colleagues in other helping professions. They borrowed theoretical constructs and clinical methodology from these disciplines. Many books by clergy and religious emerged in the 60s dealing with the application of personality theory and counseling techniques within religious settings. Most of the literature focused on the *intrapersonal,* as ministers sought to enrich their understanding of the human person through the utilization of the scientific and clinical method.

Today, however, a review of the literature reveals an attempt to utilize the clinical and scientific method to study the *transpersonal* dimension of the human person, i.e., the relationship of the individual to God, along with the interrelationship of the transpersonal with the intrapsychic and the interpersonal. Recent annual convention programs of the AAPC and Division 36 of the APA reflect this emerging interest. At the 1982 APA meeting in Washington, D.C., the presidential address for Division 36 was entitled "Experience of the Other: Personal and Transpersonal Considerations." At the 1982 AAPC convention in San Antonio, programs on "spiritual direction" and the "use of ritual" in the counseling process indicated a growing professional awareness that a holistic understanding of the human person frequently requires an exploration of the client's relationship to God.

There is a growing awareness today of the convergence of a holistic counseling which includes the "transpersonal" dimension of the human person with the art of "spiritual direction" arising out of the Church's long spiritual and mystical tradition. K. Culligan, in a chapter entitled "The Counseling Ministry and Spiritual Direction," commented:

> Although its name and methods derive from the past, spiritual direction harmonizes with new forms of counseling which have emerged in the Church following the advent of modern therapeutic psychology. If we view our counseling ministry as the Church's attempt to help all her people grow in all their relationships, then spiritual direction, which concentrates on the person's relationship with God, coordinates with other specialties such as psychotherapy, group therapy, marriage and family counseling, crisis counseling and career guidance where the focus is on the person's relationship with self, others, things or events. In this view the spiritual director is a counselor in the Church whose primary focus is helping persons grow in their relationship with God through prayer.[5]

Spiritual direction, a strong tradition in Roman Catholicism, especially within the religious communities of men and women, has enjoyed a notable resurgence of interest in the past ten years as religious communities rediscovered their roots and unique traditions. An important part of renewal in spiritual direction has been an effort to incorporate the insights of contemporary personality theory and the many advances in the field of counseling and psychotherapy. This is reflected in the rich literature on contemporary spiritual direction in traditional journals. It has also resulted in the foundation of the journal *Human Development,* which is dedicated to "interpreting the wealth of information in psychology, medicine and psychiatry impacting on the work of persons engaged in spiritual guidance and counseling."[6]

More recently there are signs of the beginnings of interest on the part of the general pastoral counseling movement to incorporate the Church's rich spiritual direction tradition into the preparation of pastoral counselors. This attempt at an integration of spiritual direction within the total preparation of pastoral counselors was noted at the 1983 AAPC convention in a workshop entitled "God's Action; Our Response," which dealt with the practicum training in spiritual direction and an application of the clinical case-study method to the training of spiritual directors. The spiritual direction practicum, as described, was similar to the traditional counseling practicum in that sessions were recorded for critique in individual and small group supervision and for study in interdisciplinary case conferences. It differed, however, in that the primary focus in the counseling practicum was on the intrapsychic and the interpersonal, while in spiritual direction the primary focus was on the transpersonal, specifically, the individual's relationship with God.

From pastoral practice to theological articulation

Pastoral counseling from its inception has been an arena for innovative practitioners who have attempted to employ the clinical method to enrich ministry. In the best spirit of pragmatism, they have drawn from the contemporary helping professions whatever appeared to work, bypassing whatever seemed ineffective. The functionalism of the ACPE movement has influenced many pastoral counselors. Seward Hiltner, in 1975, while acknowledging the contribution of ACPE to "functional competence," urged ACPE to "relate its insights more profoundly to the theology of the church." He commented to a European audience:

> I am afraid that neither I nor my successors are going to push the movement to relate its insights more profoundly to the theology of the church. If catastrophe hit the movement, it might realize that to gain theory is not to lose function. But short of that, or of some truly charismatic interpreter who can show our current onesidedness, I am afraid that you Europeans are going to continue to be justified in regarding American CPE as theologically uninterested and unsophisticated. There is one other possibility: If you, starting from theory, can actually relate theology to what emerges from CPE, then you may influence CPE leaders here. If you can, you will be genuine prophets not only for Europe but for America as well.[7]

Hiltner's critique in 1975 could also, for the most part, apply to the AAPC at that time. Although the critique continues to have validity today, there is growing awareness of the need for pastoral counselors to reexamine their theological and ministerial roots. In "Recovering Lost Identity," the lead article in the March 1980 *Journal of Pastoral Care,* Thomas Ogden eloquently called pastoral counselors to this task:

> The task which lies ahead is the development of a post-Freudian, neoclassical approach to Christian pastoral care which has taken seriously the resources of modernity, but which has also penetrated its illusions, and having found the best of modern psychotherapies still problematic, has turned again to the classical tradition for its bearings, yet without disowning what it has learned from modern clinical experience.[8]

Today there is a growing articulation both by grass-roots practitioners and by professors of theology and pastoral care of the religious underpinnings of pastoral counseling and its relationship to ministry. The recent book *Pastoral Counseling* described the pastoral counselor as "a religiously integrated person who approaches others with a sense of mystery, along with an ability to enter into communion with others in a therapeutic alliance, with the goal of reconciliation and personal religious integration."[9] In developing that description one chapter dealt explicitly with the religious and faith dimension of pastoral counseling: the counselor is a person of faith, who approaches counseling within the context of faith, with a view of holistic growth on the part of the client.[10]

From therapeutic isolation to denominational relatedness

There is a growing recognition in many churches of the need for quality counseling within the overall ministry of the Church. The contemporary response to training programs in pastoral counseling centers by clergy, religious, and lay ministers whose primary intention is in ministering as members of parish or institutional pastoral teams represents a clear realization of that need. In the first six years of the master's program of Loyola College in Maryland (1976-1982), graduates included 72 clergy, 54 religious brothers and sisters, and 47 lay persons. Of these graduates, some 85 percent are utilizing their training in pastoral counseling as pastors, chaplains, and members of pastoral teams; 15 percent are engaged in a specialized pastoral counseling ministry.

Preaching, teaching, and liturgical roles of a pastor or chaplain provide a visibility and availability enjoyed by few other members of the helping professions. Through these activities they enter into periodic contact with a large number of people. As a result it is quite natural for people to seek out the minister at times of special stress or need. Counseling is integral to the pastoral role:

> It is deeply connected with other functions of ministry. Frequently the counseling relationship is a natural follow-up to preaching and teaching as individuals attempt to integrate and to internalize the gospel message presented to them in the pulpit and through the many forms of religious instruction.[10]

The role of counseling within the general pastoral setting has implications for the multidimensional functions and relationships of the pastor, chaplain, or member of a pastoral staff. In a chapter entitled "The Counseling Pastor," the rich potential for counseling within a general ministry setting is explored. Opportunities are identified under the headings: short-term counseling, referral for long-term insight therapy, ongoing supportive counseling, spiritual direction, education for living a fuller life, developing a professional counseling staff, and empowering volunteers. As this list suggests, today's counseling minister, in addition to providing direct counseling services, has the opportunity to offer rich educational experiences that assist people in leading full and satisfying lives.

From the therapy hour to counseling outreach

After undergoing training in counseling, many ministers find that their experience in counseling has a profound impact on their style of ministering in areas other than counseling and individual pastoral care. They point to an increased "person-centeredness" in all areas of ministry. In teaching and preaching, they find themselves beginning with the human experience, identifying with the daily struggles of their people. They see themselves bringing a new awareness of the inner experience of people to the traditional practices, prayer life, and liturgical functions of their congregations. They approach their many meetings with church groups and organizations with a renewed sense of ministry, seeking to serve as catalysts in fostering the inner growth of individuals and groups as projects are organized and implemented.

As the realization of the deeper needs of people emerges at the level of the local congregation, ministers with training in counseling and other religiously oriented counselors have new opportunities to mobilize the resources of the community in order to work towards meeting those needs. Every parish has the poor, the widowed and divorced, the housebound, people struggling with addiction to drugs and alcohol, the unemployed, the depressed, the mentally ill, the suicidal, and a host of struggling people looking for acceptance, understanding, and support, as they seek meaning and purpose in life. The vast majority will not find their way into the pastoral counseling center for weekly therapy; yet these are people yearning to tell their story and to be heard.

If their story is ever to be told, however, it will require creative outreach efforts on the part of those who minister at the grass-roots level of contact. The counseling pastor and staff must extend themselves in such a way that those who need help will be encouraged to accept it. Over and over again, the therapeutic literature in the field of counseling outcomes points to the critical importance of "hope" in the healing process. For many people simply being heard within the context of a caring relationship is an experience that they will never have unless a pastoral person reaches out to touch them.

The issue here is one of pastoral *initiative* versus waiting for people to cross the office threshold. Through a ministry of creative counseling outreach, pastoral counselors at the parish level can meet the needs of people who would never find their way to the counseling office or center.

In a world of social upheaval and extreme need, pastoral counseling cannot offer a panacea for complex problems. Its practitioners, however, can be "prophetic" by communicating to the world of helping professionals the need for the poor and the disadvantaged to have their stories heard in an atmosphere of acceptance, understanding, and care. Highlighting the role of counseling at the level of the local congregation should not suggest the disappearance of the pastoral counseling center; rather it allows for a rich opportunity for specialists within the centers to take an active consultative role with pastors and other members of ministerial staffs. As one of the major challenges ahead, the pastoral counseling movement can realize its full potential by exploring how and in what context pastoral counseling can best serve the needs of a great diversity of people. Further efforts to understand the potential for counseling within the local congregation will only serve to point up the desirability of having specialists who are removed from the local scene. An effective local counseling ministry will need to call upon specialists from pastoral counseling centers not only for the referral of long-term clients but also for ongoing supervision and the conduct of educational programs. Through an exploratory and cooperative process, specialist and generalist can minister in mutual interdependence as they seek to give witness to God's acceptance, forgiveness, and healing power.

Challenge of the future

For nearly two decades the AAPC has sought to organize ministers specially interested in counseling with a view to setting standards for pastoral counseling and developing training programs. While the majority of the membership through the years has been ordained Protestant clergy, in recent years Roman Catholic priests, brothers, and sisters (.5 percent of the membership in the 1982–1983 directory) have joined the ranks of AAPC. At the nineteenth annual convention, Donald Houts, president, in his written welcome to the members, commented:

> The AAPC stands in a unique position to the faith groups/denominations, the mental health field and the society at large. How we utilize our position, manage our resources and articulate our policies, demonstrates our capacity to provide leadership to the pastoral counseling movement.

The challenges facing the AAPC and the broader pastoral counseling movement involve many of the issues inherent in ministry today, including the emergence of lay ministry within a number of faith groups. Specific challenges for pastoral counseling in the decades ahead have been alluded to under the six "emerging patterns" discussed above. The agenda includes:

1. Pastoral counselors must move beyond the adoption of theory and practice from psychology and psychiatry to include a self-conscious

awareness, appreciation for, and ability to utilize the full resources of the Church's ministry, including the ministries of preaching, teaching, organizing, and celebrating.

2. Pastoral counselors must develop a pastoral vision that moves beyond the goal of clinical competence to that of witnessing to God's loving care as people search for meaning and purpose.

3. Pastoral counselors must move beyond the intrapsychic and interpersonal dimension of the human person to include not only a sensitive awareness of the transpersonal dimension, but a growing level of expertise in spiritual direction, understood as the process of facilitating the client's relationship to God.

4. Pastoral counselors must move beyond the pragmatic and the functional to an in depth reflection on the rootedness of their ministry within the overall mission of the Church.

5. Pastoral counselors must move from marginal denominational investment to a vital pastoral identity within their own faith groups, concern for the total ministry, including new as well as traditional forms of ministry.

6. Pastoral counselors must move beyond the middle class model of psychotherapy to include the element of pastoral initiative in reaching out to the vast numbers of hurting people who will never find their way to the pastoral counseling center.

As pastoral counseling moves into the decades ahead, it will need to deal creatively with the tension of integrating clinical competence in counseling and psychotherapy with commitment to the overall ministry of the Church. In attempting such an integration, pastoral counseling serves as a bridge between the sacred and the secular, between the Churches and the mental health professions. A bridge requires a firm foundation on both of its shores.

NOTES

1. P. Kim & F. Van Tatehnove. The utilizability of the pastoral counseling response scale (PCRS). *Journal of Pastoral Care* 35(1): 81–98, June 1981.

2. Henri J. Nouwen. *Creative Ministry.* New York: Doubleday & Co., 1971.

3. W. Clebsch & C. Jaekle. *Pastoral Care in Historical Perspective.* New York: Prentice-Hall, 1964.

4. H. Clinebell. *Contemporary Growth Therapies.* Nashville: Abingdon Press, 1981.

5. K. Culligan. The counseling ministry and spiritual direction. In *Pastoral Counseling.* New York: Prentice-Hall, 1983.

6. J. Gill. *Human Development.* New York: Jesuit Education Center for Human Development, 1980 to present.

7. S. Hiltner. Fifty years of CPE. *The Journal of Pastoral Care* 29(2): 90–98, June 1975.

8. T. Ogden. Recovering lost identity. *Journal of Pastoral Care* 34, 4–19, March 1980.

9. B. K. Estadt. Profile of a pastoral counselor. In *Pastoral Counseling.* New York: Prentice-Hall, 1983.

10. B. K. Estadt. *Master's Program In Pastoral Counseling (1976–1982): A Self-Study.* Manuscript prepared for USCC & AAPR accreditation visits, 1982.

3

Psychotherapy: Basic Principles

Although we speak of psychotherapy as though it were a unitary entity, in actuality there is no single form of psychotherapy. Techniques, patients, therapists, and even therapists within any given school of psychotherapy vary widely in their styles, manners, and approaches to patients. This multiplicity of variables makes success of any individual therapy difficult to assign as proof of the validity of a particular school of thought or mode of intervention. There is more to psychotherapy than simply technique. Patients respond to diverse approaches. If psychotherapeutic success were primarily attributable to a particular technique (as each school of thought claims), then logically no other school of thought or technique should work as well. This is just not the case. Research in the past few decades has begun to shed some light on the nature of the psychotherapeutic process. We have learned that there are certain common denominators in the process of psychotherapy that cut across all schools of thought.

The following seven elements are common to all forms of psychotherapy: relationship, emotional release, cognitive learning, conditioning, identification, suggestion and persuasion, and reality testing.

1. Relationship

The client-therapist relationship should be the single most important factor in securing psychotherapeutic success. The patient-therapist relationship encompasses the unconscious, transference, and countertransference elements that the analytic tradition has clarified. It also includes conscious positive and negative realistic aspects. All of these factors combine to form the therapeutic transaction. Each person — patient and therapist — contributes something to the therapeutic experience.

What does the person ("patient" or "client") seeking psychotherapy expect of the experience? First, on some level there generally is a perceived need to change. "Something has to change." "Things can't go on like this." Even if, initially, the need for change is projected onto a spouse or the environment, some desire to alter a situation precedes the patient seeking help. This need for change must be accompanied by a second factor to begin effective therapy. That element is motivation. Motivation is that degree of responsibility which transforms the need for change from an idle wish to a possibility. Usually without these first two elements, a person will not engage in therapy past an evaluation. Third, the patient has a certain hope from the encounter. Implicitly, if not explicitly, the person has an expectancy of getting help from the therapist. This hope, the expectation of being helped, is critical to the treatment transaction. Its absence constitutes a most powerful resistance to change or cure. In one sense the patient who is seeking help endows the therapist with a help-giving potential. In another way the hope is based on the reality of the therapist's social role and participation in the whole healing tradition. Fourth, the patient also presents his or her ego strengths as well as limitations. It is out of these forces that the new functioning and the greater autonomy will hopefully emerge. Of course the patient also brings the "nature of his or her illness," or a particular constellation of symptoms, needs, and fears. The patient, in short, presents a total person — not merely a problem.

The therapist too engages his or her particular person in the encounter. The early psychoanalytic literature often read as though therapists were interchangeable, like razor blades. The major emphasis of that early period was on the nature of interpretations. The presumption was that as long as the therapist produced the correct interpretation at the auspicious moment, the patient would get better. Recent literature acknowledges other important factors in the therapeutic alliance — the "real relationship," as well as counter-transference. We have learned that therapists are not interchangeable, for a great deal hinges on the actual attributes of the therapist. Among the most important qualities the therapist must bring to the relationship are knowledge, objectivity, empathy, and integrity.

Knowledge in the therapist implies not only adequate training, but more. Training and discipline in a therapist are absolutely necessary, but so too is the capacity for "understanding." There is probably no one word for it. It is the gift of being able to apply and transcend book learning within an ongoing and developing relationship. It implies the ability to use oneself as an instrument of measure. It encompasses a self-awareness which is neither self-conscious nor self-absorbed. It is inquiring, reverent, and self-assured – all in one.

Regarding *objectivity,* the traditional model of passivity where absolute anonymity and lack of any emotional response was considered ideal does not apply here. That therapeutic stance of the therapist was meant to establish a kind of "impersonal mirror" against which patients' unconscious conflicts could be most clearly elaborated. It became a very popular model for therapists, but it did not serve the best interests of the psychotherapeutic relationship.

The therapist does need to be objective. It goes without saying that the patient is not well served if the therapist is carried away on an emotional wave – that can be destructive to the patient. Yet objectivity does not obviate humanness. Patients are surrounded by a world of family, friends, or strangers, who are either overinvolved, rejecting, or indifferent. The therapist's objectivity is the *fair neutrality* that allows the patient to be him- or herself. The objectivity that the therapist brings to the relationship is a constant, stable caring in face of the struggles of a person who is developing. It should not get in the way of the client's growth.

Experimental studies have demonstrated that qualities such as warmth and *empathy* play a significant part in the percentage of therapeutic successes that can be anticipated. Generally therapists who are warm and empathic in their relationship to patients are more effective therapists. The cold, indifferent research model, a caricature of psychoanalysis, has given way in dynamic psychotherapy to a model that allows the therapist to be human, interactive, and empathic.

The values of the therapist, although not imposed, or even consciously exposed, in the relationship, will nevertheless show. The *integrity* that the therapist brings to the therapeutic relationship is not an inconsequential factor in the outcome of therapy. Actually it is not so important what the therapist says or does not say; more important is who the therapist is as a human being.

There is, then, in all therapies, of whatever type, a basic healing relationship that creates, hopefully, both a positive transference and a good working therapeutic alliance.

2. Emotional release

Some *emotional release* (generally brought about by talking) takes place in every form of psychotherapy, be it behavioral, humanistic, cognitive, or analytic. A client is encouraged to talk about his or her person, about his or her problem. In the very process of talking, most clients experience some initial relief. In the early days of analysis, we called this the honeymoon period. For if the therapist was nonresponsive and imposed a strict analytic model, the feeling of improvement often disappeared and the honeymoon was soon over. When the therapist, of whatever persuasion, interacts appropriately with the patient, however, the process of talking often effects a relief of tension and becomes part of an ongoing therapeutic experience. Freud attributed this experience to the discharge of tensions, which he called catharsis. We know now that a more complex process takes place. The ego is much more involved. For the patient talking begins a process of labeling, structuring, and organizing the problem. The understanding or active listening of the therapist establishes a hope and an expectation of relief within the context of the therapeutic relationship. With the understanding established, one can face fears, hates, losses, etc. that were hitherto unspeakable. Initial relief becomes a paradigm for the possibility of a whole range of emotional shifts.

3. Cognitive learning

All therapies have an element of cognitive learning. In one way or another every therapist conveys his or her therapeutic objectives and teaches techniques by which he or she hopes to achieve those objectives. In one way or another, the therapist offers some explanation about how change is going to occur. Those of us who are dynamically-trained teach by tracing the client's life history. It is clear that we attribute certain problems and psychopathology to certain experiences in the course of that history. We imply that if the patient will talk about *these* matters and will understand them in relationship to present functioning — therapeutic relief will follow.

Behavioral therapy attributes all of its results to desensitization and the deconditioning process. Although theoretically behavioral therapy eschews the cognitive, even Wolpe's work on film clearly demonstrates a cognitive element. From the very beginning, he takes a careful history. He shows the patient how and why a fear developed. He explains how the deconditioning or desensitization process works. The implications are apparent: if the patient develops a program with the therapist and follows it step-by-step under direction, the therapy will have its effect. There is both a cognitive and suggestive element present in all this.

The Gestalt strategy approaches therapy from an emotive and existential point of view. A client comes to therapy with certain inhibitions, fears, or angers, which personally have never been accorded full expression. The Gestalt therapist conveys to the client that during the course of the therapeutic work together, the client will learn to express these feelings and as a consequence will feel and function better. So again, there is a cognitive (and suggestive) element.

Rogerian client-centered therapy emphasizes assiduous neutrality, expressed in its reflective method, all in the service of aiding a client's accurate perception of him- or herself. Even here, however, what the therapist chooses to reflect and what is bypassed, provides subtle clues to what needs to be learned in order to function better.

Each therapist's knowledge, way of looking at things, value system and "techniques," however subtle and idiosyncratic, contribute to the exercise of each therapy. Being involved in any therapy exposes one to a degree of cognitive explanation for the problems and the process at hand.

4. Conditioning

In behavioral therapies conditioning is, of course, overt and explicit. A certain element of conditioning is present, however, in all therapies, even if it is covert and implicit. This is true of classical analytic therapy as well as any other. By what we choose to consider neurotic, we convey a certain set of values. *Neurotic* and *nonneurotic* are really modern scientific labels for what we consider healthy or unhealthy, mature or immature, good or bad, for the patient. In the process of therapy, with its multiple and repeated interpretations, we are in effect encouraging patients to be nonneurotic, healthy, mature, or good and discouraging them from being neurotic, sick, immature, or bad (positive-negative, constructive-destructive: choose your preferred language game). So, we condition (and are conditioned) by our value-laden conceptions of what we consider positive or healthy.

There are subtle ways in which such conditioning takes place. From behind the couch, the points at which an analyst says "mm-hmm" or chooses to remain silent are subtle operant cues. In face-to-face therapies the tone of voice or the inevitable body expressions, the lift of an eyebrow, the shrug of a shoulder, the look of approval or disapproval, are all nuanced operant cues, indicating what is considered healthy or unhealthy, neurotic or mature. They act as operant conditioning responses.

Franz Alexander referred to another kind of conditioning, the "corrective emotional experience" of therapy. The new and different reaction of the therapist to the patient and his or her neurotic behavior constitutes a new experience. The more objective and mature response of the therapist conditions the patient to a different kind of emotional experience than he or she had with significant figures in the past. The therapist listens, accepts, and respects the patient and his or her efforts. Anger is not retaliated but heard out. Attack is not reciprocated, but tolerated and understood. Faulty attempts and failures are not punished, but accepted; and renewed effort and success are encouraged. These corrective emotional experiences are all operant responses.

As the patient attempts new ways of adapting to life situations, a third mode of conditioning takes place, through trial-and-error learning. These experiences are reinforced in daily life and often reviewed and evaluated in the therapeutic sessions.

5. Identification

Every psychotherapeutic process involves an element of modeling or identification. A great deal of human learning takes place through modeling. Children learn to walk and talk by observing other human beings. They are not actually taught these skills. They model themselves upon the examples they see. They practice and gradually acquire these skills. Indeed in the course of a psychotherapeutic relationship over time, patients may often acquire mannerisms, certain ways of talking, or values of the therapist, without realizing it. Some writers call this social learning; others call it identification. It is another factor in the psychotherapeutic process. Its importance has been confirmed by the more recent trend toward observing therapy sessions for training, research, or therapeutic purposes. Outside observers can see the process more clearly than the therapist involved.

6. Suggestion

Some element of suggestion and persuasion, whether implicit or explicit, plays a part in all therapies. Behaviorists who say there is no suggestion in desensitization or reciprocal inhibition therapy simply are failing to see the persuasion and suggestive elements involved. An outside observer can see them clearly. Similarly, therapists of the cognitive school say there is no element of suggestion, only cognitive interpretation, in their method. On the contrary, suggestion does take place in cognitive therapy. This is not to say that cognitive interpretations are ineffective. They can be, and often are, powerful and helpful in therapy. But to see any therapy in unifactorial terms, to attempt an explanation in terms of a unitary element, ignores the multiple facets of the patient-therapist interaction. Some therapists tend to downgrade its importance because it can be so easily and destructively misused by faith healers and charlatans.

7. Reality testing

In all therapies there is a certain degree of reality testing. Learning theorists refer to this element as rehearsal; educators call it practicing. A patient learns new attitudes, new ways of coping in therapy. These new techniques have to be taken out of the therapist's office and into the world at large, where they have to be applied and practiced. Beginnings in any learning tend to be tentative, fragile, and easily given up, so the therapist plays an important role in encouraging the patient to persevere in the new attitudes and to apply the new techniques of coping. Some discouragement and difficulty is inevitable. The therapist must reinforce the hope and the continued expectancy in the possibility of change and the value of renewed efforts. Continued practice brings satisfaction and graduated successes fortify the new learning. The testing of new knowledge and techniques takes place most successfully within the context of a consistent, benign, empathic, emotional support system provided by the therapeutic relationship.

Although all seven elements are present in every form of therapy, more or less emphasis is placed on one or the other, at times determined more by the talent and personality of the therapist, and at other times more by the technique and theoretical stance employed. Analytically oriented therapy places strong emphasis on cognitive aspects via interpretation. Beck highlights this factor in his cognitive approach. Behaviorists, as stated earlier, emphasize the conditioning factor. The humanistic and existential orientations, along with the Gestaltists, place their main trust on achieving emotional discharge. So-called reality therapy rests heavily on conscious persuasion. Transactional analysis gives the relationship and reality testing equal weight. And on it goes. Each therapy has its distinguishing and individual character, but also shares common principles with all the others.

Now, let us face a hard question. Does psychotherapy work? Does it do any good? Although this is a difficult question to research, recent studies have been carefully constructed and involve one- to five-year follow-ups. There is clear evidence in these studies that more improvement took place in individuals who received treatment from an experienced psychotherapist than in individuals who were untreated, although supported by waiting-list contacts. Granted that we are still dealing with rather crude measurements, these replicable studies indicate that psychotherapy does have positive effects. We do not, however, have clear research evidence that any particular school of psychotherapy is superior or more effective than another. The rate of success seems to be related more to the quality of interaction between the patient and therapist than to a particular school of thought. Despite the lack of research evidence supporting one school over the other, there are hosts of clinicians fiercely devoted to their particular theoretical approach. This faith itself is probably not without some effect in the overall picture, but claims to "the one and only psychotherapeutic truth" are clearly myopic and arrogant.

There is some evidence that certain conditions and symptoms are more responsive to one type of therapy rather than another. For example, certain symptomatic disorders such as phobias, especially of relatively recent origin, are best treated with behavioral approaches. Deep-seated characterological problems seem to respond better to analytic or dynamic therapy where the emphasis is on the relationship over an extended period of time. Certain types of inhibited and emotionally restricted people may work more effectively in an emotive form of therapy. There is still a great deal of work to be done to find and fully understand the quickest and most effective methods of intervention.

The questions about effective and economical means of psychotherapeutic intervention pose important considerations. These are not questions of simple efficiency, convenience, or economy. The issues involve human resources and human suffering, as well as time and money.

Although historically the earliest analyses were not terribly long (six months to a year), they were intense, with five to six sessions each week. As psychoanalysis developed, its duration lengthened to periods of five or six years, with four or five sessions each week. Currently a ten-year analysis is not considered unusual. This mode of treatment and psychic exploration makes sense for those intensely involved in the treatment of others, i.e., the training or teaching in areas of psychological development. It makes sense for those who are motivated and are suitable candidates for this extended type of treatment. Like each treatment modality, it is not for everybody or for every psychic stress. Like all techniques, if misapplied it can do harm.

Over a period of years, a body of experience has accumulated indicating that a great deal of psychic growth and development can take place in relatively brief periods of time, utilizing various modes of intervention. A study by the American Psychiatric Association established that the vast majority of psychiatrists, including psychoanalysts doing psychotherapy (not including formal analysis), saw their patients on an average of once or twice a week from six to ten months. This means that currently most psychotherapy patients are seen on an average of thirty-six times a year. Behavioral therapists, marriage and family therapists, as well as therapists employing many other techniques, tend to contain their goals within the perimeters of twenty to forty visits annually. A great deal of effective work and growth takes place within these limits. Naturally treating more complicated character disorders takes longer no matter which therapy is used. Economic stress and the involvement of third-party payers are among the real considerations that pressure each school of therapy to assess its effectiveness and efficiency. The challenge of cost containment has contributed to the exciting discovery that the dynamic therapies can work effectively in shorter periods of time. It has taught therapists the need to choose patients carefully and modify their techniques appropriately. Patients chosen for brief therapy must be distinguished from those patients who really must have long-term therapy.

Psychoanalysis and long-term therapies provide a kind of luxury: there is time to assess and discover. Both patient and therapist can afford to wait and see what is behind, underneath, and around the edges of each psychic phenomenon. Short-term therapies do not have the luxury of time. Assessment, selection, focus, and intervention must be made quickly. Short-term therapy is not easier because it is brief. Harm can be done and mistakes made in a short time as well as over the long haul. In a limited time there is less opportunity to pick up the pieces. Moreover, since a precise assessment is demanded to select the correct candidate and focus for brief therapy, more therapeutic experience and greater acuity are desirable in the therapist.

To make a good assessment and selection of a candidate for short-term therapy, a good *history* of the client is indispensable. The better the history, the more focused the intervention can be. The history taking is the first step in the therapy — establishing the therapeutic relationship. It will tell the therapist two important facts. First, it will tell the therapist whether or not the patient has ever had any really *meaningful relationships* with another human being in the course of his or her life. There should be someone: parent, sibling, dear friend, teacher, relative. If there has not been such a relationship, we are probably dealing with a person who suffers from severe ego damage, perhaps a borderline personality or a narcissistic disorder. Such patients are not amenable to short-term therapy. To succeed in short-term therapy the patient also must show a capacity to be somewhat at home with feelings and to relate to the therapist in a meaningful way. If there is no echo or experiences in the person's background to build on, it is unlikely that this can be produced in a short time.

Second, the history will reveal the *ego integrative capacities* of the patient. It will show how the person has coped in the past with stress and crises: what in his/her life experience has there been to build with, and what at the moment needs to be learned and developed?

The ideal analytic patient used to be described in terms of the acronym YAVIS — young, attractive, verbal, intelligent, and successful. That is true, but such a person is also the ideal patient for short-term therapy. What these traits indicate is a person with relatively good ego strength. Chronological age is not really as important as *flexibility*. We have learned that many older people can profit from psychotherapy. Diagnosis per se is not the critical issue because some very serious conditions can profit from brief intervention if that intervention can focus on the right pressure point with a person who is willing and ready to change.)

Another factor crucial to short-term therapy is *motivation*. Although necessary for any therapy, it is important here because change is demanded in a short time. There should not be just the desire to rid oneself of the symptoms, but also an awareness by the patient that certain dynamic changes are necessary in the way he or she is coping with life.

Focus

Short-term therapy is focused therapy. As classical analysis developed, it widened its focus. Psychoanalysis is a theory of personality, a research method as well as a mode of therapeutic intervention. As the theory of psychoanalysis expanded and the concepts developed, the therapy expanded too. The focus shifted from the amelioration of symptoms to a total revamping of the personality. Experience with briefer therapies is teaching us that work on the focal conflict can bring long-term results. As the patient learns to cope more effectively with the focal conflict, long-term changes and personality shifts quite equivalent to what can happen in long-term analysis can often occur. There are many avenues to growth. No treatment modality, however, gives a guarantee of success and permanent health. Life is an open system that demands continued learning and coping. Psychoanalysts, who subject themselves to the most arduous training analysis, often have to go back for further analysis in later life. Franz Alexander often said that good analytic results require a good patient, a good therapist, and good luck. Bad luck in life can sometimes negate the best therapeutic efforts of both patient and therapist. Length of treatment and expanded range of focus in itself is no guarantee of the effectiveness of treatment.

In short-term therapy attention is focused on what seems to be the person's central concern or conflict. The problem may be one of loss, or reaction to loss, or a problem of autonomy — heirs to conflicts over separation-individuation. The focal conflict may be rivalry (with father) or overdependency (on mother) or competition (with a sibling) — heirs to oedipal conflicts. However we conceptualize it, the focal conflict is one that runs through the whole pattern of the individual's life. By highlighting it, by relating all of the material to this axis, by ignoring other aspects of neurotic behavior, we take a focus. This conscious and active process often achieves quite rapid change. Interpretations rest on what Karl Menninger calls the "triangle of insight," an awareness of how the conflict in the *current life situation* has echoes in the *historical past* as well as in the *therapeutic relationship*.

The sharp focus of brief therapy demands greater activity on the part of the therapist. The therapist does not enjoy the luxury of a "wait and see" attitude, appropriate to longer therapies. He or she participates in structuring the focus and assumes some responsibility in maintaining it. This means that the therapist has some informed and educated decisions to make. This activity on the part of the therapist in not allowing the focus to drift creates a certain amount of tension. On the other hand, it is supportive in that the therapist conveys a sense of caring, interest, and involvement.

Time limit

The limitation of time creates a dynamic pressure on the therapy just as the focus does. Setting a time limit, whether it be a rigid one of twelve sessions a là James Mann or a more flexible limit of twenty to forty visits, establishes certain expectations. From the very beginning there is an awareness that this process is not to extend indefinitely. It establishes an urgency. It reinforces the need to maintain the focus. It discourages an inordinate amount of dependency and regression. There is a deliberate effort to encourage automony and foster independence. The time limit itself implies a confidence in the ability of the patient to do something about his or her life. It reflects the therapist's belief that the patient can make it on his or her own and fosters a more realistic valuation of therapy as but one resource among many to aid growth and development.

All therapies of whatever duration aim at aiding the process of growth, strive to remove the obstacles to development, and foster a sense of self-determination. Psychotherapy participates in the tradition of healing, which opens ways to satisfaction, meaning, and hope for patient and therapist alike.

REFERENCES

Bergin, A. E., & Lambert, M. J. The evaluation of therapeutic outcomes. In S. L. Garfield & A. E. Bergin, eds. *Handbook of Psychotherapy and Behavior Change,* 2nd ed. New York: John Wiley & Sons, 1978, 139–90.

Frank, J. Common features of psychotherapies and their patients. *Psychotherapy and Psychosomatics* 24, 368–71, 1974.

Luborsky, L., Chandler, M., Auerbach, A. H., & Cohen, J. Factors influencing the outcome of psychotherapy: A review of quantitative research. *Psychological Bulletin* 75, 145–85, 1971.

Marmor, J. The nature of the psychotherapeutic process, (ch. 23), *Psychiatry in Transition.* New York: Brunner/Mazel, 1974, 296–309.

Marmor, J. Short-term dynamic psychotherapy. *American Journal of Psychiatry* 136 (2): 149–55, Feb. 1979.

Marmor, J. *Psychiatrists and Their Patients: A National Study of Private Office Practice.* Washington: Joint Information Service of APA & NAMH, 1975.

Sloane, R. B., Staples, F. R., Cristol, A. H., Yorkston, N. J., & Whipple, K. *Psychotherapy Versus Behavior Therapy.* Cambridge: Harvard University Press, 1975.

Strupp, H. H. The therapist's contribution to the treatment process: Beginnings and vagaries of a research program. In H. H. Strupp & L. Luborsky, eds. *Research in Psychotherapy.* Washington: American Psychological Association, 1962, 25–40.

Strupp, H. H. *Psychotherapy: Clinical, Research, and Theoretical Issues.* New York: Jason Aronson, 1973.

Strupp, H. H. Psychotherapy research and practice: An overview. In Garfield, S. L., & Bergin, A. E., eds. *Handbook of Psychotherapy and Behavior Change: An Empirical Analysis,* 2nd ed. New York: John Wiley & Sons, 1978, 3–22.

4

The Pastoral-Therapeutic Stance

JAMES W. EWING

> Why are you cast down, O my soul,
> and why are you disquieted within me?
> Hope in God; for I shall again praise him,
> my help and my God.
>
> Psalm 42:12

The minister is intimately acquainted with the cry of the soul in times of stress, psychological disorientation, and alienation from life. This intimacy arises out of his or her own personal experiences with these feelings and the understanding that new life is born out of suffering. The minister is aware of the essential religious character of life and finds in the therapeutic relationship a way to help psychological distress and fragmentation of the soul. This sensitivity is particularly crucial in our current cultural time when, as Paul Tillich observed:

> [the person] experiences the present situation in terms of disruption, conflict, self-destruction, meaninglessness, and despair in all realms of life. . . . The question arising out of this experience is not . . . the question of a merciful God and the forgiveness of sins; nor is it . . . the question of infinitude, of death and error; nor is it the question of the personal religious life, or of the Christianization of culture and society. It is the question of a reality in which the self-estrangement of our existence is overcome, a reality of reconciliation and reunion, of creativity, meaning and hope. [1]

The past fifty years of dialogue between the pastor and the psychiatrist have helped set the framework for the pastoral-therapeutic stance. This stance puts the pastor into a relationship with other persons in both the conscious and unconscious dimensions of their lives. The central awareness is that in human experience religion and psychology are inseparable. This chapter describes the pastoral-therapeutic stance taken by clinicians who by role, training, skill, and propensity are attuned to psychological and religious processes in people. From this perspective the pastor "listens" for pathological processes and the struggle of the soul. The pastor-therapist is a person who professionally functions as a minister *and* as a psychotherapist. He or she integrates these two identities in the relationship the pastor establishes with those persons engaging his or her skills as a therapist. He or she stands in the midst of the ambiguity that fills life and in that position can elucidate both psychotherapeutic insight and religious meaning. This integration engenders not only an identity but also an integrity for those who practice this ministry.

Images of the pastor-therapist

At the beginning of the twentieth century, psychology separated itself from religion and philosophy to free itself from control by religious dogma and philosophical assumption. Psychotherapy grew up under scientific assumptions and appealed to its science for its authority. Religion both embraced and resisted this necessary emancipation of psychology. Consequently, religion seeing its power in culture diminished has struggled to develop a viable relationship with science. This split between religion and science has not yet been healed, although multiple efforts have been made to bridge this gap. One effort has been the dialogue between the pastor and the psychiatrist. Their dialogue, framed so as to evolve a new relationship between psychotherapeutic and pastoral understanding, has contributed significantly to the identity and integrity of the pastoral-therapeutic stance.

The pastoral-therapeutic stance receives its identity from its attempt to unite psychological healing and religious meaning, so that the pastor-therapist can address the whole person. Thus, there may be psychological problems that can be helped by a religious response or a religious yearning that is expressed in a psychological symptom. In bridging these two authorities of psychotherapy and religion, the pastor-therapist can be guided by certain metaphors — internalized images — that reflect the identity and integrity of the pastoral-therapeutic stance. Three images are useful: bridge-dweller, mediator, and shepherd.

A bridge-dweller is someone who lives on a bridge. The bridge-dweller image explains the pastor-therapist position vis-a-vis persons and institutions. A bridge is a connection between two separated places; it is usually suspended so that space surrounds it; and it allows people to pass over the space that separates the two places. The bridge-dweller position of the pastoral-therapeutic stance connects the separated identities and authorities of psychotherapy and religion, building a new entity between them. The pastor-therapist is a bridge-dweller who belongs to both religious faith and psychotherapeutic science, while at the same time not belonging fully to either. His or her pastoral therapeutic stance creates a new reality by "living-on-the-bridge" where psychotherapy and religion combine into one healing response toward persons and institutions.

Such a pastoral-therapeutic stance makes its own unique contribution to healing, when it seeks to bridge disparate realities. Therapeutically, it seeks to align those internal bridges of a person (or patient) which connect conscious and unconscious life. What we know of psychological personality structure and religious symbols allows us to understand the conflict or stress a person is suffering. If the conflict is resolved through the pastor-therapist's intervention, then change takes place both in the development of healthier personality and of more adequate "God-symbols" (i.e., ideas and expressions for relating to God) that allow internal meaning and direction to shift. Psychological structure and religious symbols intertwine so that one intimately affects the other. Psychological resistance to change inhibits religious change and vice versa. The pastoral-therapeutic stance intervenes in both processes to enhance psychological as well as religious change. The bridge-dweller image helps the pastor-therapist maintain a faithfulness to this interplay of psychotherapy and religion, and it intercepts the resistance and defense that a person generates from psychological conflict and religious inadequacy.

The bridge-dweller maintains the capacity of living between psychology and religion while at the same time embracing the validity of both. The pastor-therapist functions out of both understandings and is called to master both fields. He or she can find commitments and colleagues in both places, but the effort is to live on the bridge between them. The tensions, strains, and discoveries of living between the psychotherapeutic and pastoral disciplines demand a guiding image in order to stay faithful to the new and uncharted effort. Such an internalized image of the bridge-dweller is confirmation of the effort itself.

Yet this image is vulnerable to the powerful forces of established concepts and techniques of both religion and psychology. Even more so, such bridge-dwellers are susceptible to the anxiety of being on the edge of creating something new. The uncertainty, the risk of error, and the misunderstandings by established colleagues can erode the identity and integrity of the pastoral therapeutic stance. The confirmation, however, of this position comes from suffering persons when they make the necessary integration of their psychological and religious processes. A persistent and open dialogue between religion and psychiatry provides much support and inspiration to such bridge-dwellers.

A second internalized image of the pastor-therapist as mediator responds to the rapid change within our culture. The image of mediator expresses the purpose of the pastoral-therapeutic stance vis-a-vis processes of transformation. "Mediator" represents a variety of meanings, all of which may have bearing on the purpose of the pastoral-therapeutic stance. For our purposes, however, the mediator takes part in the process of transformation that allows a person to move from one stage to another. As a pastor, the therapist directs the stirrings of change in the person which can be focused unconsciously through the transference of those feelings to the therapist and religious symbols, and consciously through the tangible awareness of the relationship to the pastor-therapist. Thus, the patient can experience a personal transformation, which is fundamentally a religious process. The pastor uses counseling as a psychological and religious passageway.

In our era of violent and far-reaching changes, the grounding of existential life is deeply shaken. Alienation, fragmentation, and disorientation characterize the way many people think about modern life — and even their own lives. This is the condition of living "between the ages," i.e., between one period of history and the next. On a personal level a person experiences it when passing from one stage of life to the next. In this often tumultuous flux, individuals seek out a reason — a mediating focus — to make sense of these changes. Pathological symptoms reflect their frantic response to find such a mediating focus within persons. After all, they have been unable to locate such centers of value in the culture around them. The yearning of these persons for a mediating symbol helps transform such suffering into health. The pastor-therapist as mediator allows for transformation to take place.

This image of mediator is consistent with the image of the bridge-dweller. Personal transformation is a process that calls for dwelling in an in-between state. On a personal level, the minister who dwells on the bridge suffers the unmooring of those conflicts and inadequate meanings that his or her patients find. Whether moving through a developmental stage or risking entry into a strange land of new meaning, the mediator becomes involved in the delicate balance between leaving a former stage or place in order to enter a new, uncertain reality.

The bridge-dweller and mediator are two images that allow us to appreciate how the pastor deals with the anxiety and struggle within persons they help. A third image is that of shepherd. The pastor-therapist as shepherd has a long and rich history in the Judeo-Christian tradition.[2] The image of shepherd expresses the purpose of the pastoral therapeutic stance vis-a-vis the need for nurture, dependence, and protection. In the intensity of psychological conflict and the struggle of the soul for meaning, the shepherd establishes an assurance that he or she will be present in the midst of change. Such faithfulness often is tested when the patient hides behind internal defenses that deflect the pain. Such faithfulness can also test one's own diligence in the times when the pastor-therapist must allow the patient to work through this dependence without losing the sense of self. The pastoral-therapeutic stance offers a kind of wisdom that acknowledges a profound acquaintance with suffering and its movement toward growth and satisfaction. These characteristics of the pastor-therapist as shepherd, gleaned from the pastoral responsibility of the nomadic shepherds, provides that sense of respite and hope at times of exhaustion and being overwhelmed by the constancy of the change and flux within the life of the patient.

Praxis of pastoral therapy

In order to be effective, the pastoral-therapeutic stance must be mediated through some structured experience. The organization of this therapeutic process into some form or structure also makes possible the identity and integrity of the pastor-therapist. There are three basic but interrelated structures that organize the skills for effective therapy and counseling: the clinical process, the settings of practice, and the training of the pastor-therapist.

THE CLINICAL PROCESS

The clinical process for the pastoral-therapeutic stance is organized by the shape of both the psychotherapeutic and the religious processes. The psychotherapeutic shape is derived from the practice of psychotherapy, which has been heavily influenced by a Freudian understanding of transferences and counter-transferences as well as psychological defense mechanisms. The religious shape comes from the practice of religious worship, which has a specific liturgical rhythm. The organization of the clinical process combines the therapeutic relationship with the religious relationship of worship. It can hardly be seen as otherwise, for it takes shape between a pastor or minister and the person seeking help, who may indeed be someone from the community.

Thus, the clinical hour reflects both therapeutic and "religious" forms. The structure of the hour follows a natural flow that contains the power of therapeutic and religious change. A pattern evolves which is guided by transferences and counter-transferences and religious worship. For example, the beginning of the hour contains a statement of condition or intent, yields to a report or explanation of behaviors or feelings, and appeals for acceptance or judgment. In religious terms these three steps are not unlike a penance service, which begins with an invocation, moves on to confession of sins, and ends with absolution. In the clinical hour, the pastor-therapist explores the inner dynamics of the situation with the patient and the functioning of the transferences and counter-transferences.

In these proceedings the pastor-therapist makes quiet interventions (i.e., makes comments or asks further questions) from the observations and moves on to communication and confrontation with the person (patient). The hour ends in recognition of what has happened. (The sequence of such a clinical encounter may remind some of the way a worship or Scripture service unfolds.) The intention of the hour is to explore the unconscious and conscious realities that function within the person in the hope that these bring healthy personality change and enhancement in religious meaning. Therapy and religious worship happen simultaneously in the flow of the relationship between the person (patient) and the pastor-therapist. Therapeutic work takes place in religious form, and religious work takes place in therapeutic form. The dual roles of pastor and therapist blend into one as the psychological and religious changes become part and parcel of each other in the person being counseled.

This therapeutic and religious rhythm not only applies to each hour but exists over a series of hours. A block of hours may be spent invoking, confessing, absolving, interpreting, expositing, offering, and blessing. The organization of the entire therapy allows the patient's deeper hurts, conflicts, and pains to emerge. As the inner life of the person connects with itself in new ways through the transferences and counter-transferences, new and unexplored symbols of meaning emerge which enable the integration of life experiences.

THE SETTINGS

The pastor-therapist works in settings that identify this ministry with both religious and health-care institutions. Hospitals, clinics, local churches and synagogues, pastoral counseling centers and interprofessional health-care teams provide the organized settings for practice. However, how these places are managed and how they are funded also express and shape the pastoral-therapeutic stance.

To a large extent the policies and practices of religious and health-care institutions determine the setting for pastoral therapy. In both settings the pastor-therapist is guided by professional competence. Members of religious institutions are accountable to the communal authority of the faith group. Thus a pastor-therapist is governed in his or her work by the structure and authority of the religious organization. The religious institution in which the pastor-therapist works usually is conscious that the pastor-therapist is a representative of the religious community and brings that authority to the clinical work. The actual form of governance in the organization varies considerably and depends upon the religious group. It can be a board of directors or advisory committee, but it can also be under the direct control of a religious hierarchy or congregation. Regardless of the specific form of this management, the pastor-therapist and the setting of the therapeutic practice are by definition governed by a community of faith that authorizes such an activity.

In health-care institutions the overriding consideration is the accountability of its personnel to whoever is responsible for the quality of health care. The core of the organization is the professional staff that assures sound health-care practice in diagnosis, treatment procedures, continuous care, termination, and record keeping. The pastor-therapist, by working in a health-care institution, complies with its policies and in turn is accountable to professional expertise. The actual form of that accountability varies according to the specific administrative and management procedures of the particular setting; nevertheless, the governing authority for decision making resides in the professional expertise. This usually takes the form of consultation, training, education, and reflective observation.

Thus, the organization of the pastoral-therapeutic stance in the settings of practice are shaped by religious communal authority and professional expertise. Religion and psychotherapy, then, provide a coming together of two different issues of governance which have a profound impact on the structure in which it is organized. The institution that takes a pastoral-therapeutic stance needs in its organization the visible influence of religious communal authority and professional health-care expertise if it is to be faithful to the identity and integrity that lies between psychotherapeutic and religious process. How the setting of practice is operated and managed has profound impact on the organization of the pastoral-therapeutic stance.

The economics of the setting also has profound implications for the organization of the pastoral-therapeutic stance. How a pastor-therapist is funded and supported depends upon the religious institutions and professional practice of health care. Religious institutions are in part financially supported by donations and gifts, regardless of services received by the donors. Health-care institutions are funded largely by the fees set for services rendered. Religious practice and professional practice are in conflict in economic principles. The pastor-therapist by nature of ministry is religiously and ethically committed to provide service regardless of the person's ability to pay. The pastor-therapist by nature of professional expertise provides service according to professional fees. To reconcile these two economic outlooks, many institutions have adopted an arrangement that includes fee-for-service according to the person's ability to pay, inclusion of benefits for services based upon health-care insurance, and contributions from the religious communities to underwrite the cost of service not covered by fees and insurance. This model represents the uneasy alliance between the nature of ministry and the nature of professional health-care practice. The viability of the pastoral-therapeutic stance to embody itself in a form faithful to its substance depends upon the economic policies of the organization of the setting. No definitive economic policy has yet evolved which does reflect the emerging new discipline of pastoral therapy. In the short run the economic functioning of the settings in which the pastor-therapist practices has made tentative compromises to provide sufficient recognition of the issues involved, but the economic policies for the long-range embodiment of the pastoral-therapeutic stance have yet to evolve.

EDUCATION AND TRAINING

The education and training of the pastor-therapist is a third structure that involves the organization of the pastoral-therapeutic stance. It is a sequential process in which the training for pastor is followed by the training for psychotherapist. In both of these tracks, the individual follows the course set out by the academic graduate school, the professional school, and apprenticeship. Over the years education and training have more and more focused upon the professional school, which has adapted the apprenticeship system of organized supervision. This education and training result in the endorsement (ordination) for ministry and certification by professional associations. The right to practice is not granted by the educational institutions per se but by the judgment of the authorized religious institutions and examination by peers in the profession, and the regulation for training ultimately rests beyond the formal educational institutions. So, the training of pastoral therapists lies in a variety of educational experiences that lead toward the faithful embodiment of the pastoral-therapeutic stance.

The educational experiences are organized in a number of ways, depending upon the religious and psychotherapeutic understandings. In either case, there must be a viable interplay between the religious and psychotherapeutic processes that integrate both disciplines for the practice of pastoral therapy. No singular structural model has yet evolved; instead, a sense of what needs to happen in any model is gradually being defined. The prospective pastor-therapist needs to master the body of knowledge that is both theological and psychological, pastoral and psychotherapeutic. He or she must know the professional techniques that define expert functioning in the field. And he or she must develop a self-understanding and awareness that is based upon personal religious faith, personality functioning, and vocational identity. Academic and clinical processes, intellectual knowledge, and experience must interact constantly in the education and training of a pastor-therapist.

The dynamic of the pastoral stance

The dynamic of the pastoral-therapeutic stance provides the source of energy for its identity/integrity and organization. This dynamic arises out of the exchange between the "pastor symbol" (i.e., the pastor as symbol), the pastor-therapist, and the person seeking help (or patient).

The pastor symbol comprises the roles fulfilled by the pastor. The pastor is the representative of God so authorized by the religious community. The meaning of pastor is manifested through the images of bridge-dweller, mediator, and shepherd. These aspects of the pastor symbol are present in the pastoral-therapeutic stance through the substantive interplay between religion and psychotherapy, its embodiment in the clinical process, the settings of practice, and training of the pastor-therapist. This role of the pastor as "pastor symbol" is separate and distinct from that of the pastor-therapist and the person seeking help.

The pastor-therapist, who is first of all a pastor, is the one authorized by ministry and psychotherapy to practice the pastoral-therapeutic stance. The pastor-therapist functions within the pastor symbol to the extent that he or she is faithful to the images of the symbol. This faithfulness is manifested in the capacity to function as pastor or minister within the transferences and counter-transferences and to engage in the religious meanings evolving in the person.

The person (or patient) is the one who seeks help because of a felt psychological conflict, situational stress, or struggle of the soul. He or she brings to the relationship the ambivalent mixture of unconscious and conscious processes of a life that is caught between conflicts of personality organization and the struggle of the soul.

These three roles may be set against each other as polarities. These polarities compose the dynamic that produces the energy for the pastoral-therapeutic relationship:

Pastor Symbol ⟷ Person
Person ⟷ Pastor-Therapist
Pastor-Therapist ⟷ Pastor Symbol

In the pastor symbol vs. person polarity, the pastoral-therapeutic stance connects with the yearning in the person for a pastor figure. This is the yearning for new life, transformation, and nurture. The pastor symbol awakens these yearnings as the struggle of the soul reaches out for hope and sense of meaning. In return, the person gives substance to the pastor images as bridge-dweller, mediator, or shepherd from the specifics of his or her own unique individuality. The result of the interaction between these images and personal substance is an energy of the spirit.

In the person vs. pastor-therapist polarity, the specific transferences and counter-transferences evolve from the unconscious life of both person and pastor-therapist. These exchanges precipitate the unique personality organization and conflicts inherent in the personality structures of both. A very specific relationship emerges between the two people, so that therapeutic intervention in the unconscious processes leads to change and conscious awareness.

In the "pastor-therapist vs. pastor symbol" polarity, the pastor images guide the pastor-therapist in functioning as the representative of God on behalf of the religious community. The pastor-therapist "administrates" the pastor symbol (as the priest administers the sacrament), and in the act of administration the images become known within him- or herself. The pastor symbol empowers the pastor-therapist to live his or her own images as bridge-dweller, mediator, and shepherd.

Each of the three polarities always stands in relationship with the others. A triangular dynamic produces the energy for psychological and religious change. This triangular dynamic allows therapeutic and religious forms to blend:

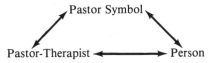

The energy of the pastoral-therapeutic stance is generated out of this dynamic (allowing, of course, for various resources of religious and psychotherapeutic understanding to enter into it for the sake of health and salvation, i.e., wholeness and meaning). The substance of such a dynamic emerges not from the pastoral-therapeutic stance itself but from within the very specific relationship of the pastor symbol, the pastor-therapist, and the person. This relationship deals with the concreteness of the unique interaction. It can include specific understandings of psychological theory, technique, and religious belief. The triangular dynamic is the energy source that enlivens and makes possible the interplay between psychological and religious processes (identity/integrity) and the embodiment of these processes (organization).

This triangular dynamic of the pastoral-therapeutic stance is based upon certain assumptions about the nature of personality and religion. It assumes that the human personality does function with dynamic energy understood according to the depth psychologies as explored by Freud and Jung. It assumes that the human being does create symbols that express meaning which transcend the specific psychological understanding of life and function to provide an integration and transformation of life experiences. It assumes that human beings are God-creating creatures in the sense that values cluster in certain centers of meaning which provide explanation through myths, stories, and legends. And it assumes that human beings create communities in which they develop a sense of belonging, attachment, loyalty, and fear. These assumptions form a perspective through which the triangular dynamic of the pastoral-therapeutic stance is understood.[3]

The value of the pastoral-therapeutic stance

The pastoral-therapeutic stance has a value by its presence within the work of ministry and psychotherapy. It focuses the interplay between psychological and religious processes that occur within persons. Human life yearns for wholeness and transcendence. The pastoral-therapeutic stance allows us to reach out to these persons who experience the fragmentation and alienation of our culture. It has emerged within religious and health institutions as an essential form for the healing of psychological conflict and religious struggle. Its value is present in three ways: the pastor symbol, the interpretation of life, and the courage to live with the ambiguity of life.

The pastor symbol arouses the unconscious dimensions of the human struggle toward the images of the pastor. This deep urge within the human seeks not only therapeutic correction but also religious meaning. The pastor-therapist draws to him- or herself this desire and is able to interpret it both as a pathological perception and a yearning for transcendent meaning. The pastor symbol not only attracts such deep responses from the individual, but also stands within religious tradition as the basis for communal authority. The value of the pastor symbol is its own existence within the context of psychotherapy and religion at a time of intense cultural and personal change.

The pastoral-therapeutic stance provides an interpretive framework for connecting the symptoms of disease and the malaise of meaning. The interplay between psychological and religious processes within persons allows for the exploration of such a connection. The specifics of this connection remain unknown in many important ways, but the pastoral-therapeutic stance provides an interpretive possibility that introduces and values such a possibility. Questions of health and of existential meaning can open the way to therapeutic as well as religious understandings. The very dialogue begun between psychiatry and religion is but a step toward the interpretive understanding of this relationship between disease and meaning.

At an emotional level, the pastoral-therapeutic stance assists in the courage to live with life's ambiguity. This courage is energized through the existence of the triangular dynamic of the pastoral symbol, the pastor-therapist, and the person. It is an existential hope, more than a specific religious creed or psychological theory. It understands anxiety as a signal that life is seeking its own fulfillment. In the midst of such ambiguity, an important value is gained in accepting the internal fragmentation as the starting point that leads toward greater health and resolution of the struggle of the soul.

The vision of the pastoral-therapeutic stance

The pastoral-therapeutic stance offers hope for transformation in persons and in the culture. This historic period of rapid change befuddles the human mind and imagination. But the vision held out by the pastoral-therapeutic stance is a source for an imaginative creativity of life as it moves toward its new day. Imagination is the capacity to envision new possibilities and to give shape to change. Vision keeps alive the resourceful creativity of imagination. In the pastoral-therapeutic stance this vision is active in the clinical process, the struggle for a new paradigm for the relationship between psychotherapy and religion, and the recognition of new realities.

Within the clinical process vision engages the person in a dialogue with his or her present reality. As this present condition is perceived and felt, it becomes the occasion for change. The direction for that change and the capacity to choose among options of behavior and feeling are guided by the imagination. An active imagination is a vital therapeutic tool in assisting suffering persons to connect the hidden fragments of the psyche. It also assists the person in transcending the present reality in the hope of reaching a new reality. The pastoral-therapeutic stance stirs the imagination to develop a new vision of life that encompasses a new integration of the self and a new relationship of the self to emerging realities.

In the relationship between psychotherapy and religion, vision offers imaginative possibilities in the development of a new paradigm that would unite the two. Intellectual discovery through reflective understanding of clinical observation and through research leads to new ways of seeing, hearing, and perceiving the interrelationship between religion and psychotherapy. This discovery is in process and projects itself ahead over the next decades. The elements of such a new paradigm are in current efforts such as the dialogue between religion and psychiatry. The actual consequences of work by the pastor-therapist is producing a history, the directions of which are yet unknown.

Vision requires imagination and imagination stirs excitement that energizes the new discoveries. Vision as the source of imagination allows the recognition of new realities when they begin to appear. Processes are in motion that are urging toward new realities. The pastoral-therapeutic stance, as currently perceived, is one of these. The sense of something new, something only becoming, needs the power of recognition. This is true not only in individual persons seeking newness of life, but also in the work of psychotherapy and ministry. Without vision, the happenings of new understanding only lie dormant and inaccessible. The vision of the pastoral-therapeutic stance creates new possibilities by maintaining the resource of imagination as past, present, and future connect in the movement toward new realities.

NOTES

1. Paul Tillich. *Systematic Theology,* vol. I. Chicago: University of Chicago Press, 1951, 49.
2. Seward Hiltner has given much attention to the image of the pastor as shepherd, i.e., S. Hiltner & L. Colston. *The Context of Pastoral Counseling.* Nashville: Abingdon Press, 1961.
3. Two specific works are helpful in this regard: P. Tillich. *The Dynamics of Faith.* New York: Harper & Row, 1957. H. R. Neibuhr. *Radical Monotheism and Western Culture.* New York: Harper & Row, 1960.

REFERENCES

Hiltner, S., & Colston, L. *The Context of Pastoral Counseling.* Nashville: Abingdon Press, 1961.
McNeill, J. T. *A History of the Cure of Souls.* New York: Harper & Row, 1951.
Neibuhr, H. R. *Radical Monotheism and Western Culture.* New York: Harper & Row, 1960.
Neibuhr, H. R. *The Purpose of the Church and Its Ministry.* New York: Harper & Row, 1956.
Tillich, P. *Systematic Theology,* vol. I. Chicago: University of Chicago Press, 1951.
Tillich, P. *The Courage to Be.* New Haven: Yale University Press, 1952.
Tillich, P. *The Dynamics of Faith.* New York: Harper & Row, 1957.
Williams, D. D. *The Minister and the Cure of Souls.* New York: Harper & Row, 1961.

5

The Diagnostic Interview

HERBERT S. GASKILL

This chapter outlines the kind of information psychiatrists require before they can begin to understand the emotional problems presented by a client. There are precautions, however, for anyone whose privilege it is to deal with distressed people. First, these problems are never simple, even when they appear to be. Second, they require careful observation and listening for nuances, for often these hint at the real trouble involved.

For practitioners, diagnosing by intuition is the most rapid way of arriving at wrong conclusions. People do not always react as we wish they would nor do they stay in pigeonholes or categories. Their problems are individual, and if we are to be of help, we must first listen, collect necessary data, and then try to understand the things that really trouble them and underlie their problems.

The personal exchange: Evaluation and history-taking

The diagnostic interview has many forms, and there is no single correct way to obtain a patient's psychiatric history. Each counselor has an individual style and should follow it; each counselor functions most effectively when utilizing those interview techniques that are congenial and relevant to his or her personality. At the same time the therapist must often adapt technique to the needs of a particular client. Each person who comes for psychiatric assistance has individual problems and attitudes that influence the way he or she presents the self and communicates immediate and past history to the counselor. To clients the discussion of life history is an intense emotional experience, often accompanied by a variety of feelings — guilt, anxiety, relief, pleasure, etc. Consequently, counselors should be empathic, recognizing differences in style and feeling. They should adjust interviewing to maximally facilitate the client's presentation of the necessary information.

Any communication between a patient and a doctor is considered privileged, that is, it is not discussed or in any way disclosed outside the consultation room. This consideration pertains to any therapeutic relationship and most particularly to a psychiatric one, irrespective of the therapist's particular discipline. Thus, the consultation room itself should be arranged to ensure privacy. It should be impossible for the occupants to be overheard. Interruptions should be kept to a minimum, for nothing is more disconcerting to an anxious and fearful client than repeated telephone calls or other needless interruptions. Both counselor and client should be comfortably seated. The former should be relaxed in order to give undivided attention to the client and be free in order to listen to the content of the client's thoughts and to observe nonverbal behavior, particularly emotional responses or their absence. The client, too, needs an atmosphere that is relaxed and conducive to the free discussion of problems.

Finally, there is the matter of time. Two individuals who have never met before need sufficient time to establish a relationship that permits the client to develop trust and confidence in the counselor. The latter should indicate in advance the length of the interview. An hour is generally found to be a useful unit; however, as with other techniques, the counselor can be flexible — any one of a number of factors may necessitate arranging a longer or shorter session. If the initial interview seems to warrant it, a second meeting can be scheduled.

There are a variety of ways to conduct the diagnostic interview, and each has its advocates. Some therapists use a highly structured interview; others rely on an associative method. While the latter has its usefulness, it is certainly more difficult for the beginner; furthermore, it may not elicit the necessary information and may transform the diagnostic interview into therapy, when therapy is not yet intended. An effective method lies between these extremes. It involves structuring the interview around certain broad, general topics, but permits the client considerable latitude in developing his or her story.

Necessary information for considered judgment

Psychiatric history-taking serves a number of functions. Most importantly, it provides counselors with information to diagnose the particular symptom complex or type of personality problem and to formulate a basic evaluation of the client. In addition, it enables them to make initial estimates of the client's need for, and ability to use, psychotherapy or other methods of treatment. It permits them to decide whether their particular treatment skills are suited for this particular individual. For example, a nonmedical therapist who decides that hospitalization and/or drug therapy is the best therapeutic approach would refer the patient to a physician or might conclude that such considerations as length of treatment, severity of the illness, or somatic complications rule him or her out and thus refer the patient elsewhere.

During the interview counselors should assess the clients' motivation for treatment, the nature of their expectations of treatment, and their conception of the psychotherapeutic process. Motivation can vary from clients who clearly realize that they have a psychological problem and are eager to attack it to individuals who do not recognize any problems and come only because they have been forced to. Although it is easy to dismiss the latter type, particularly today when the demands for therapy exceed treatment resources, the counselor may be able to motivate such a person to become a client. In any case it takes patience and understanding to establish a therapeutic relationship. For example, some clients expect a magical cure; others unconsciously seek an infantilizing relationship with the counselor—which in fact would increase their dependence rather than lead to a resolution of the problem. Again, clarification and discussion of these issues are important. For some, the procedure will end their interest and commitment; for others it will make treatment possible.

Putting a biography together

History-taking involves much more than merely gathering important data about the individual's life history. Expert diagnosticians are good observers and use all the information that the various senses can register: the client's appearance and dress; affects or lack of emotional reponse; the way he or she communicates, both verbally and nonverbally; the type of relationship that is established with the counselor; what is said and what is omitted; the use of symbols, their meanings and reactions evoked. Each observation is relevant to the total personality-picture.

The art of biography as practiced by psychiatrists is a recent and all too often meager production, when compared to those of the creative artist. All the great creators of literature have had this unique capacity to communicate intuitively, but nonetheless explicitly, the important character traits of their heroes, so that we recognize the unity between their behavior and their psychological motivations. Whether it be the Greek dramatists or more modern writers such as Shakespeare, Dostoevsky, or Hawthorne, they grasped the importance of genetic, dynamic concepts as they relate to psychological motivation.[1] This led Freud, who introduced these ideas into our scientific heritage, to recognize their earlier contribution in his comment that "the creative writer cannot evade the psychiatrist nor can the psychiatrist the creative writer" (Freud, 1906). Osler no doubt had much the same thought in mind, when he recommended that each physician have a ten-foot bookshelf of great literature at his bedside (Osler, 1905). While the purposes of the creative writer and the psychiatrist are not identical, their subject matter is. The models they have left us are readily at hand (Stone & Stone, 1966).

The truly creative artist often conveys information intuitively or indirectly without the reader's being fully conscious of the picture that has been created.

> The writer can indeed draw on certain qualities which fit him to carry out such a task: above all, on a sensitivity that enables him to perceive the hidden impulses in the minds of other people, and the courage to let his own unconscious speak. But there is one circumstance which lessens the evidential value of what he has to say. Writers are under the necessity to produce intellectual and aesthetic pleasure, as well as certain emotional effects. For this reason they cannot produce the stuff of reality unchanged, but must isolate portions of it, remove disturbing associations, tone down the whole and fill in what is missing. These are the privileges of what is known as "poetic license." Moreover they can show only slight interest in the origin and development of the mental states which they portray in their completed form. In consequence it becomes inevitable that science should concern herself with the same materials whose treatment by artists has given enjoyment to mankind for thousands of years, though her touch must be clumsier and the yield of pleasure less. (Freud, 1910)

Consequently, for counselors who need to diagnose the illness as accurately as possible in order to plan treatment, a more formal and detailed biography is necessary. When data are available, the history should include the following general categories of information:

1. The history of pregnancy and birth, including any known facts concerning hereditary and constitutional endowment and defects.

2. The physical, psychological, and social climate that served as a background for the client's development, particularly the parents, siblings, educational experience, and cultural influences in the family.

3. The strengths and stresses that have either facilitated or distorted past development.

4. The current stresses confronting the individual and their relation to his or her past.

5. The ways in which the client's current adjustment is inappropriate or maladaptive, reasons for the use of inappropriate solutions, similar patterns in the past.

Each individual is unique. While it is true that everyone follows, with varying success, the same developmental sequence, the particular circumstances under which an individual develops are unique and contribute significantly to success or failure. An only child has a very different family environment from that of a child with siblings. The fact of never having had to share the parents with rivals, reasons for the parents' not having had additional children, and parental attitudes toward the only child are potent developmental influences. Similarly, the oldest child who is the first to go to school occupies a different position from the siblings who follow. Consequently, specific information relating to such questions is important.

The mind has been aptly called the primary mode of achieving adaptive behavior. From infancy on learning is cumulative and becomes part of the total personality. The past is always part of the present, and present behavior must be viewed in terms of past life-experiences. Heredity also plays a large part in development, and psychiatry seeks to expand the current knowledge of all genetic factors. Even intelligence, which is largely hereditary, may be influenced significantly by the environment, which either enriches or fails to encourage intellectual development. Other aspects, such as the strength of the drives or the particular lines of ego development (Hartman, 1964), undoubtedly have innate influences, although ways of determining the definitive contribution of heredity are still not available. While human beings do not have innate instinctual patterns of behavior, they do have culture. In many ways culture substitutes for instinct (Dobzhansky, 1962). Each culture and subculture hand down certain traditions that act as patterns for guiding large segments of behavior. Importantly, culture (like instinct) has an adhesive quality of resisting change, although this may seem less meaningful today in this period of rapid cultural change. Consequently, the general and familial subculture in which the patient grew up should be described.

Beginning the process: the first interview

Usually clients come for help because of an acute, immediate problem. Thus, after the initial courtesies have been exchanged, a general question about the circumstances precipitating the request for consultation serves as an appropriate starting point. The interview could begin with the question: "When you called for an appointment, you said that something was disturbing you which you wanted to talk about. Tell me, in as much detail as you can, the nature of your problem and/or symptoms, when they began, what seems to aggravate them, and what seems to ease them. Any thoughts you have about what might have caused them are also important." Counselors then can sit back and see what is forthcoming from clients. In general, it is wise to let them tell their story in their own way and without interruptions. They may need encouragement in the form of a brief comment, a smile, or a nod from time to time. When clients have finished, counselors may want to summarize what was heard. Not infrequently clients can become more objective when listening to their story and can add previously forgotten details or make pertinent corrections. While eliciting information about the present illness, counselors mentally organize the details and note clients' emotional responses and other nonverbal cues. Counselors should ask questions about any aspects of the history which are unclear. It is important to get this information in as much detail as possible during the first interview, because it is usually presented with less distortion than during subsequent meetings, when clients tend to be more influenced by what they think the counselor wants to hear. Furthermore, clients have been seeking an opportunity to unburden themselves and are eager to discuss problems as fully as possible; doing so with a sympathetic and attentive therapist provides tremendous relief, and the client communicates more freely and with less anxiety under these circumstances.

When the history of the present illness is completed, the counselor can make certain important judgments about the nature of the problem, for example, the acuteness or chronicity of the illness. With some clients it takes only a few minutes to reveal that the problem is one of long-standing. In such cases the essential factor is that clients consider themselves ready to take constructive steps to solve their problem. With other clients the immediacy of the problem is equally apparent, and it becomes important to try to understand what the circumstances were — both external and internal — that precipitated the psychological decompensation.

Chronicity raises questions about clients' motivation for treatment. Why have they suffered so long without doing anything to alleviate the situation? There may be reasons such as lack of finances and/or time for treatment, knowledge of someone else's "bad" experience with psychotherapy, etc. While occasionally having a certain validity, such excuses are more often rationalizations; usually less obvious and more irrational anxieties are the basis of such procrastination. The ability to trust other people is a crucial factor (Erikson, 1964, pp. 274ff.). Many individuals, particularly those who need psychiatric help, have been so traumatized in their relationships with others that only with great reluctance do they decide to seek psychiatric help. Usually, damaged parent-child relationships interfere with the development of the capacity for trust. Other clients are afraid that they will become too dependent on the counselor; yet such individuals intuitively recognize this fear as an unconscious wish. Whatever the reason for the delay, it is important to explore it fully in the initial phases of therapy so that a therapeutic relationship can be established.

The history of the present illness also reveals clients' interpretation of what has happened to them, i.e., whether they ascribe the present difficulties to external events or to their own psychological conflicts. While it is true that certain life-situations (e.g., some cases of combat fatigue) are sufficiently traumatic to trigger neurotic reactions, this is generally not the case. While external events may be the precipitating factors in a neurotic conflict, the fundamental difficulty lies in the activation of intrapsychic conflicts that make it impossible for individuals to deal with their current life-situation. A view of personal problems as being caused by a malign fate has significant therapeutic implications: it gives evidence of relatively little psychological mindedness and will necessitate additional preliminary therapeutic work to help the client develop it.

The question of note-taking during the diagnostic interview often perplexes neophyte counselors. Again, no absolute rules apply. However, since this first interview is crucial in establishing an interpersonal relationship that will lead to a therapeutic alliance, counselors who devote a major part of their attention to note-taking risk losing contact with the client. It seriously interferes with rapport and often gives clients a sense of distance rather than the closeness they anticipated. Furthermore, as has been suggested earlier, counselors' ability to use all of the senses to observe the client, while at the same time associating freely with the information being presented, will be significantly hampered by note-taking. (The counselor, of course, can jot down occasional names, ages, and dates with which to refresh the memory when summarizing the material after the client has left; such brief notations generally do not adversely affect the interview.)

Extensive note-taking may raise another problem. Clients are always concerned about others' access to these notes. If they ask about this, they have a right to expect this to be dealt with realistically. Such questions, like many others in the course of therapy, have both realistic and fantasy implications. In the latter case they are generally due to neurotic anxieties. From the beginning therapists should always approach such questions with an open mind, appreciating both the realistic and neurotic connotations. Consequently, in the initial phase, when trust is often least, this can suggest additional concern to clients, thus limiting the freedom of their communications with possible distortions in the history.

DEVELOPMENTAL HISTORY

Once the presenting illness has been satisfactorily explored, the counselors should elicit information about the developmental history by asking a series of specific questions or by asking a more general question that allows clients to present the material in their own way. An example of the latter is:

> Would you tell me as much as you can recall of your development, beginning with your earliest memory and bringing us up to the present time. I want to know about your family, your home, your schooling, your health, including illnesses and operations, and your various activities, including sports, dating, and other interests. Anything you have been told about your birth and early development is also important.

This may seem like a major assignment, but clients' organization and presentation of the material reveal a great deal about the kind of persons they are. In addition to the information they give, the omissions are also important because such omissions do not occur by chance but have meanings that will become evident as therapy progresses. The emphasis clients place on certain events and relationships, and brief allusions to other aspects, are also relevant and ought to be explored at an appropriate time during the course of therapy; the same applies to their earliest memories. Early memories (prior to age six) often give leads to important aspects of early life-experiences. Sometimes these memories are "screen" memories involving considerable distortion (Freud, 1899). Such distortions are valuable, since they hint at clients' interpretation of early life-experiences. The paucity of memories, particularly when it extends beyond age six, also bears diagnostic significance. Some clients will recall very little of their childhood and appear to have a global amnesia for all events in their lives prior to adolescence. Such massive repression suggests that major difficulties and anxieties involved in growing up necessitated "forgetting" much of the past—it is a poor prognostic sign, will prolong therapy, and make it more difficult.

For clergy, as for family physicians, the past history may be unnecessary. Pastors who have known parishioners for many years (sometimes from birth) may already have much or all of the information about their past history readily at hand. It may seem redundant under such circumstances to request a detailed past history, and pastors can limit their questioning to what is unknown or unclear. However, a thorough review may help the counselor in establishing a perspective and giving the client an opportunity to look at him- or herself more objectively and to see relationships unnoticed in the past. Talking about relationships and events constitutes a modality different from that of just thinking about them. Some clients, in listening to themselves, develop new insights. This is suggestive of psychological mindedness and is a good prognostic sign for therapy.

FAMILY HISTORY

Significant developmental information begins with the family of origin: description of parents and siblings, their ages, health, personalities, and the client's relationships with them. Counselors should ask about family members' educational, cultural, and religious background; illnesses; economic and vocational achievements; the relationship between the parents, including separation and divorce; the parents' attitudes toward discipline and child care; and their personal habits, goals, and ideals. Did the parents show any favoritism? Did the client relate more to one parent than to the other? If so, which one? Counselors should obtain information about any stressful periods or changes in the client's relationship with either parent while growing up (especially during adolescence) and whether emotional emancipation from the parents occurred. And they should inquire about adult relationships with the parents and siblings.

Counselors should discuss circumstances surrounding the death or the divorce of parents, including the client's reactions to and interpretations of these events. Meanings and implications will vary with the client's age at the time of occurrence and the sex of the parent who is lost. For example, a child who loses a parent at age five may have a totally different reaction if it occurred at age ten, or even at fourteen. In general, the older the child, the less crippling the event will be in terms of later ego development. The child's developmental phase at the time of the loss also has importance for the counselor (Fleming & Altschul, 1963). For a boy of five (the age at which the oedipal conflict, with its intense rivalry with the father, is at its height), the father's death will have different psychological implications from the same loss at age ten (the latency period). Circumstances and the client's reactions to the remarriage of the remaining parent are important. Finally, if the client had been adopted, the counselor should know the age at adoption, the age upon learning about it, reactions to the information, and fantasies about real parents.

With regard to siblings, counselors should determine the ordinal position of the client, as well as age at the time of birth of the other children. Reaction to the new arrival and any regressive behavior on the client's part at this time should be noted. They should have information about severe illnesses or death of siblings that can have important conscious and unconscious meanings for the child. Discussing a sibling's birth and relationship to the client often affords an unforced way of gaining information about the latter's sexual development. Counselors can ask: was the child aware of the mother's pregnancy? What was the family's attitude in communicating such information to the child? When did the child become aware of sexual differences, and what was the reaction? Was there mutual sex play with the siblings? If the parents knew of it, how did they react?

SCHOOL HISTORY

The next critical period in the client's life is the entry into school. While socialization starts in the preschool period, its first major test occurs at the beginning of school. The child's ability to tolerate separation from home and mother without undue anxiety is the central issue. (This is obviously two-sided, since those children who develop school phobias are responding to the mother's usually unconscious wish to hold onto the child (Johnson, Falstein, Szvek, & Suendsen, 1941). Such mothers cannot tolerate separation from their children and feel threatened by the growing independence and initiative of the child.) The child's memories of school and emotional responses to teachers and pupils critically influence development. So, counselors should recapture the client's initial reactions to starting school, and they should obtain a detailed history of the entire education, including academic achievement, areas of concentration and interest, and any discrepancies between goals and attainments. In regard to the latter, it is important to know about particular circumstances that interfered with the achievement of these goals. At the same time, counselors can discuss the family's general attitude toward education, their emphasis on grades, and the relationship of these factors to the child's intellectual endowment and motivation.

In addition, information about childhood peer relationships, attitudes toward teachers, discipline, and authority, learning difficulties, participation and achievement in extracurricular activities helps counselors assay total school performance and provides clues to the client's general level of energy and ability to sustain his or her interests. School adjustment also may indicate the ability to make realistic decisions regarding primary and secondary motivational goals.

ACCURATE HEALTH RECORDS

Counselors should not overlook the client's health record, including both physical and neurotic illnesses. The record of physical illnesses should include: infectious diseases, allergic reactions, frequency of colds and other illnesses, injuries, and operations (and indications for the latter). The child's or adult's use of illness and convalescence may reveal an underlying psychopathology. The person who has repeated minor illnesses with prolonged periods of invalidism often has a limited capacity to surmount any type of object loss or separation. He or she tends, under such circumstances, to respond through regression and withdrawal, which may involve physical illness. This pattern is often unconsciously encouraged by parents and/or physicians who failed at the outset to recognize its psychological importance. Repeated injuries or polysurgery suggest an accident-prone individual who suffers from a neurotic sense of guilt and is constantly seeking "punishment." Counselors should inquire about pronounced character traits—those of the very good and quiet child as well as those of the delinquent. The inventory should include such specific neurotic reactions as enuresis, phobias, speech disturbances, temper tantrums, and sleepwalking. In discussing these, the counselor should note the ages of onset and cessation, and any stresses that might have occurred at that particular period.

VOCATIONAL PATTERN

Counselors should also review the client's vocational record. Is it commensurate with education, or were there unusual circumstances that interfered (e.g., military service requirements)? What is the client's job record, e.g., frequency of change of employment, the reasons for such shifts, the attitude toward and satisfaction from work, the relationship with employers, etc.? The client's own judgments about his or her progress, or lack of it, suggest how realistic the client is about self-evaluation. Some people project all of their problems onto the environment, while others constantly underestimate their abilities or create situations that invariably lead to their downfall. Repetitive and compulsive patterns of behavior imply significant psychopathology.

Military service can be an important experience for many men and women. Date of induction, length of service, branch of service, stresses incurred, circumstances under which the individual entered the service, meaning of the separation to the client and family, adjustment to the service, and readjustment to civilian life are important parts of the record. Long-lasting and troublesome psychological aftereffects have been observed following the Vietnam conflict. These dramatic reactions are part of what has come to be called post-traumatic stress syndrome.

COURTSHIP AND MARRIAGE

Counselors' summary of the client's current family situation should include a description of the spouse and their relationship. The courtship and circumstances leading up to the marriage may disclose facets of the personality which are less obvious in other relationships. In the marital relationship, transferences — stereotyped reactions that are carry-overs from the infantile past — are more likely to appear and unrealistically influence the patient's behavior toward the partner (Kaufman, 1947; Gaskill, 1959). The extent to which transference reactions dominate the relationship often indicates the client's maturity and skill at reality testing, i.e., objectivity. None of us is without hostages to the past, but the degree to which they encroach us on and distort current object relationships is crucial. So counselors should be aware of the number of children, whether they were planned or not, the client's reaction to new family members and the subsequent course of their relationships, relationships with both the client's and the spouse's families, and even living arrangements and economic circumstances.

HISTORY OF SEXUAL ADJUSTMENT

Sexual adjustment is a vital part of the marital history. Discussion of sexual development and adjustment may create a great deal of anxiety in certain clients; counselors need to exercise real tact, so that the client can be free and comfortable about this behavior. If counselors use circumlocutions to phrase questions or if they show embarrassment or imply judgments in discussing sexual matters, they only further intensify the client's difficulties. Clergy have an additional and complicated problem in exploring this aspect of behavior. Religion is the primary source of moral judgments about sexual mores, and the client cannot help but be aware of this. Consequently, the rabbis, priests, or ministers must clearly differentiate between the roles of counselor and minister. Generally, they will find it useful to define their role as counselors to the client before starting the interview; indeed, they may have to do this repeatedly, since the latter will need reassurance about this new role of the pastor. Because sex is an anxiety-laden subject for most people, counselors should allow considerable latitude in discussions of it. Forcing them prematurely may interfere with the therapeutic alliance and prevent counselors from getting adequate information.

Some of the client's sexual history may be revealed in discussion of sibling relationships; in talking about parents, clients may indicate how they imparted or failed to impart sexual information. If not, counselors can begin with current sexual adjustment in marriage and go on to explore earlier development, including sexual behavior during courtship and dating, and masturbation (attitudes and reactions to it, age of onset, how long practiced, whether solitary or mutual, nature of fantasies, etc.). In adolescence sexual experimentation is common. Consequently, counselors should get as much specific data as possible about the nature and persistence of the practice. For many children, there are two peaks of masturbation, the first around age six, at the height of the "family romance," and the second in adolescence, with the upsurge of sexual feelings accompanying the hormonal changes occurring at puberty. If the masturbation was discovered by the parents, counselors should ask how they handled it. The parents' reaction and particularly the methods they used to discourage masturbation, may have long-term effects on the child's later sexual development, attitudes, and behavior.

A child's curiosity about sexuality normally becomes very active from about age four to seven. Families vary widely in their handling of the child's sexual curiosity. Although the general cultural climate tends to encourage a realistic and healthy approach, some parents still believe that by making sex a taboo subject, they ensure the child's remaining ignorant and uncontaminated. However, it usually happens that the child gets information (and misinformation) elsewhere. Moreover, such parents tend to have major or minor sexual psychopathology that is acted out in the family; such behavior further complicates the situation for the child. Very rigid parental attitudes usually are indicative of problems that can be handled only by excessive control. A client should also talk about additional siblings born during this period and his or her awareness of mother's pregnancy — what was he or she told about conception, pregnancy, and birth? Some individuals have no memories relating to such important events. While we know that the infantile amnesia tends to block much of what happens prior to age seven, when such amnesia includes events from ages three to seven, it tells of more massive repression.

If the client is a woman, the counselor should take a detailed history of her menstrual functioning, beginning with the onset of her menstruation. A number of questions can be raised. What were the circumstances under which it occurred, had she been prepared for it by mother, and what was mother's attitude? (Did mother view it as a burden and threat, did she intensify her restrictions on her daughter's activities?) When was the menstrual cycle established, what is the current status of the menstrual cycle, are there any physical or psychological symptoms or reactions associated with various aspects of the cycle? More particularly, are there swings of mood or variations in sexual drive associated with the endocrine fluctuations during the various phases of the menstrual cycle

(Benedek, 1952)? The endocrine changes during the course of each menstrual cycle affect a woman's sexual interest and responsiveness. Conception, pregnancy, and parturition are important phases in a woman's life. Her psychological and physiological responses to pregnancy reflect her psychological attitudes to femininity and motherhood. Certain women have psychological complications relating to the birth of the baby, particularly mood changes in the postpartum period. Occasionally a woman develops a postpartum psychosis. A counselor can ask: what was her reaction to the baby? Did she feel confident about her ability to provide the necessary care for the baby or was she anxious and fearful? Of equal importance, the counselor should know about the baby's response to the mother's ministrations. The feedback from the infant in the mother-infant symbiosis can either reinforce or sap her confidence in her abilities (Benedek, 1952). Even those instances in which the mother's abilities are in no way contributory, for example, when the infant is ill, may carry psychological implications that deplete her self-esteem. It is also necessary to inquire into the husband's relationship to his wife throughout the pregnancy and postpartum periods. His attitudes toward the pregnancy and the new member of the family will affect his wife. Does he support her and cater to her needs, or does he withdraw and deny her necessary emotional support?

Mid-life is another developmental phase in a woman's life. A number of physical symptoms of varying severity may accompany the gradual or rapid cessation of the menses and the associated endocrine changes. In addition, a woman usually reacts psychologically to the termination of her generative functioning. Some women feel useless and unattractive; for others, release from the fear of pregnancy may increase their sex interest and permit them to enjoy sexual relations more fully. Her particular psychological reaction often reflects a woman's estimation of her functions as a mother and wife and its relationship to her ego ideal. Her conscious or unconscious view of herself as a failure may precipitate a depression or other psychological reactions that affect her relation to her husband. Both her fantasies and his actual response to this change are significant: if a real or fantasized rejection and loss of his love occurs, she may become anxious and depressed. Thus, a woman's adjustment following the menopause, as well as her reactions to mid-life generally, should be investigated.

Although there is no parallel endocrinal upheaval, similar psychological reaction often pertains in men between the ages of forty-five to fifty-five. At some point during this decade, the man begins to become aware of his decreasing physical vigor. At the same time he realizes that much of his life is behind him, and as a result he assesses his accomplishments in terms of his youthful expectations and ambitions. The greater the discrepancy between these, the more likely he is to suffer a mid-life depression of varying magnitude. Consequently, the counselor should explore this critical phase of life in the man for possible evidences of psychological decompensation.

MANAGEMENT OF AGGRESSION

An area that is often overlooked is the individual's ability to handle aggression and hostility. We know a great deal about sexual behavior, both normal and deviant, but we are still traversing a dark continent when we talk about aggression. One has only to read any daily newspaper, with its lurid accounts of crime and war, to see that the species *homo sapiens* has made very little progress toward understanding the well-springs of aggressive behavior and the mechanisms for channeling this drive along constructive lines. In general, there are only four mechanisms for modifying aggressions (Hartman, Kris, & Lowenstein, 1964):

1. Aggression may be displaced to other objects.
2. The aggressive impulse may be restricted in terms of goal.
3. The aggressive energy may be modified through neutralization or sublimation of the drive energy.
4. The aggressive drive may be modified as a result of fusion with the sexual drive.

The capacity to form permanent relationships with others depends on the person's ability to tolerate frustration. Characteristically, varying degrees of anger and withdrawal of love accompany the small child's frustration. Mature, adult relationships do not display such archaic evidences of ambivalence. Unfortunately, such an ideal state of affairs does not always result in (chronologically) adult relationships. All too often, this type of ambivalence is most clearly seen in marital relationships.

Displacement is a common mechanism for dealing with hostility, for example, the man comes home angry at his boss and takes it out on his wife. Under certain circumstances, if the object chosen is suitable, displacement may involve no limitation in the full discharge of aggression. On the other hand, displacement as illustrated in the above example does not solve the real problem and usually creates only additional difficulties. Many instances of "man in search of a target" are responsible for much of our social tension. Discrimination against minority groups represents a discharge of individuals' unresolved aggression in behavior that to some extent has become culturally condoned.

Another misuse of aggression is its denial through reaction formation, in which persons unconsciously control aggressiveness by becoming unduly kind and oversolicitous in situations in which they should experience anger. Such rigid defenses not only rob individuals of energy but also render them relatively helpless, since they are unable to recognize a situation that demands aggressive action. Certain other individuals manage aggression by turning it back on themselves. Self-defeating behavior takes many forms, including various psychosomatic syndromes; the ultimate in destructive behavior is suicide. Such behaviors need to be carefully evaluated. When aggressive drive energy is adequately modulated through neutralization and/or fusion, individuals have adequate reservoirs of energy to apply to constructive activities and to sustain interests. Unfortunately, those child-rearing practices that encourage such a development are all too frequently not sustained and encouraged because of adverse social, economic, political, and educational conditions in large segments of our population.

RECREATIONAL INTERESTS

Counselors should also find out what individuals do for pleasure and recreation, which is a vital part of the necessary balance between work and play. While a utopian world would unite pleasure with work, few people ever achieve this ideal. Western industrial society places a high premium on production techniques that deprive individuals of creative pleasure in their work and make them rely more heavily on avocations to renew energies. Consequently, an inventory of nonprofessional activities becomes important. This should include their relative place in daily life, the types of satisfactions derived from them, and the degree to which they permit expression of creativity and individuality. Obviously, at one end of the spectrum are those hedonists who make pleasure their only goal and, consequently, never really achieve it, while at the other extreme are those individuals who cannot relax and who get sick when they are not working. Ferenczi (1960) aptly subsumed these under the "Sunday neuroses."

RELIGIOUS AFFILIATION

Another aspect of life fundamental to the counselor's summary is the client's view of religion. An individual's religious commitment, nominal or sincere, is a vital part of his or her everyday life. Some persons participate actively in Church affiliations that directly influence their behavior. For others, Church membership may be less important, but an ethic and moral code may still significantly impinge upon their behavior.

Like all aspects of human behavior, religious activity can undergo neurotic distortions and lead to compulsive and more or less meaningless behavior due to excessive neurotic guilt: its extreme form is scrupulosity. However, for most individuals, religion is a resource that can be called upon to mobilize important strengths when facing crises.

DREAM AWARENESS

Neurophysiological studies (Aserinsky & Klietman, 1953; Snyder, 1966) have found that dreaming is a nightly occurrence for everyone, but that some people either are unaware of dreaming or cannot recall dreams. A casual inquiry as to whether the client remembers any recent or repetitive dreams may yield insight into unconscious processes (it may be more effective to ask about dreams at this initial counseling phase, when the dream censorship is less alert, than later) (Freud, 1953). A dream that immediately precedes the diagnostic interview may say more about the patient's unconscious attitude toward therapy than his or her responses to questions. The same type of insight may be drawn from dreams that occur immediately following the initial interview. Often they describe clearly the patient's reaction to the counselor and the initial problem or problems that will have to be dealt with in treatment.

MENTAL FUNCTIONING

So far I have said nothing about the client's mental status. In any diagnostic interview there needs to be an evaluation of the central nervous system's functional capacity. In certain types of organic brain disease, such as senile dementia, delirium, brain tumor, or mental deficiency, clients may show various degrees of abnormality in cognitive functioning. In the toxic-organic syndromes, the underlying changes in the central nervous system may be reversible or irreversible; in either case, they will tend to show cognitive disturbances. Under this heading falls the *sensorium,* with particular reference to the state of consciousness and any degree of clouding of consciousness.

Counselors may want to note other mental functions, for example, disturbances of memory; orientation to time, place, and person; reasoning ability; judgment; ability to perform simple mathematical problems; ability to concentrate on the current task; and general intelligence level. While this information can be obtained by asking specific questions, in most instances the counselor will be able to evaluate these functions on the basis of the client's performance during the course of the interview. In certain instances where a person is unable to cooperate effectively with the interviewer, it may be necessary to question the client directly about these areas to arrive at an appropriate diagnosis.

In psychotic clients, counselors should be aware of aberrations in mental functioning, such as hallucinations, delusions, ideas of reference, misinterpretations; beliefs that one is being persecuted or grandiose beliefs regarding identity, power, wealth, and destructiveness; ideas of self-deprecation and worthlessness or great sinfulness and self-accusation; ideas of poverty or illness; ideas about unreal conditions of the self or the environment, as well as hypochondriacal concerns about bodily illness. While eliciting such information, counselors should watch the appropriateness of the affect accompanying the thoughts as well as their presence or absence. In the case of delusions, one should ascertain the tenacity or degree of doubt with which the patient holds to them. Finally, one should determine whether the client has any insight into the fact that he or she is ill.

In most instances in which clergy find themselves dealing with either toxic-organic syndromes or frankly psychotic clients, they should arrange a psychiatric consultation or referral. Such cases often need immediate hospitalization and provisions of various types of somatic therapy that they are not prepared to undertake. In certain organic syndromes, delay in proper therapy may cause irreversible pathology. In the psychotic client, there is an ever-present danger of injury to self or others; such a danger makes immediate evaluation imperative.

The preceding paragraphs have outlined the major areas that should be explored in the diagnostic interview. The critical reader will naturally ask whether it is possible to inquire into such diversified areas in one interview, even if an hour has been allocated to it. While increasing experience will enable the counselor to use the interviewing time more efficiently, in most instances one session will not permit a review of all the subjects suggested above. How many interviews should be devoted to diagnosis? No absolute rules can be laid down. Counselors' style, the particular conditions under which they are working, clients' needs and ability to contribute effectively must be considered. With those occasional clients whose anxiety is extreme, counselors may have to forego taking a full history, and the entire interview may have to be centered on the presenting problem and limited to dealing wth the acute crisis. Because of the emergency nature of the situation, counselors may do best to conclude with arrangements for treatment or referral at this time. The history can then be obtained at a later date in the course of therapy. However, most cases are not emergencies.

In situations that allow for additional sessions, counselors must decide on an appropriate number of diagnostic interviews. In general, two or three interviews (usually two) work out most satisfactorily. When the diagnostic interviews take place over a longer period of time, the original purpose is lost sight of and frequently the interviews (although inadvertently) become psychotherapeutic. This has certain unfortunate consequences. Clients may not have wanted to undertake treatment and thus be deprived of the opportunity to decide for themselves after learning what is involved in psychotherapy. Instead, clients should be given a clear idea of what treatment involves in terms of method, time and energy, commitment, and cost. Otherwise, they may feel trapped, having become ensnared by disclosing too much and perhaps having developed a relationship with the counselor from which they feel powerless to extricate themselves.

Concluding the first interview

Assuming that the diagnostic interview will be limited to two sessions, counselors have to decide how to handle the interruption as well as the structuring of the second interview. In general, it is wise not to be too rigidly scheduled when making the diagnostic interview. Flexibility permits greater latitude in deciding when to terminate the interview and enables counselors to cover the important subjects during the first session, in view of the clients' anxiety and stress and the need to introduce subjects at the most appropriate point. Extra time also allows counselors to jot down important notes at the conclusion of the interview, review the information, record additional data or opinions, make an initial formulation of the problem, and plan for the next session. By summarizing the session, they get greater perspective on the data collected.

Having decided to bring the initial interview to a conclusion, counselors can say: "You have told me a great deal about yourself, but obviously there are gaps that occur to both of us. I would like to see you again to continue our exploration." Clients, not infrequently, will be relieved at this break; but having revealed so much of themselves, they naturally are concerned about the counselor's evaluation and the nature of the problem. In most instances they will accept a comment indicating that the counselor recognizes the desire for a diagnostic formulation, but believes that the time has not yet come for a definite opinion. Occasionally, it may be necessary to go further than this to relieve tension. After arranging for the next appointment, counselors may want to make additional comments that include information about the structure of the next interview and certain suggestions about tasks the client can perform until the next meeting. How the client responds to these suggestions and the degree to which he or she is able or unable to comply with these requests may give additional diagnostic information.

During the concluding remarks counselors may ask the client to think about the interview, note whether important areas were not covered, and offer to bring these up at the beginning of the next hour. The concluding remarks also include any corrections or additions to the material discussed. Since counselors have already questioned the client about dreams, they may want to suggest that the client bring in any remembered dreams that occur between the two interviews. They can also ask the client to discuss subsequent reactions to the interview. These may provide further information about how realistically they can appraise the situation and their role in it. Some clients are unable to produce anything realistic, but will respond in a way they think will please counselors. Some give evidence of an overloading of positive or negative reactions, which may indicate the beginning of transference reactions. To correctly evaluate such comments requires objectivity on the part of counselors, since they must be able to determine when the client's comments are realistically based and when they are unrealistic and have their roots in the past. Finally, counselors should say that in addition to outlining the nature of the problem, they will want to discuss the client's ideas about psychotherapy.

Structuring the second interview

After the initial exchange of greetings, counselors should sit back and give the client an opportunity to initiate the interview and discuss the various items outlined at the end of the last hour. In the event that some or all of these are omitted, counselors should bring them up and observe the client's response to such questions. They should keep in mind specific reasons why these were left out and the client's reaction to the fact that he or she ignored these suggestions.

Following this, counselors should continue with the areas of the history not covered in the previous interview, making sure that adequate time be left at the end of the hour to formulate the problem and give their recommendations. If they indeed recommend psychotherapy, the client should be asked to respond. If agreement and willingness are indicated to undertake treatment, the client should be asked to discuss what he or she knows and thinks is involved in the psychotherapeutic process. These days, relatively few clients are completely naive about psychotherapy; nonetheless, many of their ideas involve major or minor distortions.

Counselors should then indicate their areas of agreement and disagreement, making explicit what they consider to be the basic aspects of the psychotherapeutic process. It is generally wise to limit these statements to the basic essentials, since the relationship will evolve naturally along the lines that are best suited to the patient and the therapist (Sharpe, 1950, pp. 28ff.). At the same time they should agree upon a baseline that can be referred to when specific problems arise later. In addition, such discussion further assists the patient in deciding whether to start therapy, considering all that this commitment implies.

If the decision is made to accept the recommendation for psychotherapy, the client and counselor should decide the frequency and length of interviews and agree upon a suitable time for the therapy sessions. They make a mutual commitment to maintaining the interviews on a regular basis. In arranging the time of the appointment, the realistic problems of the client and counselor should, whenever possible, be taken into account. The fee should also be relevant to the economic circumstances of both parties. Neither the client nor the counselor will be comfortable unless this decision reflects the needs of both.

Therapist's homework

Once the client has left, counselors should organize the historical material gathered in the diagnostic interviews in a meaningful way. They can do so by using the outline of subject matter enumerated above. But this method has one disadvantage: it makes it easier to overlook the interrelations of the different aspects of the history as they occurred in time. Use of a chronological developmental sequence may draw out the dynamic connections between seemingly unrelated experiences that had a close temporal relationship to each other. For example:

	Year	Age	
July 7	1960	0	Birth – client is first child.
November	1962	2½	Toilet training is completed.
January	1963	3	Father is drafted, leaves home. Baby sister born – client regresses to infantile behavior – frequent soiling during day and at night occurs.

In this illustration it becomes apparent immediately that the birth of the sibling and the departure of the father for the service are sufficient traumas to precipitate the regression in the child's behavior.

Once material has been organized to their satisfaction, therapists should make a diagnostic formulation. First, they should arrive at a genetic-dynamic diagnosis. The genetic category includes the important life-experiences, particularly early childhood events, that had important bearing on the development of the patient. Initially, the infant has no capacity for channeling drives and only acquires it through learning under the guidance of parents. Gradually, a widening circle of individuals will contribute to learning, but the early experiences, when the child is most impressionable, will center mainly on the relationships with the parents. The instinctual drives furnish the energy, at least in large part, and are the motivational forces that seek specific kinds of satisfaction. These dynamic forces are modified in part by the maturational changes that occur in the instinctual drives as the child grows and also by learning, which modifies the expression of the drives. Thus, certain dynamic patterns become characteristic of each individual and must be identified. Such a genetic-dynamic diagnosis gives a picture of the individual's psychological structure and should explain why the precipitating factors that initiated the personality decompensation were effective. A descriptive clinical diagnosis should also be included.

The Diagnostic and Statistical Manual of Mental Disorders (DSM, III, 1980) offers five axes around which the information may be structured. Axis I organizes *Clinical Syndromes* and Axis II the *Personality Disorders:*

> Axes I and II comprise the entire classification of mental disorders plus Conditions Not Attributable to a Mental Disorder That Are a Focus of Attention or Treatment. The disorders listed on Axis II are the Personality Disorders . . . and the Specific Developmental Disorders . . . the remaining disorders and conditions are included in Axis I.

Axis III includes and takes into account *Physical Disorders or Conditions* that are "potentially relevant to the understanding or management of the individual." Axes IV and V are considered supplementary to the official diagnosis, but are included as useful considerations for planning treatment and may have prognostic significance. Axis IV rates the *Severity of Psychosocial Stressors;* it

> provides a coding of the overall severity of a stressor judged to have been a significant contributor to the development or exacerbation of the current disorder. An individual's prognosis may be better when a disorder develops as a consequence of a severe stressor than when it develops after no stressor or a minimal stressor.

Axis V is listed in the *Manual* as the *Highest Level of Adaptive Functioning Past Year* and

> permits the clinician to indicate his or her judgment of an individual's highest level of adaptive functioning (for at least a few months) during the past year.

This information frequently has prognostic significance, because usually an individual returns to his or her previous level of adaptive functioning after an episode of illness.

Pastoral counselors may find it useful to organize the material around the multidimensional themes offered by Paul Pruyser in the following chapter. His seven categories: awareness of the holy, providence, faith, grace-gratefulness, repentance, communion, and vocation, take into account the theological perspective of counselor and client and avoid some of the difficulties of medical language and categories.

Therapists should evaluate the patient's reasons for presenting him- or herself at a particular time and the motivation for psychotherapy. In the process they often can identify the problems that must be dealt with in the initial phases of therapy. Such predictions can be extremely helpful in anticipating resistances that will complicate the development of the therapeutic alliance. Finally, therapists should state their initial therapeutic goals, at the same time recognizing that they may have to be modified as additional material becomes available and as their understanding of the patient increases.

The last statement implies that no matter how detailed the history taking has been, omissions as well as incorrect data will turn up as the psychotherapeutic sessions unfold. They will result partly from conscious or unconscious distortion, which is to be expected in the initial stages of such a relationship. Trust—basic trust in Erikson's sense—is achieved only through increasing experience in the therapeutic relation. No matter how anxious or guilty the client is, he or she still carries certain inhibitions in communicating to an individual viewed as an authority and an analogue of parents. The client has to learn to expose him- or herself even though criticism is expected and to refrain from censoring material that will unquestionably elicit judgment. The patient's task is made more difficult when counselors also serve as the client's minister. In such instances it may be too much to expect parishioners, who have always seen their clergy as the epitome of moral judgment, to immediately accept the latter in their new role, as being able to listen in a noncritical way and to accept clients' problems as behavior to be understood rather than judged. Consequently, much testing will ensue until trust is established. The other aspect of treatment which contributes to the development of new data is the gradual penetration of repressions. Generally, as clients proceed, they recover additional memories. The new data will necessitate reformulations of the material and perhaps modifications of the therapeutic goals. As counselors gain new insights and decide on new goals, they should note these changes.

The diagnostic interview tests all of the counselor's skills, but at the same time always provides challenges and opportunities for discovering new or different patterns of adaptive or nonadaptive behavior relating to psychological development. Each individual has a unique personality, despite his or her similarities to other people. While each person has to face the same conflicts in the course of development, the particular environmental circumstances and life-experiences under which these are resolved are always unique. Consequently, a person's psychological interpretations of events, the meanings assigned, are (all in all) his or hers alone. The combination and relationship of individual and universal human experience make people — and counseling — continually interesting and confront the counselor each time he or she seeks to explore the pattern of a new client's psychological configuration.

REFERENCES

American Psychiatric Association. *Diagnostic and Statistical Manual of Mental Disorders: DSM III,* 1980.

Aserinsky, S., & Klietman, N. Regular ocular periods of eye motility and concomitant phenomenon during sleep. *Science* 118, 273–74, 1953.

Benedek, T. *Studies in psychosomatic medicine: psychosexual function in women.* New York: Ronald Press, 1952.

Dobzhansky, T. *Mankind Evolving.* New Haven: Yale University Press, 1962.

Erikson, Erik H. *Childhood and Society,* 2nd ed. New York: W. W. Norton & Co., 1964.

Ferenszi, S. Sunday neuroses (1910). In *Further Contribution to the Theory and Technique of Psychoanalysis.* London: Hogarth Press, 1950.

Fleming, J., & Altschule, S. Activation of mourning and growth by psychoanalysis. *The International Journal of Psychoanalysis* 44, 419–431, 1963.

Freud, S. Screen memories (1899). In *Standard Edition,* vol. 3. London: Hogarth Press, 1962, 303–22.

Freud, S. Delusions and dreams on Jensen's Gradiva (1906). In *Standard Edition,* vol. 9. London: Hogarth Press, 1959.

Freud, S. A special type of object relation made by man (1910). In *Standard Edition,* vol. 11. London: Hogarth Press, 1957.

Freud, S. The interpretation of dreams. In *Standard Edition,* vols. 4 & 5. London: Hogarth Press, 1953.

Gaskill, H. S. The physician-patient relationship. In Association of American Medical Colleges *Report of the Second Institute on Clinical Teaching,* n.p., 1959.

Hartman, H. Psychoanalysis and developmental psychology. In *Essays on Ego Psychology.* In *Papers on Psychoanalytic Psychology: Psychological Issues* monograph 14. New York: International Universities Press, 1964, 44-112.

Hartman, H., & Kris, E. The genetic approach in psychoanalysis. In *Papers on Psychoanalytic Psychology: Psychological Issues* monograph 14. New York: International Universities Press, 1964, 7-26.

Hartman, H.; Kris, H.; & Lowenstein, R. M. Notes on the theory of aggression. In *Papers on Psychoanalytic Psychology: Psychological Issues* monograph 14. New York: International Universities Press, 1964, 56-85.

Johnson, A., et al. School phobia. *American Journal of Orthopsychiatry* 11, 702-11, 1941.

Kaufman, M. R. The patient-physician relationship. In *Teaching Psychotherapeutic Medicine.* Cambridge: Harvard University Press, 1947, 63-78.

Osler, W. *Aequanimitas.* Philadelphia: P. Blakiston's Son and Co., 1905.

Sharpe, E. G. *Collected Papers on Psychoanalysis.* London: Hogarth Press, 1950.

Snyder, F. Toward the evolutionary theory of dreaming. *The American Journal of Psychiatry* 123, 121-36, 1966.

6

The Diagnostic Process in Pastoral Care

PAUL W. PRUYSER

During decades of interaction between clergy and the clinical disciplines of psychology and psychiatry, the overwhelming emphasis has been on augmenting and perfecting the pastors' healing skills and on conveying to pastors useful knowledge about normal and abnormal psychological conditions. The vicissitudes of the human life-span and an understanding of the successive life-themes and growth-tasks appear to have been of major interest to practicing pastors who pursued clinical pastoral education in order to deal skillfully with the foibles and personal problems of their parishioners. During or after the seminary years, many pastors studied personality theory, gained familiarity with descriptive psychiatry and psychiatric syndromes, acquired counseling skills, and learned the techniques of various forms of individual, marital, family, or group psychotherapy. Undoubtedly, these borrowings from other professions' knowledge and skill have enhanced these pastors' sense of professional competence and, to all likelihood, have been to the benefit of their problem-laden parishioners.

Trends that endanger the integrity of pastoral ministry

Having been a sideline participant in clinical pastoral education for many years, mostly as a consultant psychologist to training programs, seminary faculties, and individual ministers, I am concerned about some attitudes and trends that have the effect of endangering pastors' professional identity as well as the authenticity and autonomy of ministry. Let me put my observations succinctly, well aware of risky oversimplification.

1. On the whole, ministers tend to act from a passionate ethical desire to be helpful to their people. They tend to engage with zeal in a great variety of helping relations, and their conscience propels them to undertake tasks of sometimes extraordinary difficulty. Their dedication to meliorism may bring them close to a professional stance that could be described as *furor therapeuticus,* which runs the built-in risk of producing disappointment, if not professional burnout.

2. The sociology of professions shows crisscrossing curves of ascent and descent of the popular esteem or relevance attributed to the professions at any given time. As one profession rises in esteem or prominence, other professions appear to lose esteem, undoubtedly for a complex mixture of good and bad reasons, but nevertheless with powerful effect on any profession's self-esteem. Certain professions achieve dominance at certain times, with the result that their basic and applied knowledge, their techniques or skills, and their language games are being emulated by members of other professions whose status is (again for a mixture of good and bad reasons) under a cloud. Many observers of the professional scene have noted that as dynamic psychiatry and psychology became prominent from the late 1940s through the 1970s, the practitioners of pastoral ministry felt themselves confused, seated themselves at the feet of psychiatric Gamaliels, and sought to raise their professional self-esteem and enhance their professional skills by absorbing psychological knowledge and skills. With a touch of imperialism, the psychological disciplines began to consider ministers as "first-line mental health workers" and showed some eagerness to help ministers become "better" at this function.

3. The discovery by ministers of useful knowledge and skill to be gleaned from the psychological disciplines, as well as the steady spread and intensification of formal clinical pastoral education, laudable enough in their own right, have led, among other things, to an increasingly strong conviction voiced by many pastors that the basic theological disciplines as taught in seminaries have little to offer in guiding them to make wholesome and effective interventions in the lot of their troubled parishioners. All too often pastors began to substitute psychological-mindedness for theological-mindedness, sometimes to the point of doubting the relevance to their pastoral work of the theological disciplines, the Church tradition, and the religious language conventions. To put it somewhat starkly, the new knowledge overtook the relevance of the old knowledge, and the practicing pastor's professional self-esteem began to be measured by his or her psychological expertise.

It is a sad commentary on the integrity and authenticity of any discipline or profession when its members suppress their own basic and applied sciences or doubt their applicability to the tasks of healing, guiding, and sustaining that they face daily. What might be done to stem the tide of such intraprofessional alienation? What might be done to foster in practicing pastors a sense of professional authenticity and specificity as they function in overlapping and interacting networks with other helping professions?

A perspectival view of knowledge and professions

No human endeavor is without philosophical assumption. Scholars and professionals tend to hold worldviews that guarantee for their own endeavor an acknowledged niche that promises safety, respect, status, or durability. Such views vouchsafe the worthiness of their undertakings, specify the uniqueness of their knowledge, and demarcate their difference from other disciplines. In the course of our education, most of us become attached to certain models that are supposed to guide or anchor our conceptions of our own disciplines, usually with some defensiveness toward or concern over the ambitiousness of other disciplines by which we may feel endangered.

Some very traditional but still reigning models are in need of brief review.[1]

One of the most abiding models holds that each discipline occupies a bounded space in a large field representing *all* knowledge and/or has privileged access to a peculiar substance culled from an envisioned pool of allegedly real entities. Spatial and substantive thought of this order appears to be an entrenched habit from which even highly educated persons are not free, despite the obvious fact that reality does not lend itself very well to spatial divisions and analysis into bits. For instance, where does "soma" stop and "psyche" begin? The simple spatial view is essentially a territorial view that begs for border raids and territorial defense. A modified spatial model is the pyramidal one, in which disciplines are assigned to the bottom section, middle ranges, or the top of a hierarchy that supposedly reflects corresponding orders of reality. This leads to vying for a place at the top and concomitant denigration of "lower-order" disciplines that allegedly deal with the less than "really real."

The layer-cake model appears to be very popular. In that order three cake layers are stacked to represent, from the bottom upwards, such assumed entities as body, mind, and soul or spirit, each addressed by quite different disciplines. Reality, either as experienced or upon reflection, is not comparable to a system of layered entities. Perhaps the most presumptuous of all is the onion model, which regards most disciplines as peripheral peels that can be discarded to eventually reveal a pith or core that is the truest representation of reality's essence—with the innuendo that one's own discipline is of course affiliated with just that desirable core. All these models beg for animosity between the disciplines, but even worse, by their neat designs appear to be a far cry from the intricacies of reality. We need a model that can do justice to the process character of reality, to the historical forces of division of labor and specialization of functions that have produced the proliferation of disciplines and professions, and to the inventiveness of the human mind that is constantly creating diverse forms of knowledge for its own purposes. I propose, leaning on Whitehead,[2] James,[3][4] and Meland[5]—a perspectival model according to the following diagram:

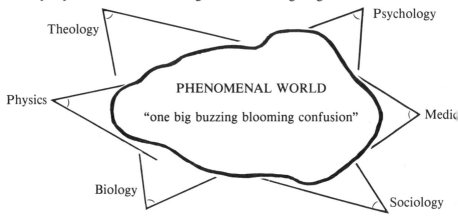

The observable reality that is our common ambience presents itself to the newborn, according to James, as "one big buzzing blooming confusion," with which we are slowly coming to terms by the unfolding of our cognitive and emotional capacities and by instruction. The confusion in which we start gets replaced by an evolving order produced by culturally transmitted ordering principles inherent in the human mind itself as it operates on the chaotic self-presentation of the phenomenal world. We acquire a knack for placing the chaotic manifold into a certain perspective, putting it into a light of our own choosing, focusing on it from a certain angle, and thereby getting some grasp on it. Each discipline should be regarded as a special point of view or unique perspective on the original chaotic manifold that bombards the senses. By the time any playfully entertained perspective has become a formal discipline or profession, it has gained a marked degree of internal consistency, has acquired a stylized tradition, possesses a canon of procedures and rules, and has invented a unique vocabulary by which to describe the data and processes in which it is interested.

A crucial and noteworthy feature of the perspectival model is that without perspectives there are no data. A sensory chaos only produces confusion, not data. In other words: nothing is anything in particular unless "it" is put into a perspective and is subjected to a set of mental operations. Each perspective (i.e., discipline, profession, form of knowledge) creates its own data, elicited from the phenomenological chaos. Another important implication of the perspectival model is that each perspective (discipline, profession, etc.) deals with reality and that it does so *on its own terms,* without having to be beholden to any other. Each discipline is autonomous and responsible only to itself for its plausibility, viability, integrity, relevance, and heuristic promise for more and better knowledge or its capacity to make meliorative interventions in man, nature, or culture. With these several virtues, the perspectival model is fit to deal with James's insistence on pluralism and its experiential justification, namely, that human experience is multiform, multifaceted, and astoundingly rich in nuances that no philosophy should be allowed to rule out. Moreover, the perspectival model is more likely than any other model to promote mutual respect between the disciplines and to foster interdisciplinary collaboration.

Professional identity

Most pertinent to the purposes of this chapter is the portrayal of any organized discipline as consisting of a more or less cohesive combination of one or more basic sciences, one or more ancillary sciences, certain applied science features, a special language game, and when the discipline has become also a profession, a set of skills or techniques that are no longer intuitive, but backed by theoretical reflection and transmitted under tutelage.[6] Education for ministry and the praxis of pastoral work rest on such a package, which has attained its shape through centuries and is constantly being reshaped by the exigencies of the discipline's situation in the world and of its professional endeavors.

Though textbooks tend to promote the impression that disciplines start with basic science and gradually branch out into applications and skillful interventions, members of the helping professions are surely aware of the enormous impact of praxis on theory. Professional helpers are always under pressure to "do something, now" — with guidance from their basic theory if available, without such guidance if must be. The needs of their customers are urgent and their own zeal to help forces the practitioners to make at times a bold move. If the latter turns out to have been effective or inspired, a rationale for it is drawn up which eventually finds its place in the discipline's basic and applied science divisions. In other words some of these professions' basic theory is not a product of pure contemplation but the fruit of attempted transformations by practitioners addressing concrete cases that pose some unforeseen novelty. A considerable part of theological knowledge is indeed a kind of transformational knowledge, formulated to be in the service of ministry whose task it is to help change persons from an undesirable condition A to a more desirable condition B. Like other professional helpers and change agents, ministers are in the transformation business. Their professional work is to be guided by their knowledge of the accumulated lore of their discipline, augmented by selective reliance on ancillary sciences suited to their ministerial tasks and purposes. All helpers should be clear about the nature of the transformations to which their discipline aspires. Physicians seek to move persons from sickness to health. Ethicists seek to move persons from brutish self-interest to reverence for others and a broad concern for everyone's well-being. Pedagogues seek to replace naiveté by sophistication. Theologically grounded transformations seek to replace sin by virtue, alienation by reconciliation, damnation by redemption, arrogance by a sense of creatureliness, nihilism by faith.

Professional identity, then, consists in being identified with a chosen perspective and acquiring skill in systematically "looking at all things" from within this perspective. It entails reliance on one's basic sciences; respect for the perspective's relevance, potency, and explanatory power; skill in using the discipline's transformational propositions and procedures, and versatility in using the discipline's particular language game.

Professional identity does not prescribe the wearing of blinders for the propositions and procedures of other professions. All the helping professions stand much to learn from each other and are indeed accustomed to all kinds of cross-fertilization that have occurred in their diverse histories. But the use of other perspectives or disciplines as ancillaries to one's own should not lead to identity diffusion or confusion. Ministry is a potent and rich profession that has much to offer to mankind. Millions of people with personal problems turn first or exclusively to their clergy for help or enlightenment. Ministers alone in our society have two enviable professional prerogatives: the right of initiative and the right of access.[7] Most ministers have good conversational, instructional, and interpretive skills. They are known as accessible and helpful people. Last but not least, they share with their parishioners a non-technical vocabulary of ordinary religious language that abounds with stories, symbols, rituals, and other widely understood lore. Moreover, despite some trappings of office, the minister's relation to anyone is essentially egalitarian in the sense that both parties in a pastoral helping-process defer to an unseen third party of greater ultimacy, authority, and power than can be claimed by either the helper or the person to be helped.

The diagnostic task in attempted pastoral transformations

Logic demands that professions seeking to bring about transformations in the lives of their clientele should have means for diagnosing their clients' present condition and should think highly of their members' diagnostic task. Physicians should know illnesses; educators should know the cognitive capabilities and limitations of students. Ministers should have means for making pastoral-theological assessments of the persons who seek their help so as to derive from such assessments the ends and means for their melioration. When not preceded by a diagnostic evaluation, certain interventions may miss the mark, others may entail risks, and all of them are only shots in the dark.

Ministry does have a diagnostic tradition of its own, based on theological considerations and leading to pastoral interventions; this tradition is part of the history of the "cure of souls." The *Malleus Maleficarum*[8] (1487) is a diagnostic manual written for priests of that time to guide them in their role as exorcists. What Catholics call moral theology is a special discipline that evaluates acts, intentions, and dispositions of people, so as to enable a fitting pastoral response to the presenting situation. An "examination of conscience" is part of the sacrament of reconciliation. "Spiritual direction" involves a consideration of motives. Jonathan Edwards' *A Treatise Concerning Religious Affections* (1746)[9] is to a large extent a diagnostic work in which the author examines the reliability of "signs" of any person's religious state. Kierkegaard's works can be considered as one protracted attempt at relentless self-examination, aimed at throwing light on what the "man of faith" is to think, feel, do, and be. But even apart from this venerable pastoral diagnostic tradition, there is the weightier observation that people who seek pastoral counsel are likely to have already been engaged in an informal self-diagnostic process that has led them to the conclusion that pastoral expertise is needed to pursue that self-evaluation in greater depth or with more precision.

The question "What do troubled people seek of pastors?" has often received rather superficial response; from my inspection of pastoral verbatims and video-taped counseling sessions as well as my clinical knowledge of troubled people, I have the growing conviction that people turn to pastors—correctly—because they want to have the opportunity *to look at themselves and their problems in the light of their faith and their religious tradition,* with the help of an expert in just this perspective. By the time any person is reaching out for professional help, he or she has usually become aware that a problem is multifaceted and may well need multiperspectival clarification. If so, it is all the more important that each of the co-opted experts use the tools of his or her trade and satisfy the customer's wish for selectivity. Giving stones — even precious stones — for bread does not still hunger.

At this point a reader may object that pastoral examining (diagnosing) runs the risk of being authoritarian. I side with this objection, and I surmise that this risk is one of the reasons why pastoral-diagnostic work has gone out of favor and why seminarians are by and large not receiving instruction in that pastoral task. In addition I do not emulate the diagnostic attitudes that appear to prevail in other helping professions, which are indeed often quite authoritarian. For a better alternative I take my clue from psychoanalysis, whose technique involves a constant appeal to the patient to be his or her own diagnostician (with the assistance of an expert) and analyze his or her own case. [10] The ideal diagnosis in all professions is a self-diagnosis leading eventually to a cooperatively formulated prescription, as described by Cousins in *The Anatomy of an Illness as Seen by the Patient*. [11] It is time for all helping professions to recognize that their clients and patients are always engaged in self-scrutiny anyway and are entitled to formal assistance, if need be, in this endeavor. In any helping process the client's initiative, activity level, curiosity about the self, and thirst for betterment are to be enlisted and stimulated.

Guidelines for pastoral-diagnostic explorations

In many helping professions a careful diagnosis is half the cure. This is especially so when the diagnostic work avoids the pitfall of yielding a mere typological label, but eventuates in a dynamic formulation of the problem and the problem-laden person, done in such a way that both can be addressed and the best possible solution found commensurate with the person's own inner and external resources. To be conducted in this spirit, pastoral-diagnostic work requires, in the first place, an attitude of immense curiosity about and interest in the troubled person, coupled with keen observation. It involves compassion with the person's plight; ability to "hear" the not-spoken, the not-yet-spoken, or even the unspeakable; interest in complexity; acceptance of irremediable ambiguity; capacity to distinguish between surface and depth in the person's self-presentation and communication, and, above all, some control over one's own *furor therapeuticus*. But such work requires also a belief in the potency of some basic concepts — in this case theological concepts — to highlight individual differences and thus to serve as guidelines for sizing up the particular factors that operate in the concrete case at hand. To be diagnostically useful, the chosen concepts and guidelines should produce empirical differentiations. They should have phenomenological aptness and richness and be amenable to interview situations. They should derive from the pastor's transformational knowledge base into which have gone a great many historical precedents in pastoral intervention.

In this section I offer some guidelines for consideration by pastors interested in doing diagnostic work. But I do so with the caveat that these guidelines are the thought-product of a psychologist trying to think theologically and making an effort to empathize with pastoral helping situations. What I am attempting here should have been undertaken by pastoral theologians and practicing pastors in the first place, and I am well aware of the provisional status of my recommendation. The subject matter is worthy of a whole book that I hope someone will write; I have devoted a whole chapter to it in my own *The Minister as Diagnostician,* [6] which in part rests on my previous work in psychology of religion. [12] [13] In being invited to contribute to the present volume, I can only make some concise and tersely worded statements.

If I were a pastor faced with persons seeking my help in personal problems, I would first explore whether my parishioner or client has any *awareness of the holy* and how this awareness affects his or her sense of *creatureliness.* For what kinds of beings, powers, ideas, or values does the person have a feeling of reverence, and on what does he or she "utterly" depend? Does the person know awe, bliss, and humility, and in what situations? Is there any self-abnegation, a sense of mystery, or acceptance of one's contingency? Some seemingly humble souls are arrogantly demanding and insist that their God will deliver to them exactly what they (mis)take him to have promised. What are the person's *idols* for whom sacrifices are willingly made — in time, money, energy, or devotion? Exactly what and where is the divine, if any, in the person's life and world view?

I would also be very curious about the person's sense of *providence,* the more so since pastoral interview situations are often loaded with tragic happenings, leading the client to ask: "What can the divine intention be? Why am I besieged? Why me? What have I done to deserve this?" Abstract notions about the divine purpose are one thing — what everyone wants to know is the divine intention toward him- or herself, on account of which this theme is a fertile one for exploration. Some people are so beset by malevolence in their lives or have such a bleak world view that the very thought of any benevolence anywhere, let alone toward themselves, cannot dawn on them. Because I believe that pastoral care may be described as "providential care mediated," it stands to reason that the dejected person, disappointed in providence, is likely to have less than full trust in the pastor too, wondering at first whether the pastor is indeed willing or able to help him or her, deems the person worthy of help, or in turn believes in a benevolent provider as a transcendent source of help. Or else, belief in providence can be smothered by feelings of great personal competence and self-sufficiency, in which case there is not even any need to consider providential guidance.

Tied in with attitudes toward providence is the *important distinction between hoping and wishing:* the hoper is concerned with global benefits such as life, freedom, deliverance, and salvation; the wisher is concerned with specific things such as money, rain after a drought, social esteem, or the death of his enemies. The hoper tests reality; the wisher engages in magical thought. The hoper is an eschatologist, who lets God be God; the wisher is only an apocalyptist, who seeks reversals of his fate and the fulfillment of his revengeful fantasies. All such personal variations on the theme of providence throw considerable light on what people believe God has promised to them: a well-furnished mansion in heaven or "only" his abiding presence and an understanding of their plight.

Third, I would want to explore with the person what *faith* means to him or her, subjectively. Is the person a hearty yea-sayer to life, ideals, and reality, or a critical, cautious nay-sayer full of ifs, buts, and howevers? Does the person have courage to be, and does this courage energize actions and give enthusiasm and stamina? Or does the person remain lukewarm and prone to "bad faith" and without true engagement in anything? Is the person anxiously possessive about *his* or *her* faith: "My faith is leaving me in the lurch," or "My Bible tells me that . . ."? Many personal horizons have been narrowed rather than widened by what some persons describe as "my faith." Many personal relations have been restricted to intercourse only with like-minded, like-believing, like-instructed, and like-molded people in a small world, beset by fear of strangers and a precarious hold on "faith."

Sooner or later, a pastoral-diagnostic interview must deal with *grace.* The pastor is bound to meet troubled people on just that plane of experience where grace is of dynamic importance. When guilt feelings are expressed, grace is not necessarily just around the corner. Some people are refractory to grace, no matter how freely or "irresistibly" offered. Others appear to *demand* forgiveness without assuming any responsibility for their foibles or sins. Does the person feel in need of grace at all and even concede to occasionally feeling grateful when luck comes along, or does he or she present him- or herself as a completely self-made person, who owes nothing to others but sees everything as his or her "good right"? Some people, in contrast, have been drilled all their lives to be "so thankful . . ." to everybody that their protestations of genteel obligedness make a mockery of the patent misery of their situation. Their forced gratitude lacks honesty and spontaneity; it is at heart a grim business. In the end attitudes toward grace elucidate appropriate or inappropriate feelings of merit or entitlement.

Closely linked with all the previously presented themes is *sense of repentance, sorriness for sin,* or *willingness to repent.* Does the person present him- or herself as an agent in the problem situation faced, or does the person abrogate all responsibility for it? Is there a feeling of a need to change or only a wish for circumstances to be altered? Some persons present themselves only as victims of fate, not responsible or accountable for their misfortune. Others, in contrast, present themselves as hyperresponsible and as the sole agents of their predicaments, burdening themselves with guilt feelings when in fact their outward behavior appears to be nearly impeccable. They consider themselves great sinners, sometimes to the point of naming themselves with some secret glee "the greatest of all sinners" in league with the devil. Their scrupulosity compels them to make endless confessions without resolution. Blind to their own perverted pride (which they are not ready to confess), they hold themselves beyond forgiveness. Some throw the burden of repenting on others: "If my divorced wife could only say that she is sorry, I would feel better."

A sixth theme worth exploring is the person's *sense of communion:* with whom or with what, if any? Does the person feel embedded in the chain of being or set outside it? Separation, alienation, isolation—these painful feelings are frequently voiced in pastoral interviews. Suffering tends to isolate the sufferer; in other cases the estrangement is self-engendered or willed, but leads to unanticipated consequences. Feelings of bitterness are often keenest toward other members or factions of the local congregation and, in some cases, toward the denomination's national leadership. Such bitterness is all the more painful for persons who guiltily know that believers should be forbearing, kind, and charitable. Ideological similarities and differences can play a decisive role in patterning the sense of communion: some seek communion in close face-to-face groups, and some feel kinship with distant others. Disappointment in people may enhance attachment to animals.

If I were a pastor, my theology would prompt me to be especially alert to any person's *sense of vocation,* i.e., the willingness to be a zestful participant in the scheme of creation and providence and to live with a sense of purpose. In this context vocation does not refer solely to what one does to earn a living, but describes a fundamental attitude toward life as a task to be shouldered with energy, enthusiasm, and melioristic zeal, while keeping a watchful eye on the demonic element in human nature and human affairs. The capacity to live one's life as a journey or pilgrimage gives meaning to the whole life span and aids in the acceptance of inevitable tragedies. Depressions and overly cautious attitudes undermine this capacity and make life grim. The sense of vocation or its absence can significantly affect a person's life-style: those who have it appear to live in an expanding psychic economy that allows them to be open to a wide range of experiences, to assimilate much from their world, and to enjoy much of it — very different from those who live in a shrinking psychic economy that leads them to caution, hesitancy, and the rejection of much that comes along in life. Control is the watchword in the latter case, with an eventually stifling effect. Maybe humor is a sign of the presence of a sense of vocation, inasmuch as humor is not afraid of the imagination and does not disdain playful tinkering with the opportunities that life offers.

These guidelines illustrate the kind of pastoral-diagnostic work that can be germane to the profession of ministry. Undoubtedly my own theological orientation has affected my choice of variables somewhat, and the reader should therefore feel free to augment, alter, or replace the selection and formulation of these guidelines. There should be ample room for experimentation — as long as the adopted guidelines have the capacity to bring out individual differences and allow the pastoral diagnostician to size up the unique qualities of the person who is seeking help. Even more important than allowing the pastor to assess the person, the guidelines should operate in the diagnostic interviews in such a way that the troubled person becomes engaged in sizing up him- or herself. For that is, at the deepest level of intention, what problem-laden persons are after when they choose to place themselves and their situation in the perspective of their faith and its tradition.

The pastoral use of ancillary disciplines

Just as linguistics and archeology may be co-opted as ancillary disciplines in the pursuit of biblical scholarship, and just as elocution enters as an auxiliary skill into the art of preaching, pastoral work with troubled individuals or groups can greatly benefit from knowledge accrued in psychology, psychiatry, social work, and other helping professions. Pastors interested in working with troubled persons are well advised to avail themselves of clinical pastoral education and to acquire interviewing and helping skills under supervision. But the use of ancillary disciplines and skills in any profession should be subordinated to the profession's basic goals, fundamental premises, intrinsic orientation, and vital interests — in a word, to the profession's specific *raison d'être* in a world full of other professions. The troubled person seeking help from a pastor wants the genuine article and not a substitute or ersatz or watered-down version of something else. Although troubled persons may not be able to state clearly and fully what they want, they should be granted at least some intuitive foreknowledge of what they are seeking — sufficient to judge whether or not they eventually got what they sought.

Can the "genuine article" that people seek from pastors be described? Does a theological focus in pastoral counseling or other forms of pastoral work provide special content, satisfy special needs, and facilitate special transformations? Does a perceptible theological perspective in pastoral work vouchsafe the pastor's unique professional identity and confirm the legitimacy of the troubled person's special quest for a *pastoral* helper? I would certainly hope so. But more important than my hope in these matters is the conviction of an experienced, skilled, and well-trained pastor, my colleague Dr. Richard Bollinger,[14] who holds that a theological focus in pastoral work entails at least the following opportunities for troubled people:

1. To arrive at a deeper awareness of the human condition by discussing the tragic aspects of life, the idea of courage, the meaning of suffering, and to be moved from self-centeredness to a concern for others.
2. To be helped in articulating moral concerns such as dealing with loyalties, responding to unfairness, atoning for misdeeds, assuming responsibility, making choices, and shouldering inevitable duties.
3. To be given a chance to sort one's religious and ethical beliefs and to study how these beliefs do or should affect actual behavior; to scrutinize whether intentions and behavior are indeed congruent with the affirmed beliefs or whether there is much disparity between beliefs and acts.
4. To be comforted in personal tragedy and to be aided in celebrating life's important transitional moments, whether joyful or sad; to receive blessings, to be embedded in community, and to be affirmed in one's worth or one's creaturely significance.
5. To engage appropriately and with a sense of being understood in religious language; to avail oneself of the religious guidance inherent in biblical or traditional stories, sayings, poetry, and other lore; and to be moved by the symbolism of rituals.
6. To be able to witness, even if only in the privacy of the pastor's study, to the tenets of one's faith; to express intentions and hopes; and to feel reconciled.

I have nothing to add to this impressive list, except to ask: Where else can a troubled person find such opportunities for exactly this kind of self-diagnosis, self-discovery, and self-healing?

NOTES

1. Paul W. Pruyser. *The Psychological Examination*. New York: International Universities Press, 1979. ch. 1.

2. Alfred North Whitehead. *Process and Reality: An Essay in Cosmology*. New York: MacMillan, 1933.

3. William James. *Psychology: Briefer Course*. New York: Henry Holt & Co., 1892.

4. William James. *A Pluralistic Universe*. New York: Longmans, Green & Co., 1911.

5. Bernard E. Meland. *Higher Education and the Human Spirit*. Chicago: The University of Chicago Press, 1953.

6. Paul W. Pruyser. *The Minister as Diagnostician: Personal Problems in Pastoral Perspective*. Philadelphia: The Westminster Press, 1976.

7. Paul W. Pruyser. The use and neglect of pastoral resources. *Pastoral Psychology* 23, 5-17, Sept. 1972.

8. J. Sprenger & H. Kramer. *Malleus Maleficarum*. Trans. Montague Summers. New York: McKee, 1928.

9. Jonathan Edwards. *A treatise concerning religious affections*. John E. Smith, ed. In *The Works of Jonathan Edwards,* vol. 2, Perry Miller, ed. New Haven: Yale University Press, 1959.

10. Paul W. Pruyser. The diagnostic process: touchstone of medicine's values. In *Nourishing the Humanistic in Medicine: Interactions with the Social Sciences,* W. R. Rogers & D. Barnard, eds. Pittsburgh: University of Pittsburgh Press, 1979, ch. 10, 245-61.

11. Norman Cousins. *Anatomy of an Illness: As Perceived by the Patient*. New York: W. W. Norton & Co., 1979.

12. Paul W. Pruyser. *A Dynamic Psychology of Religion*. New York: Harper & Row, 1968.

13. Paul W. Pruyser. *Between Belief and Unbelief*. New York: Harper & Row, 1974.

14. Richard A. Bollinger. Notes for workshops on "The Minister as Diagnostician," periodically given at the Menninger Foundation, Topeka, Kansas.

PART TWO

Life Stages:
Development and Stress

1

Good Beginnings: Separation–Individuation

J. ALEXIS BURLAND

T he human infant at birth is physically and psychologically immature. Certain life-sustaining physiological processes are operant,
certain interactional behavior patterns are in evidence which allow for
primitive communication with the environment; but the newborn cannot
sustain its own life. D. Winnicott stated: "There is no such thing as an infant" (1960, p. 39, footnote), by which he meant the infant cannot exist
without what he called the "facilitating environment"—i.e., maternal
care. The infant can exist only as part of a dyad.

This fact of nature has far-reaching consequences. Psychological
development proceeds as a result of the interaction among inherent constitutional factors and this facilitating environment. Each individual
human infant is born with certain levels of activity, certain sensitivities,
assets, limitations; and each is born with a "pre-programmed" maturational timetable. But the degree of the realization of any one infant's
potential and the ultimate shape of the adult psychological equipment
will reflect the adequacies, inadequacies, and unique characteristics of
the dyadic partner's nurturing skills. There used to be a debate between
those arguing that nature is paramount and those arguing that nurture is
most important; in fact, it is the confrontation between the two that
determines development.

As a result the infantile past remains a most significant determinant of
present mental activity. The very structure of the adult mental apparatus
reflects the infantile past. Further, when developmental challenges are

less than adequately resolved, issues related to them remain as "unfinished business," so to speak, and continue to exert an influence on mental activity beyond their initial presentation. The past is relived, and the present is experienced partially as part of the past, as our mental structures perform in their characteristic manner and as we continue to strive to achieve mastery over as yet unresolved past challenges.

It was one of Freud's earliest discoveries that behind any neurosis in the adult is what he termed the infantile neurosis—that adult wishes, anxieties, and relationships, particularly when in conflict, are reexperiencings of wishes and anxieties from early childhood and of the relationship with the primary objects, i.e., the parents. He had in mind the oedipal configuration, of course, but the same holds true for the dyadic events that precede that developmental challenge.

Psychosexual development, with its by now familiar oral, anal, and phallic-oedipal stages, traces the unfolding of the inherent human instinctual forces and their impact upon the developing mind. Since it was elaborated by Freud and his associates at the turn of the century, other aspects of early human psychological development have been charted. So-called ego psychology, for instance, embodies the theory of the step-by-step development and eventual functioning of that part of the mind which mediates between internal needs and external reality.

Separation-individuation theory recounts certain other aspects of psychological development, basing its conclusions not only on clinical data, the usual source of the formulation of hypotheses relevant to psychological activity, but also on data obtained from the direct longitudinal observation of "normal" mother:infant dyads throughout the formative years of early life. The particular aspects traced by Margaret Mahler in her research include the establishment of the initial mother:infant loving bond and then the step-by-step process by which the infant grows psychologically out of that dyad and into individuality. Among other things, this complex process involves (1) the differentiation of basic psychological structures, (2) the creation of a sense of self, (3) the establishment of a "basic mood," (4) and the development of a capacity for object relationships. Although this process begins in the first three years of life, and much must be accomplished at that time if psychological development is to proceed successfully through future stages, it reverberates throughout later years as part of the life process. The intensity and nature of those reverberations have a significant impact upon mental function.

Separation-individuation theory attempts to recount the developmental process from the vantage point of the infant's subjective experience;

this is in spite of the fact that the terminology often has an interpersonal reference. This parallels, of course, the very nature of the mother:infant dyad, with its implied lack of differentiation (at first) between the infant and the mother. The theory does describe the dyadic process as observed from the outside; these are the observational raw data themselves. But these data are then interpreted, and conclusions are reached as to what that data can tell us about what is occurring within the infant's psyche — in particular, what are the developmental consequences of the dyadic experience. This requires not only sensitive and empathic observation, over time, and of many dyads but also a base of psychoanalytic theory upon which to build and with which to integrate newer concepts.

The hypotheses derived from these observations of infants are then tested and fine-tuned against clinical data obtained in work with older children, adolescents, and adults. Reverberations of these early experiences are noted in the subjective stages of patients, their moods, their perceptions of themselves and their worlds; in the reliving of them in current relationships, in particular within the transference; and in the very character and stability of the mental structures developed during them. It is precisely this clinical usefulness that serves both as validation of separation-individuation theory and as rationale for its existence.

The observational data

NORMAL AUTISM

The newborn appears to live experientially within his or her own body, responding to internal stimuli and the waxing and waning of tension and needs as they alternate with times of satiation. Mahler calls this initial phase of development "normal autism" because of this self-absorption. Within days of birth, as has been confirmed by more recent research, the newborn's perceptual apparatus awakens and increasingly responds to visual, tactile, and olfactory stimuli. This shift from self-absorption to beginning communication with external reality is fostered by the ministrations of the mother; the more responsive, empathic, and consistent the care — in particular, the more loving it is, the more rapidly and fully the shift in the newborn occurs. The normal autistic phase starts to diminish and is replaced within days of birth by the second phase of development in Mahler's schema, the normal symbiotic phase.

SYMBIOTIC PHASE

This phase peaks at about six months, with the establishment of a unique and intense loving attachment between the infant and the mother. It is readily seen in the beaming and excited smile and laughter reserved for mother alone, and readily evoked by her stimulating the infant, by talking, tickling, fondling, and playing "cootchy-coo" games, even while attending to the baby's diapering and feeding needs. The affective tone of this interaction is contagious, and almost anyone observing it feels moved by it.

One can also observe the consequence of less than "good enough" mothering. Significant neglect gives rise to failure to thrive, a condition characterized by cessation of physical growth, apathy, unresponsiveness, and, at its extreme, death. Developmentally one sees delayed smiling, poor communication, and a failure in the shift described above; that is, the infant remains to a greater extent responsive to internal stimuli at the expense of increasing receptivity to the external world. A good symbiosis fails to develop. If the neglect continues and if they survive, such children are quite asocial and interpersonally unrelated; large numbers of such children have been observed among the more impoverished inner-city families, for example.

HATCHING

Another significant shift in the infant's development seems to be related to the establishment of a good symbiotic dyad. It has been termed *hatching;* it is a readily visible event, if one looks for it, and is characterized often by a rather sudden change in the infant's capacity for concentrated focus on external stimuli. It occurs usually between the fourth and seventh month of life. The infant is suddenly more alert and more goal directed in explorations of the immediate environment. It is as though their perceptual equipment had been turned on. This developmental event has great meaning for cognitive development. For children who have experienced significant neglect, hatching either does not occur, is much delayed, or is abortive; the perceptual-conscious system then does not develop adequately into a resource to use in adapting to external reality. Delayed or abortive hatching, when combined with the neglected child's lack of affective involvement with external reality, in particular, other people, contributes further to such a child's continuing selective responsiveness to internal needs at the expense of socialization and adaptation.

SEPARATION-DIFFERENTIATION

Separation-individuation describes the infant's first discovery of objective separateness and then development of a sense of separate individuality. In the first two subphases of this process, which co-exist during the second half of the first year of life and extend into the middle of the second year, groundwork is laid for the development of autonomous and self-reliant skills. The term *differentiation* refers to certain aspects of cognitive and perceptual growth. What one sees, as a consequence of hatching, is the infant's increasing explorations of the world. Faces are a favorite subject for the child's study in this subphase. So-called stranger reaction, which occurs at about seven or eight months, reflects the infant's new awareness of persons other than mother. The infant may simply stiffen, or cease smiling, only then to examine seriously the face of the non-mother; or the infant may get so upset as to scream in fear until the mother can supply needed comfort and reassurance. The infant also invests much energy in experiencing the tastes, feel, smells, and sounds of the world, often scanning back and forth between the familiar — especially mother's face — and the less familiar. As the latter become more familiar with time, the infant's domain widens. The familiar scene is of the nine- or ten-month-old, safely ensconced in mother's lap, leaning against her bosom, eyes and ears focused on whatever activity, bright lights, sounds, or whatever fill the room.

PRACTICING

At the same time the maturation of the neuromuscular system makes possible the development of such skills as sitting, crawling, standing, and finally walking. The second subphase of separation-individuation has been termed *practicing,* as it is characterized by the infant's almost hypomanic exercise of these newly discovered, musculo-skeletal capacities. The affective tone of these activities is striking and contagious; picture the fourteen-month-old toddler, with fat bowed legs and a sagging diaper, arms extended and waving with glee, screeching and chortling with a sense of omnipotence, waddling across the room, seemingly impervious to collisions with furniture, quick to recover from falls, seemingly oblivious to mother's presence or often anxious warnings or efforts at setting limits. One says "seemingly oblivious" because an interesting phenomenon is observable at this time: if the mother leaves the room, the toddler's activity level starts to wane, and often the facial expression changes from hypomanic self-infatuation to something that resembles a kind of depressed effort at holding on to the image of the now absent mother. When the mother then returns, the toddler finds the way over to her, makes contact — touches her leg or skirt, for example — and seemingly refueled, returns once again to high-energy practicing activities. One can see from this how much the hypomanic affect, this sense of omnipotence, is reliant upon the toddler's confidence in mother's continuing love. In fact, even when mother does not leave the room, the energy level of the practicing toddler does over time begin to lessen, and a passing contact with mother is needed. One might say there is an invisible umbilical cord maintaining the dyadic connection; in this way the symbiotic attachment can be seen to be an essential launching platform for the continuing development of skills for self-reliance.

RAPPROCHEMENT

Toward the end of the second year, there is a striking change in the toddler's affect with the arrival of the next subphase of separation-individuation. The child is suddenly no longer oblivious to falls and injuries, no longer merely intermittently in need of contact with mother. Maturation of the central nervous system and cognitive development have proceeded to the point where the toddler can now differentiate between who he or she is and who mother is; separateness has been discovered. The hypomania of the practicing subphase now is replaced by some degree of whiney and unhappy dependency, with clinging and shadowing of mother. Some parents find this change so startling that they take their child to their pediatrician, concerned about the infant's mental health.

Intensely uncomfortable moments occur; more typically they involve the toddler's arms being sadly held up, pleading to be picked up and put into mother's lap, only then to push angrily against her, demanding to be put down; but then, once put down, the arms go up again; the anger is replaced by desperation and the demand to be picked up is again voiced. "Pick-me-up," "put-me-down" cycles can go on for many minutes, with increasing distress on the part of the child, and, not surprisingly, the mother. These often have to run their course and conclude only when the child has no more strength to continue. One can see then a very early internal conflict between the toddler's sudden discovery of vulnerability and aloneness, the desperate need to reestablish the safety of the symbiotic dyad now seemingly gone, and the still fragile but nevertheless important sense of self that pushes him or her into the assertion of autonomy. The child alternates from one assertion to the opposite, unable, at least at first, to find a comfortable middle ground.

This internal conflict is also shown in a particular behavior known as darting away. When mother is in the room, and watching, some toddlers will suddenly rush into some dangerous or forbidden activity — e.g., poking at electrical outlets, pulling on percolator or toaster cords, or racing to the edge of a landing — such that mother will have to run after and swoop up the child in her arms while he or she may scream in seeming protest. But the fact that the toddler engages in darting away only when mother is present and watching indicates the game-like qualities of the activity and make clear how the toddler is finding a way to seem to be both dependent and independent simultaneously.

This third subphase of separation-individuation is called rapprochement, a term borrowed from international affairs and referring to the efforts on the part of the toddler to get together again with mother. Early in this subphase the child's mixed feelings are clear, as noted in his or her push-pull interaction with the mother. But as this subphase proceeds, the toddler grows more comfortable with separateness in large measure as development of self-reliance continues. Language development is central here; it allows for a new kind of communication, more mature than the nonverbal communication characteristic of the symbiotic dyad. The development of the child's capacity for verbal communication is predicated upon his or her recognition of the space between one's self and another person with whom there is emotional involvement and therefore motivation for interaction, a space that is bridged by words and gesture.

A very significant shift occurs as a result of the overcoming of the challenges of this subphase, namely that the support system of the child's narcissism grows less exclusively dependent upon maternal investment and more responsive to the pleasures of self-reliance and independent function. However, this shift is not without its philosophical ramifications, as the toddler's world changes from one of seemingly instant gratification and symbiotic protection (albeit with its vulnerability to the anxiety of separation) to one of challenge and potential frustration in a dynamic balance with the opportunity to achieve mastery.

CONSOLIDATION OF INDIVIDUALITY AND THE BEGINNINGS
OF EMOTIONAL OBJECT CONSTANCY

The separation-individuation phase is concluded by the subphase originally given the meaningful but cumbersome label of "on the road to object constancy." The last two words refer to the developmental accomplishment of the child's capacity to enter into stable and loving relationships with people perceived as fully separate and independent individuals. This subphase is characterized by the continued resolution of the challenges set in motion by the discoveries of rapprochement. It is worth pointing out that these last two subphases of separation-individuation overlap with early phases of the phallic-oedipal phase of psychosexual development, so that sexual curiosity and the discoveries resulting from its gratification interact with early identity formation, as the child's sense of separate individuality unfolds.

In summary, the newborn is first brought into a unique and intense dual unity with the mother. Using that dyad as a launching platform, some degree of mastery over unfolding cognitive and musculoskeletal capacities is next achieved. Discovery of separateness then challenges the toddler to resolve the conflict between regressive yearnings to return to the lost symbiosis and the narcissistic rewards of autonomous function. Successful resolution of this conflict involves developing a capacity for a new, more mature kind of relatedness between separate individuals, with speech and gesture increasingly replacing nonverbal empathic tuning in. By way of a loving attachment to the mother, the self-absorbed, helpless newborn has become, by age three, a fairly self-reliant, loving, verbal child with a capacity to separate from mother comfortably in exploring a world wider now than the nursery.

The two developmental lines, of separation and of individuation, do not always unfold at a similar rate. For instance, some children can be seen to discover their separateness before they have achieved a sufficiently stable sense of their self-reliance to help them weather that storm, and for them the rapprochement subphase can be quite stormy, with an even greater need for the mother's stabilizing and supportive participation.

The literature is rich with more detailed recountings of the basic observational data, in particular, of course, those articles by Margaret Mahler listed in the bibliography. But one cannot recommend strongly enough that every opportunity be taken to observe under-three-year-olds directly, to see firsthand the developmental phenomena described in separation-individuation theory, preferably with some awareness of the hypotheses concerning the psychological events that are believed to occur behind the surface behaviors.

The birth of the mind

Starting with the observational data, confirming and fine-tuning it with clinical data that evidence later reverberations of these early events, and utilizing concepts already confirmed by over a half a century of psychoanalytic research into the development and workings of the mind, Mahler has proposed a developmental sequence of intrapsychic events that can be thought of as the "birth of the mind." As good-enough mothering brings the newborn gradually from the autistic into the symbiotic phase, the initially undifferentiated psyche begins to organize itself around the regular alternations between the distress of hunger and frustration and the pleasure of satiation and gratification. To use the term coined by E. Glover (1968), *islets* of mental structure start to form, memory-clusters organized around the polarity of pleasure versus distress. By six months, at the peak of the symbiotic phase, the pleasurable memories are predominately associated with mother — with her face, her smell, her sounds, her feel — and, if all has gone well, the pleasurable islets are more numerous than the unpleasurable ones. One has, then, at six months, a largely pleasure-focused dyadic partner (the child), dependent upon continuing loving and empathic maternal input to feel good, basically trusting (Erikson, 1950), and with "confident expectation of a loving surround" (as Benedek called it). Maturation of cognitive and perceptual apparatuses, and their investment with loving feelings derived from the gratifications of the mother-infant interaction, encourage the infant to experience the multiplicity of stimuli and to become a more conscious and aware participant in his or her life experiences. With hatching, those perceptual apparatuses directed toward external stimuli make possible a growing psychological awareness of the world, while simultaneously offering the infant an opportunity to exercise and, therefore, develop still further the effectiveness of this mental equipment itself.

Perceptual, cognitive, and then musculo-skeletal development contribute to the continual growth of the mind. Memory traces become more detailed and sophisticated, separated islets of memory fragments coalesce into larger structures, so that significant people become multifaceted and differentiated from one another. The world, and the evolving self, grow larger and more complex. The infant becomes increasingly an active participant in his or her affairs, not only by means of increased self-reliance but also in the interaction with the dyadic partner. The infant initiates and determines the quality of these interactions to an increasing degree.

Anger increases as a challenge to the infant. The more he or she perceives and responds to more subtle frustrations, the more physical development makes possible its direct expression. The polarity of pleasure and distress is revealed in the elaboration of what are termed *positive* and *negative* introjects, that is, memory clusters of gratifying interactions with the "good mother," and memory clusters of painful interactions with the "bad mother." At this stage these "two mothers" remain largely split apart; when angry, the infant, in great distress, rages at the bad mother — only often within seconds, when in need or when gratified, to beam lovingly at the good mother.

In the differentiation and practicing subphases of separation-individuation, the infant's cognitive and musculo-skeletal equipment develops and with it, the ability to deal aggressively with the environment. Activities and objects, human or otherwise, are purposefully selected; needs can be arranged to be met. In the continued unawareness of human mortality, the toddler basks in a sense of omnipotence. Moments of frustration, if intense enough, can still cause distress; but the well-enough mothered toddler still maintains the illusion that should his or her omnipotence fall short, mother's power will surely do the trick, in effect, hers being synonymous with the toddler's, as the two are not yet fully differentiated.

Extreme frustration, evoking what is termed *infantile rage,* relies upon splitting for its disposition. That is, the evoked negative introject — the mental image of the bad mother that causes displeasure for the bad toddler — is projected outward onto the mother and attacked. The child's rage is often displaced onto the bad toy, the bad dog or bad cat, or the bad sibling. In some instances, the toddler takes him- or herself as the object to attack. Yet the good mother is preserved by this splitting of good and bad. If the bad is displaced, the mother herself remains the good object; if mother herself becomes the bad object, then the memory of the good mother is preserved, to be happily recalled once the rage has abated. The symbiotic bond remains still essential and operant.

With the discoveries of rapprochement, the late toddler is thrust into a world now devoid of this symbiotic support system. The so-called mother of separation replaces the mother of symbiosis. Though still perceived as omnipotent, mother is now viewed as withholding of that omnipotence that in the infant's eyes she had once shared. The illusion of symbiosis, the support of which D. Winnicott called the mother's most important function, is now replaced by what will be a lifelong process of disillusionment, and mother's task is to cushion the fall. Initially the infant refuses to acknowledge the change and denies the new realization of aloneness and vulnerability, clinging to mother as if to insist that geographic proximity would erase the painful awareness of separateness. In darting, as described above, the mother is forced to participate further in the child's life, again as if to insist that running after and rescuing the reckless child is equivalent to the persistence of symbiosis. The child's demand that the symbiosis persist relates directly to the fact that the child feels unable to survive alone; this conviction is strengthened or weakened by the success with which the mother conveys support and helps the child contain desperate rage, and it is influenced by the extent to which the child relies upon self-reliant and autonomous skill development.

This latter development plays a critical role in the resolution of challenges presented by the rapprochement phase. As indicated above, each "pick me up" can be seen as partner to a "put me down"; or, to use the words of a six-year-old patient struggling to cope with still unresolved rapprochement discoveries, each "help me, I can't" was matched with a "no, get away, I can do it myself." "Come closer" is matched with a "go away." Perceiving the world as overwhelming and seeing one's self as unable to cope with it are matched with a conviction that one has at least a chance of achieving mastery of the world and self. As we shall see, though much is accomplished during the third year of life in coping with this dialectic, the tension persists as a dimension of psychological life for many years.

The good-mother/bad-mother split is "healed" as the child recognizes —through a cognitive developmental process—that mother is but one person, with good and bad attributes. This healing comes about through a greater confidence in self-reliance, which lessens the need for a regressive return to the symbiosis and therefore diminishes the intensity of the infantile rage in the face of frustration (i.e., the process that results in individuation) and through the continuity of the loving bond with mother as a newer more sophisticated tie that exists between two separate individuals. The initial split occurred when the infant was directing helpless rage and dependent love toward the same object, i.e., mother; yet, the split made possible the ejection of the bad and the retention of the good. In achieving a relatively comfortable sense of separate compotent individuality, the split is no longer necessary.

Rapprochement finds resolution through the combined compromise of increased self-reliance, almost contradictorily supported by mother's and then father's nurturant input and through the elaboration of a network of support systems that operate in a dyadic mode (see Winnicott, 1951). That is, the launching platform of the symbiotic backup is maintained symbolically by means of security blankets, favorite toys, rituals and routines, and/or magical good-luck charms of many kinds. As we shall see, the prominence of these transitional objects depends in large measure upon the successful resolution of the rapprochement phase of development.

Clinical data and application

Dynamic, insight-oriented therapy has as its goal change through insight. That is, the process by which the desired change in a person's psychological functioning is accomplished includes, as one of its most important ingredients, an increased awareness and understanding of that person's mental life. Insight is achieved through the careful examination of three things: first, a person's perceptions, interpretations, and reactions in current reality; second, in that unique relationship with the therapist called the transference; and third, in the infantile past. The process of working through psychological conflict is characterized by the spontaneous movement of self-observation back and forth within these three arenas. As a particular defensive maneuver or nidus of anxiety is understood by the patient, it is examined in the way it works in current life, in the transference to the therapist, and in its origins and development in childhood. This examination of childhood is referred to as reconstruction, the discovery and elaboration of one's psychological autobiography. Mahler's observations of developing children have increased our knowledge of the significant crossroads and challenges of those early years, making it more possible to recognize the critical events to which our patients are making reference indirectly or obliquely. But by a similar token, the understanding of these events that is possible only when an articulate patient finds deep insight offers an opportunity to further refine our understanding of the original developmental event.

The transition from the autistic to the symbiotic phase of development is a critical developmental event; it brings the newborn into cognitive and emotional involvement with the facilitating environment which results in the capacity for meaningful relationships with others and for a relatedness to reality. It is, therefore, not surprising that later reverberations of this event reveal themselves in the areas of relationships to others and reality.

In my work with inner-city poor who are neglectful of their children, work done for over a decade involving consultation with foster care and mental health agencies, and including the analysis of a neglected inner-city child-in-care — I observed a recognizable syndrome I term the *autistic character disorder*. These children, adolescents, and eventually adults had experienced great maternal neglect and had failed, in varying degrees, to make the transition into an adequate symbiotic relationship. They remained, therefore, poorly related to others, either quite severely isolated or, at best, capable only of need-fulfilling attachments, i.e., they would invest themselves in others only insofar as such relationships gratified their wishes and only for that time during which those wishes were being actively gratified. They also remained poorly attentive to reality, learning little of the world as it is, quite contentedly projecting onto the world whatever image they might choose, and therefore remaining essentially asocial. Loving feelings were striking in their absence; for instance, when observed in families the individual interacted only negatively — giving insults, criticisms, scoldings, and complaints. In its stead hostility was the most prominent affect, either actively in the form of rages, destructiveness, or frank hostility, or passively in the form of perceptions of others and situations as hostile and destructive toward them. These children — of all ages — almost never smile or laugh; in a roomful of toddlers such as these, instead of the more expected hypomanic and gleeful screeches of delight, there is chilling silence. And finally, they are remarkably thin-skinned, unable to tolerate any frustration or pressure, and quick to collapse into wretched helplessness, with great deficiencies in their self-esteem (see Burland, 1980).

EXAMPLE ONE: A DEPRIVED CHILD

The neglected child suffering from this syndrome whom I saw in analysis offered clinical data in support of the dynamic formulation that is implied in the phrase *autistic character disorder*. Neglected and deserted by his mother, Jack came into care at age five already a behavior problem of sufficient intensity that he hardly seemed a foster-home candidate. When I first saw him at age seven — though he could smile seductively when he wished — he was what I then called mindless in his frenetic, joyless, driven search for stimulation and excitement. He monologued rather than dialogued. When, at our initial meeting, I asked him why he was in residential care, he replied with a fantastic, disorganized, and confusing narrative about a home beset by robbers who broke in to take baths, killer dogs, midget avenging angels who hid under radiators from which they emerged with swords to cut off the dogs' legs, etc. His monologue would have gone on and on had I not interrupted it after some fifteen minutes. His affect throughout was sweet, but bland and monotonous. He had made no connection with anyone, either staff or peer, in his first months of placement. He was always on the move, mostly disrupting organized activities or provoking fights with others. He swaggered as though he were "ultra-tough" and happily intimidated those he could, but he was very fearful and more prone to collapse in helpless rage-filled tears than to confront or master a challenge. Everything had to go his way, or he would collapse in despair. He was learning nothing in school, in spite of probably average intelligence (though his scores, with much scatter, averaged in the borderline range), and his disruptive behavior was sufficient to require a referral to a special-class setting. He resembled many children in the inner-city school system, clearly uneducable and barely containable.

The major thrust of the first year (or more) of treatment centered on bringing Jack into a relationship with me; it was an attempt to move him developmentally through the distance he had failed to compass in his first year of life. His initial reaction to me was determined by his developmental lag: he experienced me as an unstable self-object. That is, his image of me was fleeting, changeable, inconstant, and contradictory; in the most positive image, I was over-idealized, and he basked in my attentiveness, bragging to the other children of his time alone with me, behaving in an almost hypomanic fashion when with me. But in the blink of an eye, this perception of me could be replaced by its opposite: a rage-filled assumption that I was trying to destroy him. Generally speaking, if I seemed to comply with his demands, I was viewed in a positive light; and if for any reason I appeared to him to be frustrating, that positive image promptly deteriorated. He was left without the "good" me, with only the "bad" me to rage against. Using the development theories outlined above, this can be understood as reflecting his weak and unstable positive introjects and his comparatively more impactful and stable negative ones. His play activities were equally unstable and fleeting; their preoccupation with violence, however, was fairly consistent.

In discussing these patterns in terms of his current reality, the relationship with me, and the past, it was possible, over time, to identify his passive yearnings toward his mother and how good and loving mothering makes a child feel good and loveable, while a rejecting mother makes her child feel wretched. As this was discussed and played out with dolls, his investment in me strengthened and stabilized; he started telling the other children I was his father (although psychologically speaking it seemed clear he really meant mother). At this point, some fourteen months into the analysis, to my surprise, he suddenly hatched. He came in one day so much more alert and reality-focused that he seemed a transformed child. From that day his school work improved, his play became increasingly socialized, his relationships stabilized. Much analytic work followed, but it seemed clinically evident that the early analytic work had accomplished both the bringing of Jack into his first meaningful interpersonal connection and simultaneously a sweeping improvement in his relationship to reality. The developmental interaction between these two seemed confirmed; in other words, the establishment of a positive nurturing relationship brought forth a developmental burst of growth of a broad array of ego skills.

EXAMPLE TWO: A HOMOSEXUAL

A thirty-year-old practicing homosexual male came for help around a severe depression precipitated by the sudden angry departure of his lover of several years. In treatment, the following pattern was identified and clarified: his intense need for homosexual contact was preceded by the insidious onset of feelings of emptiness, depression, impotence, and helplessness. To undo his own uncomfortable deficiencies, his mind would turn to imaging the opposite, a tall, strong, potent, and beautiful male. He then would travel to those parts of town known to the homosexual community as "cruising" areas, where he would seek out someone who resembled as closely as possible the ideal image in his mind. In sex with this man, my patient would take into his body, orally or anally, this idealized man's ejaculation. This intercourse acted as a kind of communion, whereby he took on the virtues and power he felt so desperately he lacked.

As our work together confirmed, this pattern was symptomatic of his persistent search for a connectedness that was predicated upon his own weakness yet with an ability to obtain a sense of strength through a symbiotic-like interaction in which the other's strength became his. At one point in treatment, as these issues were being worked through, he felt driven to construct a system of mirrors so that he could observe his partner's penis as it moved in and out of his (my patient's) anus: it appeared to him as though they were fusing, then separating, then fusing. He masturbated to simultaneous orgasm to increase the intensity of the feeling of fusion. He experienced similar yearnings in the transference. He reconstructed a repeated interaction between himself and his mother: he would be on her lap, holding *Life* magazine and turning the pages, giving the names for the items his mother would point to in the various pictures and feeling an intensely warm excitement every time his mother showered him with flattery for answering correctly. He was two or three at the time; as he put it, "I peaked then; it's been downhill ever since." In his obligatory and compulsive homosexuality, this patient revealed his clinging to a pre-rapprochement mode of interpersonal interaction: he experienced first a sense of isolation and loss of nurturant input and support, then remedied this situation by regaining the illusion of safety and strength by means of a symbiotic fusion with the (maternal) source of power.

EXAMPLE THREE: A SUICIDAL ADOLESCENT

An adolescent was referred for treatment because of an attempted suicide. He had grown up with a compulsive and demanding mother and a passive, alcoholic father; his depression clearly reflected the deprivation he had experienced. He very rapidly developed a strongly positive transference, somewhat atypically for adolescents, and moved into treatment energetically and with a consistency he had never before revealed. However, as he seemed to be more and more deeply committed to the therapeutic process, his behavior worsened: his grades at school fell sharply, he used drugs more and more heavily, even to the extent of risking arrest by participating in middle-of-the-night purchases and sales of hard drugs in parts of town known for their criminal activity and heavy police presence. Not surprisingly, in light of his underlying sense of helplessness, he had many fears of the real world, and arrest and imprisonment were near the top of the list. Yet that apprehension failed to inhibit his behavior; but he also seemed to experience little conscious fear while engaging in the dangerous activities. What came out in treatment was a previously unconscious fantasy he had: that there was an ever-present "fairy godmother" hovering over him, protecting him from all dangers: this was a transference fantasy that reflected the illusion of the omnipresent and omniscient therapist-mother, a wish and hope that now, at last, he was to receive the mothering he felt he had never before adequately received. His commitment to treatment, rather than being a reflection of a therapeutic alliance, was symptomatic and regressive. Like the homosexual patient described above, he clung to the wish for a symbiotic fusion with the all-powerful mother. That this wish was assumed by him to be in fact gratified (as his behavior demonstrated) was in itself an expression of that very same wish, for in the ideal symbiotic situation, all wishes come true. In this sense, all "acting out" of behavior, that is, behavior that is in keeping with inner wishes as opposed to outer reality, speaks for a fixation to this early level of ego functioning.

EXAMPLE FOUR: A DEPRESSED ADOLESCENT

Another late-adolescent patient struggled with similar problems. He was depressed and felt a strong passive yearning for nurturant input, from his rejecting mother, his depressed and isolated father, and most other people in his life, including his college professors, friends, and, of course, his therapist. One summer he had, on his own, devised a research project in his area of study and carried it through with such success that he was invited, though still an undergraduate, to present his findings at an upcoming professional convention. Instead of feeling pride over his accomplishment, he was driven to tears, crying out in pain and complaining that he had had to do it all alone.

Such a clinical vignette points to the critical role that the challenges of rapprochement play in psychological development. As described above, once the newborn is brought into the symbiotic dual unity of parent and child, physical maturation and psychological development lead to the discovery of actual separateness and usher in a push (albeit an ambivalent one) for autonomy and self-reliance. But that ambivalence can be great, especially when the positive introjects are insufficiently reassuring and supportive in bolstering the toddler's still shaky sense of competence. Another mid-adolescent in treatment dealt with this issue in a most moving manner. It was late in his treatment, and he was looking back over our work together and philosophizing about his past, his needs, and his conflicts. Sadly he complained about the clumsiness of words as a means of communication — how much better it would have been if his thoughts were instantly known to me, without words and, further, how nice it would have been if we met not by scheduled appointment but only at those moments when he felt he needed me. These thoughts reminded him of a favorite fantasy from the past: a "money tree," always with him, that dropped into his hands exactly the amount of money he needed when he needed it. In keeping with these regressive yearnings, his presenting symptoms were an inability to function independently and achieve in school, and great insecurity as to his masculinity.

EXAMPLE FIVE: STRUGGLE WITH AUTHORITY

The rapprochement struggles are often played out around the "mother of separation," who is personified by some current person or organization, or, as we saw above, by the therapist in the transference. A young adult in treatment was a participant in the social activism of the 1960s, and was present at the famous October 1967 storming of the Pentagon by antiwar demonstrators. She said of the experience: "There in the big granite building sat all those fat cat generals, with all their medals, and not one of them cared how awfully I felt!" In reconstructing her childhood, she revealed how much that event paralleled the relationship with her parents; and it also presaged a core transference struggle that filled many months of treatment. It can be argued that most, if not all, of sociopolitical ideology, and philosophy, consists of attempts to come to terms with the bitter disillusionments of rapprochement (see Burland, 1976).

EXAMPLE SIX: PARENTAL ANXIETY

"Darting away" was described earlier as a phenomenon seen in toddlers who struggle with the conflicting wishes to remain in mother's care and, at the same time, to be autonomous. The same is a characteristic problem for adolescents so it is not surprising that darting away should be frequently encountered in this age group. One high school student found himself repeatedly in trouble because of the abuse of "recreational" drugs. An adopted child, his relationship with his parents was always one of conflict. They were elderly and anxious and from the start feared he would resent them. In response he viewed their anxiety as rejection, and over the years multiple "push-pull games" evolved between them. His current dalliance with drugs simply replayed an old pattern, although there was much initial resistance on the part of the parents to acknowledge it. They preferred to place the blame totally on the drugs themselves instead of family dynamics. They also needed the symptomatic disguise of their hostility toward this anxiety-generating child, hostility that was revealed in the mother's nearly hysterical conviction that her son would overdose and kill himself. The pattern between them consisted of the boy's leaving provocative signs of his drug use for the parents to find. When they reacted with their predictable hysteria and efforts at "controlling" his behavior, he, with seemingly righteous indignation, raged at their over-protection and intrusions into his personal life. When his parents were counseled not to allow themselves to get so upset by what was, in effect, more of an interpersonal "game" than a "drug problem," he would leave more and more blatant signs of his activities which culminated in an incident where he allegedly passed out in school from taking several of mother's tranquilizers. Though he needed to protect his fragile and unstable sense of autonomy by protesting his parents' intrusiveness, he simultaneously continued in his desperate clinging to the mother, whom he saw as remote and unavailable and whose availability he had to stimulate with threats of self-destruction. Understanding the dynamics behind this pattern made it possible to focus on the pertinent issues—the unresolved rapprochement conflict—while avoiding the trap of treating the situation as purely and simply a "drug problem."

Discussion

Growing up is a two-party system; so is psychotherapy. This coincidence accounts in part for the extent to which the therapeutic situation almost selectively evokes reverberations from the primal dyad, a fact commented upon by both Spitz and Winnicott (see their 1956 articles). The patient's distress and need, and his or her coming to the therapist for help only further serve to evoke the mother-infant mode of interaction for the patient, however, with characteristics related to each patient's particular and unique past. When the patient's problems relate to issues that arose subsequent to the separation-individuation phase of development, when early mothering was "good enough" and adequate object constancy has been achieved, the relationship aspect of the therapist-patient interaction is less prominent as an area of unresolved conflict requiring therapeutic attention. But even in these instances, the developmentally achieved capacity for relationships acts as a relatively invisible but nevertheless crucial contribution to the therapeutic process. Where this is not the case, where issues either in establishing a meaningful relationship with the therapist or in maintaining a comfortably separated and individuated position within the therapist-patient relationship arise as reverberations of as yet unfinished business from the infantile past, this aspect (rapprochement especially) of the process requires much direct therapeutic attention. In this situation separation-individuation theory can help the therapist conceptualize how the patient's past is being relived in the present. As suggested by the above clinical vignettes, the process of working through involves helping the patient see and understand his or her past in the present. The transference is naturally a significant arena where this can be played out; in fact, "good therapeutic technique," an unfortunately difficult phrase to define, can be seen to require as at least one of its ingredients the creation of a setting where such transferences can have an opportunity to evolve and be recognized.

One dimension of the relationship issue is the distinction between transference and the so-called real relationship with the therapist. Despite attempts to view the therapist as a truly "blank screen" devoid of any and all personal characteristics, a view that sometimes enhances the development of transference, the fact is that the therapist, no matter how neutral and impersonal in behavior, is a real person, with a real style of interaction. Therapy is not formless, i.e., "blank"; it has a definite form — the therapist is attentive, empathic, consistent, neutral, supportive when indicated, etc. Again, where the patient has achieved adequate object constancy and lives a socially connected and active life, the "real" qualities of the therapist remain part of the facilitating background; the therapist's real qualities are accepted and appreciated, but utilized more than discussed. Where, however, infantile relationships were not adequately developed and where, therefore, most if not all later relationships were also inadequate, these same real qualities of the therapist stand out as something unique and special, either to be feared or embraced. For instance, in the analysis of the neglected inner-city child this real relationship to the therapist was as important in fostering the resumption of interrupted development as was the transference dimension of the interaction. Here again one can use the discoveries of separation-individuation theory to understand the importance, say, of empathically tuning in on the patient's poorly verbalized distress or of the calm but stabilizing acceptance of the patient's affective distress, both of these approaches reflecting certain aspects of good-enough mothering.

Needless to say the evocation of unfinished business from the infantile past within the relationship with the therapist can contain sufficient conflict to act as a resistance rather than as simply a potentiator. This is particularly true when unresolved rapprochement issues are being relived and, hopefully, reworked, because of the dependence/independence, closeness/apartness conflicts that characterize this developmental phase. It has been said that the best thing a mother can do for her child is to bring the child up to be treatable; this somewhat flippant statement does contain a grain of truth insofar as it refers to the child's capacity to enter comfortably into a therapeutic relationship. The task of working with patients who continue to struggle with separation-individuation issues, then, can be understood as searching for ways to treat the less-than-easily treatable. For instance, the patient described earlier, who was devastated because he had achieved success on his own, struggled in the transference with similar issues. As he came to put it, "Help me . . . but don't touch me!" Or, as another patient said, "The hungrier I get, the more tightly I keep my mouth shut!" Such "pick me up—put me down" cycles are played out within the relationship with the therapist and have, therefore, a direct effect on that work itself. But, again, the early life developmental scenarios explicated by separation-individuation theory offer to the therapist a framework for understanding such situations and ways of putting into words for the patient the current issues and their past roots.

In summary, the research and writings of Margaret Mahler on separation-individuation have illuminated vast areas of early psychological development. With this knowledge, efforts at understanding the significant events from our patient's past and of recognizing the past's role in the present are aided. Further it offers approaches for discussing these events, both dynamically and as scenarios. The above recounting of the infant observational data, the theoretical conclusions drawn from it, and the clinical application are but an introduction to a topic that by its very nature can be elusive and "hard to get a feel for." It is suggested that the literature on the subject, some of it annotated below, be studied, that every opportunity be taken to observe in a knowledgeable way the behavior of children under age three and that older children, adolescent, and adult patients be observed with these concepts in mind. One's self-analysis can also be directed to explore this area.

REFERENCES

Balint, M. *The Basic Fault*. New York: Brunner & Mazel, 1979. A most interesting discussion of the problems inherent in treating those still struggling to master the developmental challenges of the first two years of life. This book was written without knowledge of separation-individuation theory, but deals with similar issues.

Blos, P. The second individuation process of adolescence. *The Psychoanalytic Study of the Child* 22, 162–86. New York: IUP, 1967. This important article discusses how individuation, which had begun during the separation-individuation phase, picks up again during adolescence and how this effects the therapy of adolescents.

Burland, J. A. Separation-individuation and reconstruction in psychoanalysis. *The International Journal of Psychoanalytic Psychotherapy* 4, 303–35, 1975. A more elaborate presentation of material discussed in this article.

Burland, J. A. Conservatism and liberalism: a psychoanalytic examination of political belief. *The International Journal of Psychoanalytic Psychotherapy* 5, 369–96, 1976. Using political writings and clinical material, this article describes the relationship between early psychological development and later socio-political orientation.

Burland, J. A. A psychoanalytic psychiatrist in the world of foster care. *The Clinical Social Work Journal* 8, 50–61, 1980. A more detailed description of the developmental consequences of maternal neglect in the inner city.

Freud, S. *Constructions in Analysis*. Standard edition 23, 255–69. London: Hogarth Press, 1964. Freud's late-in-life summary of his views on the importance of reconstructive work in therapy.

Glover, E. *The Birth of the Ego*. New York: IUP, 1968. A brief but beautifully written attempt at describing the development of mental structures in the first year of life; much of separation-individuation theory views the matter in a similar fashion.

Lax, R., Bach, S., & Burland, J. A. *Rapprochement: The Critical Subphase of Separation-Individuation*. New York: Aronson, 1980. A collection of papers— theoretical, clinical, and applied—discussing this one subphase in great depth.

Mahler, M. S. On the significance of the normal separation-individuation phase, with reference to research in symbiotic child psychosis. *The Selected Papers of Margaret S. Mahler* 2, 49–57. New York: Aronson, 1979. A discussion of the importance of the mother's loving availability to her infant for the fullest realization of the infant's developmental potential.

Mahler, M. S. Notes on the development of basic moods: the depressive affect (1966). In *Selected Papers* 2, 59–75. New York: Aronson, 1979. Describes the appearance of mood in the practicing and rapprochement subphases and its consequences for later development.

Mahler, M. S. On the first three subphases of the separation-individuation process (1972). In *Selected Papers* 2, 119–30. New York: Aronson, 1979. One of the best presentations of these subphases, with both clinical and philosophical implications detailed.

Mahler, M. S. Symbiosis and individuation: the psychological birth of the human infant (1973). In *Selected Papers* 2, 149–65. New York: Aronson, 1979. A general discussion of the significance of the first three years of life for future development and function.

Mahler, M. S., Pine, F., & Bergman, A. *The Psychological Birth of the Human Infant*. New York: Basic Books, 1975. Dr. Mahler's summation of her research and findings.

Resch, R. C. Hatching in the human infant as the beginning of separation-individuation: what it is and what it looks like. In *The Psychoanalytic Study of the Child* 34, 421–41. As its title implies.

Spitz, R. Transference: The analytic setting and its prototype. In *The International Journal of Psychoanalysis* 51, 380–85. A discussion suggesting that the early mother/infant dyad is the prototype for the later therapist/patient dyad.

Spitz, R. *The First Year of Life*. New York, IUP, 1965. This book summarizes Dr. Spitz's extensive research on a topic also researched by Dr. Mahler. Some of Spitz's terms are different, but his findings, to which Mahler makes frequent reference, parallel hers and in some instances enrich her findings by commenting upon phenomena from a slightly different perspective. An important book.

Winnicott, D. Clinical varieties of transference (1955–1956). In *Through Paediatrics to Psycho-Analysis*. New York: Basic Books, 1958, 295–99. A discussion of how adequate or inadequate mothering in the first years of life prepares (or fails to prepare) one for therapy.

Winnicott, D. Transitional objects and transitional phenomenon. In *Through Paediatrics to Psycho-Analysis*. New York: Basic Books, 1958, 229–42. A most important paper concerning one psychological means by which the infant in a step-by-step fashion tolerates separation and individuates from the mother.

Winnicott, D. The theory of the parent-infant relationship. In *The Maturational Process and the Facilitating Environment*. New York, IUP, 1965, 37–55. A summation of Winnicott's views on the mother/infant dyad. An important paper in which several terms, later used by Mahler, are first introduced and defined.

2

Childhood: Emotional Health and Illness

JOSEPH J. REIDY

The foundation for what we know about the emotional health and illness of children was laid by Freud and several other psychoanalysts, some quite well known, such as Anna Freud and Erik Erikson, and others, like Rene Spitz and Margaret Mahler, whose work is of great value but perhaps not familiar to the public. Shortly after the turn of the century, Freud formulated his theory of the psychosexual development of children, a theory which states that children have strong sexual and aggressive drives and explains how children adapt these drives to the demands of reality. Freud's theory describes the child's early relationships with parents and stresses the importance of these relationships for the course of future relationships.

The data came from Freud's psychoanalytic treatment of adults, from the memories of these patients, and from reconstructions of important events of childhood. Treatment of children by psychoanalysis and psychotherapy began in the years between the two world wars, and these treatments were sources of further knowledge of normal and pathological development. During this time psychiatry and pediatrics offered little information regarding normal emotional development, and for the most part children were not thought to be in need of treatment. Their difficulties were given labels such as stubbornness, being spoiled, or in severe cases they were considered to be depraved—conditions not considered to have an intrapsychic source. Often their symptoms were attributed to faulty rearing, to physical causes, or were the result of lax morality.

The followers of psychoanalysis eagerly applied their new knowledge to the rearing of children. In the past fifty or so years, much advice and information have been given to parents, educators, and others concerned with the upbringing of children. Some of the teaching did not produce the hoped-for results, and often this was because of the incompleteness of the knowledge at the time. More and more data have been added to the original psychoanalytic theories, and at the present time there exists a sound basis for healthy child-rearing. Unfortunately, this knowledge has not always found its way to the hands of those who raise children.

The major steps in child development are the formation of an emotional relationship with another person, loving and being loved by that person, gaining control over the aggressive and sexual drives, and the internalization of ideals and standards of conduct in the superego. Each of these steps involves conflict and anxiety, and the childhood conflicts and anxieties reverberate through the lifetime of the person. The dangers that give rise to these anxieties and conflicts are: the loss of the person with whom the relationship has been made; the loss of love; physical injury, including injury to the genitals; and the results of the actions of the superego, that is, guilt and punishment. In this chapter I wish to review some of these developmental steps, presenting not a comprehensive account of child development and pathology but selected aspects of development which I feel are of particular interest and importance to ministers.

The first and most important relationship

In the past forty years there has been an enormous increase in research concerning emotional development, in the treatment of emotionally disturbed children and their families, and in the training of professionals in child care and treatment. The earliest researches, and perhaps those most responsible for stimulating further work because of their startling, even shocking findings, were studies of children in deprived and traumatic circumstances. The most widely known of these studies are those of René Spitz of children reared in institutions and of Anna Freud and Dorothy Burlingham of children separated from their parents during war. The children suffered deterioration in their emotional development, affecting not only perceptual and cognitive functions, but in severe cases even their ability to remain physically healthy. They were disturbed in their affective life and in the development of essential ego functions, notably the ability to form human relationships.

Defects in the emotional development of the children reared in institutions—defects so serious that for many their ability to trust and love was seriously and permanently impaired—occurred because their mothers were absent. Their need for food, shelter, and medical care was adequately met, and in most child-caring institutions the employees were devoted to the care of the children (as they saw it); but infants and young children were cared for by so many that there was no single person who was always there and who provided for all of a child's needs. Because there were so many children to care for, the caretakers had little time to cuddle the children, talk to them, sing to them, or play with them. There was little stimulation or interpersonal interaction.

This occurred in other settings: homes from which the mother was absent because of mental or physical illness or because she worked; thus the infants and young children were left in the care of neighbors or in day-care facilities that did not meet their needs. It happened to children who were placed in a succession of foster homes. In all of these cases no one person did for the child the many things a mother does, which she does over a long period of time, thus forming with the child a special relationship of trust and love.

The early studies resulted in many changes in the care of infants and children, among them the closing of many institutions which did not provide a healthy environment, the introduction of better programs in those which continued, and more early adoptions. Even with these changes, today there are many grave deficiencies in the way individual families and society care for children, with serious consequences for their emotional development.

The caretaker of the child need not be the biological mother nor a woman, but for the sake of simplicity, I will refer to that person as the child's mother. Mother is the one who gives to the child most of the feeding, the holding, the loving care, particularly in the first two years of life. In so doing she becomes the person with whom the child forms his or her first human relationship. There must be a continuity in their relationship; it cannot endure long separations. She must relate to the child in a relatively consistent manner and be effective in relieving her child's distress and anxiety, and in meeting physical needs. The child comes to associate the pleasure experienced in these maternal contacts with the perception of mother as a loving person, and sees him- or herself as loved by her. Because of this satisfying relationship, the infant acquires the attitude that Therese Benedek calls confidence and Erik Erikson basic trust, and this marks the beginning of the child's sense of identity and of self-worth. From this first relationship comes the continued growth of the child's ego in all of its functions.

To understand children we no longer have to depend, as Freud did, on the memories and reconstructions of adults in psychoanalysis. The researches mentioned above involved direct observation of children in different settings—ordinary life situations, as well as stressful and traumatic circumstances. Psychoanalysis of very young children now provides us with valuable information. Treatment of adults who suffer from borderline and narcissistic personality disturbances enables us to understand more of a child's first human relationship. Persons with borderline and narcissistic disorders fall somewhere between those with psychotic and neurotic illnesses. Their personality disturbances are due to developmental arrests and defects which happened during the first two years of life.

When the infant is able to differentiate from mother about the middle of the first year of life, he or she is then able to begin the development of important ego functions, particularly those of knowing the world outside the self—"reality assessment"—and making a one-to-one relationship. These will provide the child with the foundation for the sense of self and the sense of identity. Because of the relationship with mother, the infant learns to control drives (i.e., aggression and sexuality) and expressions of feelings. Toward the end of the period of "primary psychic development"—roughly the first eighteen to twenty-four months of life—the infant achieves *libidinal object constancy*. This means that a mental representation of mother has been formed. This mental representation includes more than an awareness of mother; it includes the infant's *libidinal* feelings, that is, attachment to her, love for her. By *constancy* is meant that the representation of mother remains in the infant's mind when she is not present, and even when the infant has angry and destructive feelings toward her. When libidinal object constancy is attained, the infant has arrived at the level of development at which it is possible to tolerate ambivalent feelings toward the loved person, that is, the infant can allow in his or her mind the representation of the loved object as both good and bad, as approving and withholding approval, as loving and hating.

The clinical evaluation of a child's mental life differs from the evaluation of an adult in that we are less concerned with definable disease than with interference in normal development, interference that may result in the definable neuroses and personality disorders of later life. We are more concerned with the effect of the environment and are more likely to recommend modifications of the environment when necessary to prevent pathological development. An important cause of narcissistic and borderline personality disorders is the lack of a suitable environment for infants and young children, most importantly, the lack of an adequate mother-child relationship. Of the two conditions the borderline is the more severe and the developmental arrest has occurred earlier in life.

Persons with borderline personality disorders do not develop a coherent, stable sense of self between the ages of six and twenty-four months. They do not master the anxiety of separation from mother, and later their relations with others are similar to those of children who cling to mother and will not let her go and are angry at her for leaving. These persons are not able to find relationships that allow a realistic distance from the other person. They are dependent and clinging and tolerate poorly the separation from those to whom they are attached, yet the very closeness that they desire makes them anxious. Their anger, moodiness, and impulsiveness make it difficult for others to love them. They feel empty; when alone they are depressed. Borderline cases have not been able to maintain a libidinal object constancy and are unable to accept ambivalent feelings toward those they love. One way of handling their ambivalence is by the very primitive defense called splitting, a separation of positive from negative feelings and thoughts. They shift back and forth between feelings, unaware of the existence of one feeling while experiencing its opposite. It is normal for children to feel this way before gaining libidinal object constancy; borderline cases have never developed to the state of object constancy.

Persons with narcissistic personality disorders have also suffered from problems in their relationship with mother during the period of primary psychic development. They progressed well enough through the first year of life, but by the end of the second year, when there should be the beginning of a realistic sense of self, a firm sense of self-esteem, and a readiness for closeness in relationships, there was interference in development. One explanation is that the infant's mother, who could relate well enough when he or she was a dependent infant, could not accept the infant's self-directed and oppositional behavior occurring at this time. She may have withdrawn, leaving the infant without help in managing impulses, or she may have been severely over-controlling. The infant did not receive the needed help and became unsatisfied, seeking throughout life to gain the desired care. Adults with narcissistic personality disorders feel entitled to special consideration and take advantage of others in order to satisfy their own wishes. If mother had granted their every wish, then they feel entitled because they have always received satisfaction of their desires. If mother was a rigidly controlling or a neglectful person, then they feel entitled because they have not received what they consider their due. They lack empathy, that is, they are not able to appreciate emotionally the feelings of others. They fail to be objective in their evaluation of others, either seeing them as perfect or, if there exists the slightest flaw, rejecting them as worthless.

These and other disorders arising in the early years of life have been called by Selma Fraiberg the "diseases of non-attachment." She writes:

> the human capacity to love and to make enduring partnerships in love is formed in infancy . . . under extraordinary circumstances, when a baby has been deprived of a mother or a mother substitute through adversity or a disaster or the indifference of his society, we have found that the later capacity of that child to commit himself to love, to partners in love, and to the human community will be diminished or depleted . . . (persons who are not attached) have no significant human relationship. The narrative of their lives reads like a vagrant journey with chance encounters and transient partnerships. Since no partner is valued, any partner can be exchanged for any other; in the absence of love, there is no pain in loss. Indeed, the striking characteristic of such people is their impoverished emotional range. There is no joy, no grief, no guilt, and no remorse. In the absence of human ties, a conscience cannot be formed; even the qualities of self-observation and self-criticism fail to develop.

Effects of failures in early parenting

The parents of children who suffer from the "disease of non-attachment" may have severe personality disorders or psychotic illnesses. They may not have reached the degree of emotional maturity necessary to raise children. They may have suffered severe hardships such as poverty, desertion by a spouse, or may have had a childhood marked by neglect and deprivation. The most severe effects of the failure of early parenting come under the headings of neglect, deprivation, exploitation, and abuse.

Neglect means that the parents do not give the children the attention and care to which as human beings they have a right. These parents do not see their children as belonging to them in a personal sense or as dependent upon them for nurture, even for life. Neglect can occur when a mother becomes seriously ill physically or has a mental illness, such as a postpartum psychosis, that prevents her from relating to her infant, and when no substitute mother is provided. If the infant's parents have had a recent and severe trauma, such as the death or serious illness of another family member, the infant may be neglected and the family's attention directed to the ill member or taken up by their own grief. Some very young mothers, who have not matured emotionally, neglect their infant whom they see more as a doll to play with than as a living person needing care.

Severe and prolonged neglect can cause what is called the failure-to-thrive syndrome. These children are malnourished and may die if not given the necessary medical care. In children who survive this extreme neglect, the effect on their psychological development is often clearly evident. They are developmentally retarded, that is, they do not perform as other children their age; they are listless and show no interest in their surroundings; they do not play. If adequate parental figures are provided or if their natural parents receive prompt help, the children may have normal development. Yet the damage inflicted in these early years often leaves in these young children a permanent vulnerability to emotional stress. Later in life conflict or trauma may cause them to regress to the profound apathy they showed when they were young. As they grow into adolescence, many develop antisocial symptoms.

A second serious consequence of the failure of parenting is *deprivation*. Again, the children are not treated as humans, but become objects of their parents' delusions. Unlike neglected children, they do receive attention and care from their parents, but the parents fail to perceive their real needs and so raise them in accord with their own bizarre beliefs. Examples of this are children who are fed according to a faddish diet which may deprive them of adequate nourishment, children who are controlled rigidly and at times cruelly because their parents believe they must control their children's evil nature, or children who are raised without limitations, even to the extent of endangering their lives. Some parents will not trust others to educate their children and subject them to distorted and inadequate educational programs. Parents may have delusions about their children's state of health and take them from doctor to doctor, and as a result the children may be subjected to unnecessary medications, diagnostic procedures, even surgery. Or parents may deny serious illness in their children.

These parents perceive their children and their responsibility to them in a psychotic way, even though in other areas of their lives they may appear to be normal adults. They, and the parents who exploit their children, often feel they literally own their children. In the most extreme cases their children may show the failure-to-thrive syndrome; they may show evidence of physical violence—although here the dynamics of the parent-child relationship are different than in abused children. There are instances in which children have been isolated from other persons because parents entertained delusions about these persons, and so the children lacked important socializing experiences. The children who are deprived are often quite compliant with their parents and may adopt their parents' psychotic view of reality.

Related to deprivation is the condition of *exploitation.* Exploited children are victims of their parents' unresolved emotional conflicts, and they are used by their parents either to promote these parental unconscious wishes or to help their parents defend against them. Exploitation may take the form of pushing the child to extraordinary feats of accomplishment in physical or intellectual activities. It may occur because a child's mother cannot define the boundaries of her own self, and she may use her child as an extension of herself. For example, she may make the child her confidant in all the intimate matters of her life. Parents who infantalize their children in various ways may be unconsciously gratifying their own wishes. Parent-child incest is one form of exploitation, and there are numerous other ways in which parents use children to gratify their own sexual desires: for example, parents who take children to sexually explicit movies or parents who allow children to have access to pornography in their home are exploiting them. Exploited children are often seen as precocious, and they relate more easily to adults than to children their own age. They receive considerable gratification from their intimate relationship with their parents and from the perception of how "needed" they are by them. Indeed, they are often reluctant to give up their regressive union with their parents. This presents a considerable resistance to treatment efforts. Superficially, they may appear to be developing normally, but by adolescence their inadequate ego development and their poorly functioning defensive system become apparent. In adolescence they often act out the parental needs which by this time have become their own. Adolescent sexual promiscuity can be one form of this identification with their parents. Adolescents who have been exploited show many characteristics of persons who have a narcissistic personality disorder, and they lack the capacity to relate normally to others. If children have been used by their parents to serve the parents' unmastered aggressive impulses, they may in adolescence behave in violent and antisocial ways.

A particular form of exploitation is *abuse,* physical and sexual. Because of laws now in force in most states, child abuse has been widely publicized. On the part of the parents, the distinctive feature is their failure to master their ambivalent feelings toward their children. These parents are not able to control their anger and hatred, but at the same time they love their children. Parents and children have a strong relationship, so intense that it would seem unlikely that there would be any abuse in their relationship. Indeed, the children's loyalty to their parents often makes them reluctant to testify regarding the abuse.

Abused children are fearful of adults. They may also see themselves as bad, for they believe their parents' opinion of them. In addition to physical dangers, there are serious consequences for their emotional development. As adults, many of these children may have emotional difficulties resembling those of their parents. Boys who have been beaten and otherwise abused may use force and violence as their way of relating to others. Abused girls may grow up to be disturbed in their relationship to their peers and may tend to rely excessively on autoerotic activities, both as a comfort and as a way to discharge violent and hostile feelings.

To illustrate how childhood experiences influence mothers to neglect their infants, let me present a brief description from Selma Fraiberg's book *Clinical Studies in Infant Mental Health: The First Year of Life.* The following is taken from the chapter entitled "An Abandoned Mother, An Abandoned Baby":

> Beth was an unmarried teen-age mother. Her history was reported to us by the hospital social worker who made the referral when Trudy was 4½ months old. Trudy had been diagnosed as a "failure to thrive" baby, a baby who was being starved. Beth herself had once been a starving infant. She had been found in the streets of a war-torn country, abandoned and unfed. After an unknown period in an orphanage she was adopted at age 2½. . . . Beth was an unhappy and difficult child. She ate poorly and vomited. She was fearful and cried a good deal, but she could not be held or comforted. There were sleeping problems, then behavior problems, and eventually learning problems. She was a marginal student, rebellious and unpredictable at home. Before she was 17 she was pregnant.
>
> Beth's pregnancy and delivery were normal, and the baby was a healthy 7 pounds at birth. The baby was to be placed for adoption. . . . Instead, Beth came home with the baby, only to find that her mother refused to let her stay if she kept Trudy. Beth would not give her baby up. She applied for Aid to Dependent Children (ADC) and moved into a low-cost housing apartment. Beth was depressed, unable to take care of herself or Trudy. At 1 month of age, Trudy was eating and sleeping poorly, vomiting, and crying; she had become a vivid re-creation of Beth's own past deprivation and terror. At 2 months of age, Trudy entered a day care nursery. Group day care by day was thus added to the neglect at home. Beth was scolded and given advice by her family, the day care staff, and the pediatrician. Beth appeared sullen and defiant, and the baby's condition worsened. Trudy became increasingly apathetic. Fear for Trudy's survival grew when her weight fell toward the 3rd percentile of the normal growth curve.
>
> At 4½ months of age Trudy was hospitalized for medical examination and more adequate feeding. Beth seldom visited. After ten days of good nursing care Trudy still vomited and had not gained any weight. The primary diagnosis was "failure to thrive due to low caloric intake and severe maternal deprivation." . . . When Trudy was discharged, the hospital referred her to the Child Development Project. . . . But Beth would not meet me. Trudy

returned to the day care nursery and Beth to school . . . . Nothing changed. The sad story of Beth's own abandonment and deprivation was being replayed.

Fortunately, Beth and her baby were treated at the Child Development Center in Ann Arbor, Michigan; but this help is not available to most infants and children who suffer from the "diseases of non-attachment." Not enough people have been trained to work in this specialized area of treatment; there are only a few centers like the one in Ann Arbor, and not enough financial support for such programs.

Developmental crises

The responses of infants to abnormal environments are emotional responses in the fullest sense, different from the emotional responses of older children and adults only because the infant has fewer ways of expressing feelings. These children are irritable or apathetic, sleep or eat poorly, cry excessively, and are susceptible to infectious diseases. Most important, they slow down or stop in psychological development.

Children who are reared in a healthy environment will experience similar symptoms, although less intense, in response to developmental crises. As infants and children progress from one developmental step to the next, each step presents them with new assignments, new skills to be mastered, and new aspects of reality to assimilate. Some adapt readily to these developmental steps; others are hesitant and fearful. When children are faced with new and unfamiliar tasks, they may fear what lies ahead; they may not have confidence in their ability to master these tasks. They may show the anxiety by their behavior. They may regress in an area in which they were functioning well; for example, becoming a picky eater or wetting the bed. They may handle the fears by attaching them to external persons or things, and so they are afraid of the dark, or of animals, or of insects, or of monsters. Most behavioral symptoms the pediatrician sees in young children are caused by normal developmental stress and are not pathological. When infants or young children experience a minor stress, such as a mild illness, their behavior should be stable, that is, any regression should be slight and temporary, and they should quickly regain their lost accomplishments. A child's behavior needs to be assessed in relation to his or her developmental stage as well as in relation to the environment. At four months an infant who does not want to eat may be going through a normal struggle over the regulation of eating. If this happens when the child is fifteen months, it may mean that he or she is struggling with mother over control.

Parental reactions to developmental crises are important. Reassurance usually is sufficient for most parents; however, the beginnings of later serious difficulties, such as problems in separating, can be seen when a mother is overly alarmed at normal developmental problems and cannot be reassured.

Mother-child attachment

Although the sequence of emotional development is biologically determined, it does not happen without stimuli from the environment. Perhaps we take for granted that mother's nurturing behavior will provide this input, yet in some situations the stimulation needed for development may be lacking. In successful parent-child interaction, there is a synchrony, a mutual communication which furthers the infant's attachment to mother. From the beginning the infant gives cues to mother, cues as to needs for nourishment, protection, comfort, trust, and affection. It can happen that the infant is unable to give cues or may give mother no confirmation that her response to the cues is correct.

If the infant's mother is depressed, she may not respond to the cues, or she may fail to help the infant even when she recognizes the need. In that case, the infant may stop trying to elicit nurturing behavior from mother and may become depressed and withdrawn. A mother may respond in an exaggerated way to the infant's cues, overstimulate the child, or not allow the child to separate psychologically. An insecure mother may fear criticism if her child does not develop along with all the other children, and she may push the child before he or she is ready. Some mothers stimulate their child by too active play and so do not assist in regulation of the child's energy and emotions. The overly intrusive mother may interfere with her child's initiative to play, and she may also find herself in a power struggle with the child.

Research has been directed to the first two years of life and even to the very first moments of life because of the importance of the mother-infant attachment and the need to ensure that the helpless newborn and the mother will be given the best chance to succeed in forming their relationship. Immediately after birth, there is a "maternal sensitive period" during which mother begins to form an attachment to her infant. Immediate contact with her newborn and as much contact as the condition of the infant and mother will permit facilitates this "bonding." When this early bonding occurs, later mother-child communication is better, and in certain areas the infant develops more rapidly.

Arthur Parmalee has studied the early relationships of mothers with pre-term (premature) infants. These infants must remain in the hospital nursery, apart from mother, for days or weeks, and because of this separation the mother-infant relationship initially may be weak. Parmalee found that it is not separation alone which causes difficulties in the mother-infant attachment. Mother's own childhood experiences and the state of her relationship with her husband and other important family members influence her ability to make the attachment. The mother who feels that her mother did not love her as a child, or the mother who does not receive support from her husband and others during the period of pregnancy, delivery, and the first weeks of the infant's life is not likely to visit her pre-term baby in the nursery. When she does visit, she is not able to interact with the infant. Because problems consume mother's energy and interfere with her expression of love for her infant, there is a relative neglect of the infant.

These and other studies of the earliest mother-infant interactions do not imply that an infant's future emotional development is determined beyond possibility of change by the events of the first hours or days of life. The important finding is that it is not just maternal care—which can come from many persons—that is essential for the child's development, but maternal attachment—which can come from only one person, mother.

As a child nears the end of the second year of life, he or she has traveled far along the road of development of important ego functions. The child is aware of being separate from other persons and things, is beginning to know that things exist outside of his or her own thoughts and feelings, that is, begins to know what is "real" and what is "not real." The child can protect him- or herself to some degree against anxiety and no longer needs mother to be the protector in an absolute way. He or she can comprehend and can reason in a rudimentary way. Now talking, the child can further master reality by naming things; now walking and using motor apparatus in other ways, the child begins to master the environment and the dangers in it. In addition to this external control, there is the beginning of internal control, the forerunner of superego and conscience. The child thinks about things and actions in terms of good and bad and expects to be punished for displeasing mother and others whose love is necessary.

Effects of trauma

Patterns of interaction formed in these first two years of life influence the development of children for the later years of childhood. This does not mean that the effects of early child rearing are irreversible, for there are ways of helping children change, and there are in all children "self-

righting" tendencies. A single trauma does not usually produce permanent damage. When a single trauma appears to produce permanent
damage, it is usually found that other factors are present, such as separation, as during the trauma of hospitalization, or the manner in which the
trauma was handled, for example, an absence of emotional support for a
child to help soften the trauma of the loss of a loved one. In early infancy
severe but temporary traumatic environments do not produce lasting effects on mental and emotional development, if the infants are returned
quickly to a healthy environment. Recent research on the effects of
deprivation indicates that children who experienced severe deprivation
and suffered permanent damage were children who continued to live in
the deprived environment. Often attention is given only to the traumatic
event and it is seen as the sole cause of disturbed development and eventual emotional disorders; what had preceded or followed the trauma, or
how the trauma was handled, may be overlooked.

One must be cautious when forecasting the long-term result of trauma
or of a deprived environment. The effects may not appear for many
years. Jerome Kagan studied deprived children in Guatemala and found
that the children who experienced severe early deprivation were able to
make considerable gains and "catch up" developmentally when they were
given a more favorable environment. However, the only areas measured
in these studies were cognitive development and gross behaviors such as
delinquency. His research did not determine if these infants and young
children experienced emotional suffering at the time of the deprivation,
if they had intrapsychic conflicts, or if the lag in ego development
prevented the children from reaching their full potential. The research
did not show how these children fared in latency, adolescence, and adult
life.

Sexuality in children

Nothing Freud wrote aroused as much opposition as did his papers on
the sexuality of children. Many persons, including professionals, ob-
jected to the thesis that young children have a sexual life. Although he
used the terms *erotic, sexual,* and *libidinal* to mean more than physical
pleasure and actions, he certainly included these meanings. Not only had
children been universally considered to be passive and unfeeling, they
were also thought to be pure and innocent, lacking sexual wishes and not
capable of sexual acts. We know that, in the main, Freud was correct,
and many decades of research and treatment of children have confirmed
and refined his observations. Because there is still confusion about childhood sexuality, and especially because parents seek guidance in these

matters, often from their priest, rabbi, or minister, it is well worth reviewing some of the important findings and discussing the problems in sexual development.

The psychosexual development of children is inseparable from their relationships with others, beginning with their parents, and pathology of sexual development is one manifestation of pathology in personal relationships. The outcome of children's first sexual attachments to their parents, together with later experiences with their parents in latency and adolescence, will go a long way toward determining whether they will have a happy sexual life as adults.

Childhood sexuality is a biologically determined process of psychic development which proceeds through several stages. Sexuality, or libido, is localized in particular areas of the body during certain stages of development, and sexual pleasure is experienced as pleasure or the release of tension in respect to these areas of the body, the "erotogenic zones." These zones are the oral, the anal, and the genital; and the infant and young child use these zones for certain pleasurable activities, e.g., oral sucking and biting, anal releasing and withholding, and phallic aggression. The use of the erotogenic zones to express aggression and hostility is a common feature of many pathological states of later life, not only in a sexual manner, as in sadism, but in other ways, such as by obsessive-compulsive behavior. For the first two years of life, sexuality is expressed in oral and anal modes; but during the second year, children of both sexes become aware of their genitals, and these become important as part of their developing body, self, and gender identity. With the advent of the phallic phase of sexuality, concern over their genitals becomes the principal manifestation of anxiety.

Development up to about age three, the oral and anal periods, is also called the preoedipal period, and the years from three to five or six, the time of the phallic period, is also called the oedipal period. In the oedipal period children have several important tasks: the establishment of a gender identity, the beginning of a lifelong process of relating to others with respect to this gender identity, and forming a new relationship with each parent. By the third year, as children have separated from their infant dependence on mother and are on the way to becoming individuals, they relate more to father and other members of the family. By the time children are three their sexual identity is established; they can label themselves and others with respect to sex with a significant degree of accuracy.

They feel attraction to one parent and rivalry with the other, and they express these feelings in ways that are in keeping with their intellectual and physical development. When four-year-old children declare they will marry mommy or daddy and that they will have a baby, they do not possess the awareness which older children have of sexual love and procreation. If children in the oedipal years see parents having intercourse, their understanding of this act is limited by their experience of human relationships, and they may see it as a fight rather than a loving act. All of this is understood by those parents who realize that the capacity to express love and other emotions in a sexual way does not suddenly appear at the end of childhood or adolescence but has its beginnings early in life and, like other ego functions, reaches maturity through a long process of development. Understanding the importance of prudent handling of sex in the life of their children, they do not treat their curiosity and wooing behavior as amusing or naughty; yet they do not stimulate them by being too intimate or showing undue favoritism. They consider the child's sexual questions seriously, giving the information that is needed at each stage of development and no more information, because that would be confusing and perhaps seductive. They do not, in the mistaken notion that they are being "natural," expose their bodies to children's curious gaze, caress them in an erotic manner, wrestle with them, or let them sleep with them. This does not mean that careful parents are cold and distant and cannot demonstrate their affection in physical ways, but they are careful because they know that overindulgence, seductive and preferential treatment of their children, as well as overly repressive methods of handling their natural sexual concerns will lead to sexual difficulties and troubled love relationships in adult life.

Parents are often at a loss to know what behavior at this age is healthy and what indicates problems in sexual development. Questions about sex and birth, display of genitals, looking at other children's genitals, "flirtatious" behavior, and masturbation are common. When any of these is persistent or extreme, as when the little boy or girl seems driven to masturbate, or when a little boy keeps trying to pull down little girls' pants, it is usually a sign of problems, often problems in the parent-child relationship, and a psychiatric consultation should be sought.

Gender disturbances

There are some serious, or potentially serious, sex and gender disturbances in childhood, but before discussing them a few definitions are needed.

Sex is the term used to denote the biological state of maleness or femaleness. *Gender* is the psychological state of considering oneself to be either masculine or feminine. The term *gender-identity* has the same meaning. Gender is an assignment that children themselves make, based on comparison with others and also in accordance with the gender they feel their parents have assigned to them. *Sexual identity* is more inclusive than gender-identity, and, according to Richard Green, it has three components:

> (1) core morphologic identity — the sense of being male or female, (2) gender-role behavior — culturally dimorphic activities which typify males and females, and (3) sexual partner preference — heterosexuality, homosexuality, or ambisexuality . . . . Core identity appears to evolve and be set during the first two or three years, gender role behavior is quite dimorphic by the fifth year, sexual partner orientation begins to become manifest near the end of adolescence.

Until recent years, it was assumed that only biological forces determined a person's perception of sexuality and the important aspects of sexual behavior, and that preference for sexual partners was also biological. Not so. Gender identity and sexual preference are largely psychological states, and they result from a complex interaction of intrapsychic and cultural forces. Adults with gender identity disturbances — transsexuals, some homosexuals, and some transvestites — showed disturbances of gender identity in childhood. However, not every child who has cross-gender behavior — for example, the little boy who dresses in girl's clothing — continues to have a gender-identity problem later in life. Not enough research has been done to answer all of the questions regarding the outcome of gender-identity disturbance in childhood and the extent to which treatment influences that outcome.

If a child up to age two or three has been consistently treated as being of one sex, the child's gender identity is fixed, and, according to present knowledge, it cannot be changed. In the past, there have been cases in which a child with ambiguous genitals was falsely labeled, and there have been cases in which parents deliberately raised a biologically normal child as a member of the opposite sex. Although we say that gender identity is fixed by a certain age, that does not mean it is static. Gender identity is constantly developing, being revised, and consolidated as the child acquires more self-knowledge and bodily maturity. It is influenced by later childhood and adolescent sexual experiences and, most importantly, by the child's relation to the important adults in his or her life.

Among the signs that indicate the possibility of a gender disturbance in a boy is a dislike for his sexual organs and a preference for those of females. Another is his choice of behavior which is considered feminine in our culture: dressing in female clothing, preference for female playmates and toys, emulation of female superheroes, and effeminate mannerisms. When this behavior is persistent, the boy should have a psychiatric evaluation; it may be decided that he is in need of psychiatric treatment and that his parents also are in need of help through psychological counseling or psychiatric treatment. However, many parents whose sons show extreme cross-gender disturbances do not seek help, believing either that the behavior will disappear without causing psychological damage, or that they can change the behavior by shaming or punishing the boy or forcing him into masculine behavior. Or they do not seek help because they fear they will be blamed for the behavior of their child. Unfortunately, the forceful and shaming methods often result in the disappearance of the outward signs of the gender disturbance; but it has gone "underground," and the nature of the child's pathology has not changed.

The diagnosis of childhood cross-gender disturbance is less frequently made in girls, probably because our culture is more accepting of "tomboy" activity in girls than it is of "sissy" behavior in boys. It may be a mistake to assume that the girl who wants to dress like a boy and play with the boys rather than with other girls does not have a problem, for the same diagnostic picture that is present in boys with gender disturbances can be found in girls, and extreme cross-gender behavior in girls is correlated with adult female homosexuality and transsexualism.

The condition known as adult transsexualism is a rare but serious disorder of gender identity. According to Robert Stoller, the adult transsexual has been biologically normal, but has always identified him- or herself as a member of the opposite sex. The transsexual expects to be accepted according to gender, not according to biological sex, and will attempt to have his or her physical appearance changed by hormones and surgery. There are differences in behavior and in psychological attitudes of transsexuals, effeminate homosexuals, and transvestites. Effeminate homosexuals are biologically normal men who dress like women and prefer male sexual partners, but they identify themselves as masculine. Transvestites are biologically normal males who identify themselves as masculine, prefer female sexual partners, and at times dress in women's clothes because in so doing they become sexually excited.

As with most other disturbances of childhood, the cross-gender behavior is linked to parent-child relationships. It is usually the relationship to mother which is crucial in the development of these disturbances for both sexes; for boys, a weak, ineffectual, or absent father also influences the development of pathology. Some general dynamic patterns have been found in these relationships, although each case is different, and further research is needed for fuller understanding of these dynamic relationships.

The superego

The latency period of child development, which begins about the sixth year and continues until preadolescence, is a time of few developmental crises, and a period of growth of many ego functions, including the making of relationships outside the family (socialization), defense formation, and mastery of bodily and intellectual skills. During this period children's superego formation begins, marking the emancipation from parental standards of right and wrong. I use the term *emancipation,* not to indicate that the child's standards are in opposition to parental standards (sometimes they are), but to indicate that healthy superego formation means that children fashion their own standards. The emancipation occurs because the child first internalizes the parental standards, then modifies them in the process of making them their own.

The earliest stages of superego development come before latency, when the child obeys parental rules even when parents are absent. However, at this stage internalized parental standards and prohibitions are easily overlooked by the child when there is a chance of not being caught or punished. At this time disobedience does not cause guilt feelings, for the child is still under the influence of the developmental anxieties of the prelatency period—fear of loss of the loved person, loss of this person's love, and fear of bodily injury. This situation changes because of the pressure to solve the oedipal conflicts. To make it possible for the child to give up the oedipal wishes, a new ego function appears. At first the superego is quite rigid in order that the child can repress oedipal wishes and control masturbation. Later, in the healthy latency child and adolescent, the standards of the superego become more reasonable. Once the superego is functioning, children begin to conform to particular standards of conduct because they feel within themselves these standards are right. When they act contrary to these standards, often when even their wishes are contrary to the standards, they feel the emotional distress we call guilt.

The superego is not only the giver of laws, it is the source of self-satisfaction and self-esteem, the supplier of necessary elements of narcissism, elements which replace in part the praise and devotion of parents. To be loved and approved by one's superego becomes as important as being loved and approved by parents and other important people in one's life. If it is not loving, the superego reproaches the person, as in depression, or forces the person to adhere to an unrealistic and harsh morality, as in the obsessive-compulsive disorders.

The superego operates unconsciously, and it is only when there is pathology that we see the results of its operations. When the superego develops normally, a healthy character is formed, one which, when mature, will include personal responsibility for one's actions, feelings, and social commitment, not just an external adherence to rules. At the same time other ego functions, especially sublimations and defenses such as reaction formation, are evident. It is important that all of the psychic structures develop at approximately the same rate. If drives are too strong and the ego and superego are weak, then the personal relationships and the moral commitment needed to restrain the drives are lacking, and the control of the sexual and aggressive impulses breaks down. If drives remain primitive while the ego and superego development have gone ahead, then obsessional defenses are used to control the drives.

Many parents feel unable to judge if their children are developing normally and feel they need advice on assisting their children in developing a healthy morality. It is very easy to oversimplify these matters, and I do not presume to treat this subject as completely as it should be treated, but only to mention a few important guidelines.

Because the content of the superego, its commands and prohibitions, are derived from those which parents have inculcated in their children by word and example, the values of parents are very important in the formation of the superego. This almost goes without saying, except that adults so often fail to take into account the powers of observation of children, how impressionable they are, and how faithfully they imitate their parents. Children take their parents at their word, they make their parents' rules sacred, and they are profoundly disillusioned when they discover parental transgressions of these rules. If parents live by the rules they expect their children to follow, there is usually little confusion in the minds of the children about right and wrong. If parents expect a child to behave in certain ways, but their own behavior contradicts these expectations, or if they receive satisfaction, consciously or unconsciously, from a child's misconduct, the superego of that child will be weakened.

The beginnings of character disorders that involve the superego can often be traced to the latency years, but it is difficult to predict solely from the external behavior of latency children how they will turn out. Lying and stealing, for example, are common in latency boys, but these boys do not all become untruthful and dishonest adults. These actions are not necessarily signs of defects in the children's superego, but often indicate unconscious conflicts about their relationships to parents, sibling, or peers.

Some parents attempt to shield their children from all anxiety, but may succeed only in increasing their guilt feelings. Other parents are harsh, or rigid and perfectionistic, and the children's superego may take on these harsh, punitive, and inflexible qualities. On the other hand, if the strictness of the superego is eliminated, the children may feel very unprotected against the force of their drives. Anna Freud has called this state "the deepest of all anxieties."

Parental guidance and example are not the only determinants of superego functioning. The strength of the child's ego and of his sexual and aggressive drives are important. As the childhood ties to parents are loosened in the course of healthy emotional development, and the parents are seen as less ideal than before, the child in late latency, and particularly in adolescence, finds other superego models.

Behavior and learning disorders in school

In latency children, free of the conflicts of earlier years, have a powerful spurt in intellectual growth; but if they have not overcome early childhood conflicts and are developmentally retarded, they may experience difficulties in school. Educators have turned to psychiatry for help with some of these children, and the collaboration has produced methods and programs for aiding children with special educational and emotional needs. Enriched and discriminating school programs have helped many children to overcome their developmental difficulties as well as their learning difficulties. In one respect, this union of education and psychiatry has had a dubious result. I am here referring to the diagnostic concept of the child with *minimal brain dysfunction.*

Minimal brain dysfunction (earlier diagnostic terms were *brain-injured child* and *minimal brain damage*) is a diagnosis applied to a cluster of conduct disorders, affective states, and learning difficulties. These are attributed to "mild" or "minimal" abnormality in the brain from infection, injury, or genetic causes. One of the most frequently described symptoms is "hyperactivity." Hyperactive children manifest motor restlessness, difficulty in focusing attention, and an inability to ignore distractions; they may disturb the other children in a classroom by aggressive or noisy behavior. Although children diagnosed as having minimal brain dysfunction may have average or better than average intelligence, they may have problems in reading, arithmetic, or handwriting, in letter, number, or word reversals, as well as other learning problems. Temper outbursts and depressive episodes are also found in this picture, as well as bed-wetting and fire-setting.

This condition has been attributed to organic causes, either an infection, such as a viral encephalitis complicating one of the childhood diseases, or an injury to the brain sustained during a difficult childbirth or resulting from a blow to the head. Many of these children improved in some of their behavior and learning problems after they were given a central nervous stimulant, such as dexedrine (now replaced by a similar drug, Ritalin). Those proposing this diagnosis theorize that if infants or young children suffer *severe* brain damage they will have a recognizable neurological condition, such as cerebral palsy or epilepsy, but if the damage to the brain has been *mild* or *minimal* they will be predisposed to develop the behavior, affective, and learning disorders mentioned.

Very many children have been diagnosed as having minimal brain dysfunction, and many have had improvement in their symptoms. However, questions have been raised about this concept and information is available that has made clinicians and researchers doubt the validity of the diagnosis and the specific action of Ritalin and similar drugs. These objections have been summarized by the well-known British psychiatrist Michael Rutter.

Rutter contends that the symptoms which have been attributed to a neurological cause occur in other conditions which are due to emotional causes, and therefore these symptoms are not specific to the diagnosis of brain dysfunction. This diagnosis is often made on the basis of the symptom cluster alone when the neurological examination is negative and when there is no history of encephalitis or brain trauma. In such cases there appears little to substantiate the diagnosis. Rutter finds no clear evidence that a mild brain injury causes psychiatric and learning problems. In order for psychiatric symptoms and learning problems to be present, the injury must be severe enough to cause amnesia lasting at least seven days. Such a severe injury is not found in the history of most of these children, and so Rutter feels that minimal brain dysfunction due to trauma to the brain is "relatively uncommon." Drugs such as Ritalin given to children diagnosed as having minimal brain dysfunction have resulted in improvement in all emotional symptoms of children, even those due to non-organic causes. The only possible exception to this broad area of improvement is the symptom of anxiety. Because a group of children who show behavior and learning problems have improved when given Ritalin does not prove that these children suffer from minimal brain dysfunction.

The emphasis on helping this group of children (and it is a large group) has led to improvement in teacher training and classroom instruction, and this has helped these children. Moreover, the attention that they receive is beneficial. A large number of these children come from underprivileged neighborhoods, and it appears that many of them undergo stress from internalized conflict and disturbed family situations. In the long run, then, it is not beneficial to them if these causes of their symptoms are not attended to because of the mistaken insistence of seeing organic brain dysfunction in each of these children. Rutter states that the hyperactive syndrome is associated with the development of antisocial behavior in childhood, adolescence, and later life, and with a family history of alcoholism and antisocial personality. Many children show only superficial and temporary improvement with medication; more lasting results might come if appropriate treatment were available. Many psychiatrists have seen these children as manifesting problems of emotional adjustment and these children have improved with psychotherapy.

Children's reactions to a parent's death

When a child's parent dies, the family may turn to their pastor for help in bearing their loss and for guidance in dealing with the effect of this loss on their children. It is normal for adults to experience mourning for the dead person, but we are not sure just what is normal and healthy for children. When a loved one dies, adults stop most of their activities and withdraw to some degree from everyday concerns so that they can mourn. Mourning is a process in which the person calls to mind the memories of the loved one and by doing this is finally able to become reconciled to the loss. Mourning differs for each person, depending on the relationship to the dead person, on the conflicts one may have experienced in the relationship to the deceased, and on the defenses that are part of the conflicts.

Children do not mourn like adults, and their mourning is so different that some writers have stated that children are not able to mourn until adolescence. Not all agree with this, and it seems that most children, except for young infants, can and do mourn. However, there is one important difference. For adults, the loss of a loved one is a great sorrow, a painful and often an almost unbearable trauma. For children, the loss of a parent, particularly of mother, is also a serious interference in emotional development. If children in the mourning process withdraw, as adults do, this causes a halt in the forward movement of development, and at the worst it may produce a permanent distortion in emotional growth.

My comments here deal mostly with the effect of the loss of the mother, although some of the observations apply as well to the reaction of children to the loss of any person they love. The loss of mother has different meanings at different ages. In the early years of life, until the child can grasp the notion of the finality of death, that is, until the middle of latency, the prolonged absence of a parent has the same effect on the child as the loss through death.

In the first six or eight months of life, before the infant has differentiated him- or herself from others, he or she cannot attribute feelings to others. In reacting to the loss of the person who cares for him or her, whether it be a temporary or permanent loss, the child senses that he or she is not experiencing pleasure and not receiving gratification of needs. We do not say that the infant mourns, for in order to mourn a personal relationship is necessary. However, the infant does become apathetic and, unless an adequate substitute is provided quickly, will show characteristics of infants who fail to thrive. In the second half of the first year of life, when the child has begun to make a personal relationship to mother, the child may refuse to accept a stranger in her place. If a person cannot be found who is acceptable, the child develops characteristics of the institutionalized child, becomes retarded in development, particularly in the ability to relate to others.

By the end of the first year, when the child has made a personal relationship to mother and, even more, when, near the end of the second year of life, he or she has gained libinal constancy, the loss is experienced in a personal sense. We then can recognize some of the features of the mourning process. The child is capable of mourning because he or she has a mental picture of mother, a concept of her as a loving person, and a concept that remains even when mother is absent. At this age, and for a number of years later, the child mourns mother whenever there is a separation, e.g., if he or she goes to a hospital, or if the parents go away for a few days. This is a normal response. The child may become clinging, regress to the behavior of a younger child, show disturbances in eating and sleeping, and refuse to be comforted by another. The loss is experienced as a trauma, and the child may react by excessive fearfulness and by nightmares. Even when the child comes to accept another in place of the absent or dead parent, confidence in the relationship may never be strong; the child may show excessive anxiety about any separation. Most important are the long-term effects, the interferences with normal development. It may be more difficult for this child to resolve the normal conflicts of childhood and adolescence.

There are ways to help children master the trauma of the loss, but they cannot be "protected" from the pain of the loss. In keeping with their age and ability to comprehend, the reality of what has happened should be explained. As in other important matters, for instance, religion and sex, their questions should be answered truthfully, but they should not be given more information than they can grasp, otherwise they will be confused. Death should not be needlessly surrounded by mystery, nor should children be forbidden to talk about these matters. It is best that the explanations be given by the surviving parent or someone else close to the children, even though it may be difficult for the adult survivors to talk about their feelings. Feelings should be talked about; children should know they are permitted to be sad and lonely, to cry, and to withdraw. Often enough the adults keep information from children because it is too painful for the adults to face their own feelings, or they feel children are incapable of handling grief. Children may appear to adjust quickly to the loss, so adults may feel justified in not helping them to acknowledge their feelings. The outward appearance of calm is present only because the children have repressed painful affects and occupy themselves with activities and interests which will keep these affects repressed.

A six-year-old boy suffering from night terrors was seen at the outpatient clinic of a hospital. This condition, also called *pavor nocturnus,* is a sleep disturbance similar to the nightmare, but more severe. In this condition the child is terrified, cries out during sleep, can be aroused only with great difficulty, and has no memory of what caused the terror. This boy's mother had cancer and was dying. Although she had been in and out of the hospital several times and her physical appearance had worsened, she and her husband never discussed her illness with their children. At the clinic the psychiatrist helped the parents to tell the children about the mother's illness and impending death. Not only did the six-year-old boy's night terrors cease, but the entire family began realistically, sorrowfully, but lovingly to prepare for mother's death.

When a parent or another family member dies, it is better for children to remain in their own home, with their possessions and companions, rather than to be sent to stay at an unfamiliar place. The next best choice is for them to stay at a home which is familiar, such as a grandmother's. This applies also to other separations, for example, when a parent is hospitalized, a sibling is born, or the parents go on a trip. If it is possible for the dying person to be at home, I believe it can be not only more comforting for that person, but a help to the family, especially the children, in their acceptance and understanding of death. Participating in funeral and burial services helps the children to grasp the meaning and finality of death.

It is important that very young children who have lost their mother have a suitable person to care for them as soon as possible. This is not always easy to arrange, and very often it must be their father who provides this care, for he remains the only constant person in their lives.

Even when all these things to help children mourn are done, the loss of a person so necessary to their development will cause disturbance in development. For children mourning is not as complete as for adults; they cannot suspend their development so they can mourn the way adults can suspend their interest in the world around them. Children do not review the memories of the dead person in order to come to a resolution of feelings, or at least not to the extent adults do. They are more likely than adults to idealize the dead parent and in this way keep the parent alive in fantasy. Because of this they may not be willing to accept a substitute, even though the substitute appears quite satisfactory. If they accept the substitute, it will seem to them that they have to give up the tie with the parent who loved them, and so they will feel unloved. Also, because they have idealized the dead parent, the substitute can never equal in fantasy this parent, and so is certain to be a disappointment to the children. Adults, too, may find the mourning process painful to pursue for they cannot face the negative feelings they have toward the dead person, and they also have to idealize. The idealization prevents the mourning from becoming complete, and when the surviving parent handles feelings in this way, he or she may be unable to help the children mourn. If the surviving parent or the children continue in this way they may require help through psychiatric or psychoanalytic treatment.

These pages have discussed the principal developmental steps in childhood and the results of disturbances in these areas. The presentation has focused on the relationship of children to their parents, for this relationship is the most important factor in their emotional growth. These issues frequently come to the attention of the clergy and parents often seek their advice and help for problems of the children.

REFERENCES

Fraiberg, Selma. *Clinical Studies in Infant Mental Health: The First Year of Life.* New York: Basic Books, 1980, 222–23.

Fraiberg, Selma. *Every Child's Birthright: In Defense of Mothering.* New York: Basic Books, 1977, xi–xiii.

Freud, Anna, & Burlingham, Dorothy. *Infants Without Families.* New York: International Universities Press, 1944.

Freud, Anna, & Burlingham, Dorothy. *War and Children.* New York: International Universities Press, 1944.

Furman, Erna. *A Child's Parent Dies.* New Haven and London: Yale University Press, 1974.

Green, Richard. Atypical sex-role behavior. In *Basic Handbook of Child Psychiatry,* vol. II. Joseph O. Noshpitz, ed. New York: Basic Books, 1979, 537.

Klaus, Marshall H., & Robertson, Martha O., eds. *Birth, Interaction, and Attachment.* Johnson & Johnson Baby Products, 1982.

Klaus, Marshall H., & Trause, Mary Anne, eds. *Maternal Attachment and Mothering Disorders.* Johnson & Johnson Baby Products, 1975.

Brown, Catherine C., ed. *Infants at Risk.* Johnson & Johnson Baby Products, 1981.

Spitz, René A. Hospitalism: an inquiry into the genesis of psychiatric conditions in early childhood, *Psychoanalytic Study of the Child,* vol. I. New York: International Universities Press, 1945, 53–74.

Spitz, René A. Hospitalism: a follow-up report, *Psychoanalytic Study of the Child,* vol. II. New York: International Universities Press, 1946, 113–17.

3

Normal Adolescence

CHARLES MCCAFFERTY AND PATRICK F. OWEN

A dolescence (the term is derived from the Latin *adolescere,* meaning "to come to maturity") is a biological event, a psychological process, and a cultural phenomenon. Adults throughout the ages have shown a marked ambivalence toward adolescents with feelings ranging from approval, envy, and admiration to apprehension, dismay, and even angry condemnation. Aristotle (Kiell, cited in Mussen, Conger, & Kagan, 1979, p. 425) referred to adolescents as "passionate, irascible, and apt to be carried away by their impulses . . . . If the young commit a fault, it is always on the side of excess and exaggeration for they carry everything too far, whether it be their love or hatred or anything else. They regard themselves as omniscient. . . ." Shakespeare pleaded, "Could we but skip the years between four and twenty and one and ten when youth do nothing but fight, drink and get wench with child." Similar views have been expressed by a number of philosophers, religious leaders, and others, although Bronowski (1974) notes in the *Ascent of Man* that the common denominator in the fall of the magnificent cultures of China and Rome was their failure to pay attention to the thoughts and imagination of their younger generations.

Although adolescence is invariably a troubled and stressful time for both adolescents and adults, it is of vital importance that adolescence be seen as a positive and constructive stage in human development for both the individual and society. An appreciation of the emotional, physical, and cultural varieties of this developmental stage will help increase rapport and understanding between generations.

Historical and cultural perspective

Adolescence is in part a cultural phenomenon. The manner in which we experience it today is due in large measure to present-day economic and familial realities. Only within the last two hundred years has adolescence come to be recognized as a separate developmental stage. Prior to the Industrial Revolution of the nineteenth century, the time-period of adolescence was not clearly delineated. The pre-nineteenth-century family was primarily agrarian. Economic necessity dictated that children assume adult responsibilities comparatively early by contemporary standards (Wynne & Frader, 1979). Occupational choices offered by society and the adolescent's social sphere outside the confines of the family were quite limited. Behavioral expectations for the adolescent were more clearly outlined and vocational choices were highly influenced, if not predetermined, by the parents. Job skills, as a rule, were attained by apprenticeship and/or parental example in the home. A carpenter's son, for example, recognized at an early age that his occupational destiny lay in being a carpenter, and thus he was not faced with the stresses inherent in deciding on a vocation or a profession. Demos and Demos (cited in Wynne & Frader, 1979, p. 64) said in reference to the agrarian society of the Plymouth colony that "the child appears not so much as a child, per se, but as himself a potential farmer; he is then, an immature model of his father."

The dawn of the Industrial Age and the subsequent rise of an affluent and mobile middle class resulted in fundamental changes in the nature of society and in the manner in which adolescence has come to be experienced. The technological age has resulted in the prolongation of adolescence as more preparatory time is required before the child assumes the roles of adulthood. Of course accompanying such a development is the demand that the adolescent remain dependent for a longer period of time on his or her parents, especially if the adolescent should choose college and perhaps graduate study before reaching financial independence.

Although the time-period of adolescence is a development of contemporary society, there exists both differences and similarities in the manner in which it is experienced in various cultures. In French-speaking countries there tends to be less permissiveness with children who are supposed to be "seen and not heard." In such cultures children look forward to adolescence and early adulthood as a time of emancipation and independence. Their parents generally are more permissive with them and they endorse their adolescents' assertions of independence. There is a tendency for the reverse to be true in the United States in that we encourage independence in our children, but at the same time attempt to assert our parental authority. Spanish boys, while being encouraged to be submissive to parental authority during their childhood years, once they reach adolescence are expected to demonstrate a "machismo" and to give evidence of their masculinity in a way that might bring American adolescents into conflict with juvenile authorities.

Cultural similarities are noted as well as shown by the upsurge of adolescent unrest stemming from a common dissatisfaction with adults' attitudes toward political issues and societal values in a wide variety of cultures including the Soviet Union, Switzerland, and England. The sense of community and common interests among adolescents the world over is often reflected in their similar appreciation of rock music and blue jeans in various cultures. Mass media and rapid communication serve to allow adolescents the opportunity to identify with the causes and symbols of their peers in other countries.

Physical changes in adolescence

Adolescence is ushered in by the advent of biological puberty as pronounced anatomical, physiological, and cognitive changes begin to occur. For females, puberty begins at approximately age twelve to thirteen and coincides with the time of menstruation. Puberty in males is approximately one year later and coincides with the time ejaculation can be reached. Cognitive changes are noted as the adolescent begins to think abstractly, to use metaphor and simile, and to ponder hypothetical issues and concepts such as freedom and justice.

There are wide individual differences in the rates at which young males and females mature. It is important for parents and adolescents to realize that on any measure of maturation almost 50 percent of girls and boys mature more slowly than the median adolescent and almost 50 percent mature more rapidly (Mussen, Conger & Kagan, 1979). Boys show accelerated growth somewhat later than girls and thus during early adolescence girls tend to be somewhat taller. Boys, however, catch up quickly and their growth during middle adolescence at times becomes so rapid that they may go through a phase where they appear uncoordinated, awkward, and lacking in stamina. By age eighteen, 98 percent of physical growth for both sexes has been completed. Better nutrition and medical care as well as heredity are all thought to be important reasons for today's adolescents being taller than those of previous generations. It has been estimated that the average height for both sexes increases approximately one inch each decade.

In addition to height, boys show considerable increase in weight related primarily to the increased development of bones and muscle rather than to an increase in body fat. Penis and scrotum size increases with a coarsening of the skin in these areas, together with the appearance of pubic, facial, and underarm hair as well as voice changes. In girls there is an increase in subcutaneous fat with rounding of the hips resulting from broadening of the pelvis. Breast development usually continues for several years. In both sexes hormonal changes bring about an increase in oily secretions in the skin with 75 to 80 percent of adolescents being troubled with acne. Facial structures also mature and this is a time when boys and girls at times become preoccupied with the size of their nose and ears and these concerns play a part in the regulation of their self-esteem.

Although menstruation in girls and ejaculation in boys heralds the advent of biological puberty, this does not necessarily mean that either sex yet has the ability to procreate. The early adolescent boy's sperm may contain an inadequate number of live spermatozoa for fertility. Adolescent females do not become capable of conception until approximately one to one-and-a-half years after menstruation begins.

Psychological perspective

Although adolescence is popularly considered to span the ages of twelve to eighteen years, the termination of adolescence, unlike its beginning with puberty, is difficult to define. The particular situation of the individual needs to be considered. The college student in his or her early twenties, financially dependent and living at home, may be occupied with the characteristic problems of adolescence, whereas a married and employed eighteen-year-old man living away from home may have already matriculated into adulthood.

Adolescence is commonly divided into three principal stages (Blos, 1962; Dulit, 1975): early adolescence, ages twelve to fourteen; middle adolescence, ages fifteen to seventeen; and late adolescence, age eighteen trailing off to the early twenties. These age ranges are not firm and much overlapping exists.

Early adolescence is noted for its dramatic shift from the complacency and cooperativeness of the latency-age years (roughly six to eleven years) to emotional lability and psychological turmoil. The influence of peers and the need for group affiliations and peer-group conformity take on special importance as the adolescent starts a marked progressive shift away from his or her parents in an effort to separate emotionally, to resolve childhood dependencies, and to develop a clear sense of personal identity. The role of identification is of critical importance during this period for strong identification processes are set in motion by the adolescent's need for a measure of greater support from outside the family. Idealized friendships with peers is common, and extra-parental adults such as school teachers and coaches also play an important part as role models. The progressive shift toward greater autonomy and independence, however, is not a smooth linear process. The early adolescent, in particular, exhibits a marked vulnerability to display periodic regressive shifts in behavior as the pendulum swings back and forth between the dependent security of childhood and the threatening insecurity of the adult.

Middle adolescence is characterized by a general settling down of behavior. Compromise becomes more of a possibility, and reflective thought and a progressive shift to a higher abstract mode of thinking occurs. Emotional lability gives way to a more stable and consistent mood. Behavior becomes more predictable. The total commitment to peers, which appears so characteristic of early adolescents, lessens in intensity as they grow to feel more secure of their emotional ground. In general, adolescents become easier to live with, although their propensity to become involved in power struggles with authoritarian figures serves as a sign that the battle between dependence and independence has not yet been wholly won.

Late adolescence shows a further broadening of views, a widening of intellectual scope, and further consolidation of values. Further synthesis and consolidation of identity, particularly sexual identity, takes place. Vocational and occupational interests and choices take on increased importance as the maturing adolescent becomes more "future-oriented."

Although some young people seemingly sail through adolescence on an even keel, while others seem driven from one almost capsizing crisis to the next, all adolescents experience some measure of emotional disharmony. Probably at no other time than infancy are young people in so great need of support and understanding from their parents and the adults who populate their life.

During this period many disagreements and family misunderstandings occur over a variety of issues. However, one area—that of control and limit-setting—is one frequently heard. Commonly parents react to this question either by relaxing all behavioral controls and limits and adopting a laissez-faire attitude toward their adolescents or, conversely, by attempting to overcontrol and thereby extinguishing all signs of the normal and healthy revolutionary impetus of their young people. Both extremes are equally erroneous, for a middle-of-the-road position is called for as the young person needs both parental guidelines as well as freedom within well-defined limits to try out his or her independence.

Although the storm and stress of adolescence has been emphasized in this chapter, adolescents can and do demonstrate marked flexibility and immunity in dealing with many kinds of turmoil, including even the major upheavals which follow in the wake of a family broken by divorce—a fate which has been common in the history of presidents, artists, poets, and literary people.

In conclusion, it is remarkable that in spite of the stresses of adolescence the majority of young people ultimately make an adequate adjustment in their lives. Most develop their abilities, resolve their early vulnerabilities, enter an occupation or profession, get married, have children, and make commitments to the community which mark the attainment of full adulthood. Thus, eventually, the adult of tomorrow pays back to the next generation what they receive from their parents today.

Illustrative examples and dynamic considerations

CASE I

John was a fourteen-year-old referred because of school refusal. Academically he had done quite well until the previous six months, but there had been a falling off in his interest at school. He was also noted by his parents to have become quite irritable, withdrawn. At first they suspected drug abuse but on further inquiry there was nothing to support this. He would present physical symptoms to avoid attending school, but frequent visits to the family doctor did not reveal any physical pathology. In the doctor's office he refused to take his shirt off to have his chest examined. The school refusal progressed to the point where he would refuse to get out of bed in the mornings. He would spend most of the day in his room and he remained aloof from his usual peer group.

There were clinical symptoms of depression with some hints of suicidal ideation. The school authorities had threatened to file a truancy petition because of his extended absence.

John was admitted for further assessment to the psychiatric adolescent unit. At a staffing conference with his teachers and a counselor at school, it was noted that his absences at first had occurred on days when he had physical education classes, which involved taking showers with his peers at the school.

After he had gained rapport and a trusting relationship with his attending psychiatrist, he did eventually permit a physical examination. This was unremarkable, except for a moderate degree of gynecomastia or development of the breast tissue. In subsequent individual psychotherapy he was able to surface his anxiety and confusion about the gynecomastia. Some degree of this occurs in at least five to ten percent of boys in adolescence as part of what is essentially a normal endocrine change. The boy's depressive symptoms rapidly cleared up with reassurance that there was no abnormal sexual development and that this was merely a transitory physiological occurrence.

CASE 2

Lori was a fifteen-year-old referred from a hospital emergency room after the police brought her to the hospital following a call to her home. Lori feared that she was about to lose control and might hurt herself or her mother. Three months earlier for no apparent reason she had lost control and tore apart her mother's bedroom, doing extensive physical damage. Her mother at this time called the police and Lori had spent a few hours in a shelter home before returning home.

Psychiatric examination showed her to be highly anxious with pressured speech, somewhat loose associations, and a paranoid manner. Further assessment of the family situation showed that Lori was an only child and that her biological father had abandoned the family when she was an infant. The mother had noted that in the past year she had become withdrawn from her peers, rarely left home, and felt that neighborhood children maliciously teased her. Interestingly enough, this had reached the point where the mother had encouraged her to remain at home and, in fact, had set up a roller skating area for her in the basement of their home. Also, she had insisted on sharing a bedroom with her mother.

In light of her extreme agitation and threats of suicide, Lori was admitted to a psychiatric unit for in-patient assessment, where it was noted that there was extreme separation anxiety shown by the mother. Within the first twenty-four hours, she almost insisted on having her daughter discharged against medical advice. In subsequent psychotherapy, the dynamics became clearer. There had been a lag in normal maturation of the ego, which had been unconsciously fostered by the parent with the failure of thriving toward separation and emancipation. The smothering of the normal ego development had resulted in internalized rage against the mother, some of which had been projected in paranoid relationships with those outside the family. In this case the internalized anger, which was part of the pathological symbiotic relationship with the mother, had broken through the child's defenses. On occasions this can reach homicidal proportions or may be again internalized and give rise to suicidal risk. In extreme forms, frank psychosis may occur.

In this case separation through hospitalization, combined with psychotherapy for both mother and child, was able to correct this disturbance of normal adolescent development.

CASE 3

On the eve of his sixteenth birthday, James killed his forty-seven-year-old father with a single rifle shot. Prior to this incident both parents had been in conflict over the father's drinking problem and gambling debts. The mother had threatened to leave the home and essentially abandon the children to be supported by her husband.

The father had terminated this conflict by leaving in his car to purchase hamburgers for the family meal. While he was gone, James' mother received a telephone call from her sister, and he overheard her angrily reiterate the problems with her husband, including the fact that she was planning to walk out on the family. The mother then returned to her room. James then brought down a rifle from his own bedroom and stood by the front door awaiting his father's return. As his father entered the room, the son fired a single shot, killing him instantly.

During subsequent psychiatric assessment, the boy appeared polite, orderly, and cooperative, and appeared in no distress. He seemed normal apart from his social withdrawal and emotional aloofness from the tragedy. He was quite open and frank in describing his father's death, but related this in a matter of fact way, showing no remorse.

Dynamically, it became clear that there was much unresolved oedipal conflict between James and his parents, with an extreme dependent relationship on his mother. His internalized rage at his father, whom he saw as bringing about abandonment by his mother, was acted out with tragic consequences. Of significance also was the boy's tendency to act out the whole family's anger at an irresponsible father. It must be understood that this intra-family tension never really surfaced on a conscious level prior to this incident, and it illustrates in an unusually dramatic form some of the tensions which often exist within the parent-child triangle in adolescence.

CASE 4

Joseph, a thirteen-year-old, was left to babysit a neighbor's five-year-old daughter. The parents of the child returned several hours later to find their daughter distraught and Joseph offering less than plausible explanations. Within the next few days the child communicated to her mother that Joseph had sexually molested her. This created great panic for Joseph's parents when they were informed and the police were involved.

The above scenario is not as uncommon as it might appear and illustrates the normally poorly developed sexual-impulse control of the early adolescent. Joseph had shown no other behavioral problems in the past, and otherwise had appeared as an emotionally healthy boy. (Adolescent boys generally should not be asked to babysit at a time when their sexuality is coming to the surface and they are particularly sexually curious, while at the same time having limited, if any, developed internal controls.)

REFERENCES

Blos, P. *On Adolescence.* New York: The Free Press, 1962.
Bronowski, J. *Ascent of Man.* New York: Little, Brown, and Co., 1974.
Dulit, E. Adolescence. In George H. Wiedeman, ed., *Personality Development and Deviation.* New York: International Universities Press, 1975.
Mussen, P. H., Conger, J. J., & Kagan, J. *Child Development and Personality.* 5th ed. New York: Harper & Row, 1979.
Wynne, L. C., & Frader, L. Female adolescence and the family: a historical view. In Max Sugar, ed., *Female Adolescent Development.* New York: Brunner/Mazel, 1979.

BIBLIOGRAPHY

Erikson, E. *Childhood and Society.* New York: W. W. Norton & Co., 1963.
Group for the Advancement of Psychiatry. *Normal Adolescence: Its Dynamics and Impact* VI, report no. 68, Feb., 1968.
Heimowitz, M. D., & Heimowitz, N. R. *Human Development: Selected Readings.* New York: Crowell, 1960.
McCafferty, C., Cline D., Jordan, J. Issues in the psychiatric approach to substance abuse in adolescents. *Psychiatric Annals* II (8), Aug., 1981.
Weiner, I. B., & Elkind, D. *Child Development: A Core Approach.* New York: Wiley and Sons, 1972.

4

Problems of Adolescents

M. ROBERT WILSON

This chapter seeks to aid the reader in understanding, recognizing, and responding to psychiatric disorders in adolescents. These disorders are the principal causes of disability for this age group and afflict a significant percentage of the teenage population. Suicide, the ultimate tragic consequence of one such disorder, depression, is the third leading cause of death among adolescents today.

Contemporary pastors, well acquainted with the significant problems of *normal* adolescence, may question why this chapter concentrates upon psychiatric disorders that he or she, as a counselor, may not be able to treat. Knowing something of these problems can help ease (and explain) the frustrations involved in counseling the many adolescent patients and their parents. Pastors or parents who live in a "rational" world may find it difficult to understand why adolescents remain depressed when "everything seems to be going well for them," why model teenagers make suicide gestures, or why other adolescents do exactly the opposite of what was intended.

Just as psychiatrists must rule out organic problems in mental illness and physicians must be able to detect psychogenic disorders, pastors must be made aware of those disorders that cannot be adequately treated by counseling. The knowledge that such problems did not begin in the present and often cannot be cured by short-term counseling should ease the pastor's sense of frustration, helplessness, and even doom. Some acquaintance with such disorders will enable the counselor to be a source of guidance and comfort for the anxious parents of such adolescents.

Personality development

Understanding these adolescent psychological disorders requires knowledge of ego development both in childhood and adolescence. The three components of the personality are the ego, the ego ideal, and the superego:

— The *ego* is that part of the mind's apparatus that mediates between the person and reality. Its prime function is the perception of reality and adaptation to it.
— The *ego ideal* is that part of the personality that comprises the aims and goals for the self.
— The *superego* is that part of the personality structure associated with ethics, standards, and self-criticism. It might be best described as the ego ideal plus conscience and self-criticism.

The ego is developed during the first year of life. The ego ideal is developed during the following two years and the superego between the ages of three and six.

These three components of personality remain essentially static and preserve their original form during the latency stage of development, from age six to puberty. The appearance of puberty heralds the beginning of adolescence, and these rigid and static properties are stripped away. Matriculation into adolescence bestows upon ego, ego ideal, and superego a quality of malleability. This malleability is essential to carry out the fundamental developmental task of adolescence: the review, revision, and final affirmation of ego, ego-ideal, and superego, which, following the close of the adolescent stage of development, remain essentially unchanged and unchangeable. The review, revision, and affirmation of personality components during adolescence mirror the chronology of childhood; early adolescence (puberty–14), represents ego redevelopment; mid-adolescence (14–16) ego ideal; late adolescence (16–19), superego. Each personality component is associated with specific qualities and is responsible for specific tasks, when developed during childhood, and when redeveloped during adolescence.

The ego: development and redevelopment

Ego development is initially characterized by primary narcissism and total dependency. The word *narcissism* is derived from Narcissus, the youth in Greek mythology who fell in love with his own reflection in the water. In a state of primary narcissism, infants regard themselves as the center of the world; their needs are primary and they are relatively unaware of others except as supports to themselves. The tasks of ego development include the acquisition of a sense of self versus not-self, provided by the satisfactory and sequential maturation of the sensory pathways, and tempered by a proper blend of trust and distrust in others and a feeling of intrinsic self-worth. Freud referred to this phase of ego development as the oral stage, and Erik Erikson expanded the concept to include the task of this stage as the acquisition of a sense of trust versus distrust.

Ego redevelopment is characterized by the universal "secondary narcissism" of early adolescence and an associated rejection of dependency. Secondary narcissism occurs when adolescents have withdrawn feelings from parents and begin once again to invest totally in themselves. Adolescents gradually invest in others, particularly in peers. They protect themselves from revealing the true grief for the loss of childhood by these forms of defenses. The task of ego redevelopment is to achieve an appropriate and flexible blending of narcissism (investment in the self) and altruism (regard for the interests and needs of others.) While ego development defines "who I am" as separate from others, ego redevelopment defines "my identity."

The ego ideal: development and redevelopment

The development of the ego ideal during childhood is characterized by testing. Freud referred to this stage of development (twelve to thirty-six months) as the anal stage, referring only to the mastery of bowel control. Erikson characterized the task of this stage as the acquisition of an appropriate blend of autonomy with shame and doubt.

During the ego-ideal phase, children characteristically acquire the means of locomotion. Where they were previously carried, they can now transport themselves. They acquire mastery over bowel and bladder. They develop the ability to feed themselves. Probably of singular importance is their ability to speak for themselves, the development of language. Locomotion, bowel and bladder control, dressing, feeding, speaking are all elements contributing to the burgeoning autonomy, as opposed to the abject dependency of infancy. Yet these children must have an opportunity to make mistakes, to know limits. When they do fail, forget, make mistakes, there should be a chance for them to feel a sense of doubt or shame or embarrassment. It is the blend of the degree of autonomy plus the capacity to know embarrassment, doubt, and shame, when appropriate, that represents the satisfactory annealing of the ego ideal.

Ego-ideal redevelopment during adolescence is characterized by protesting. The task is the discovery of one's realistic location on the spectrum between the extremes of omnipotence (all-powerfulness) and impotence (powerlessness). The ego ideal of childhood is "that whom I would like to be." The ego ideals of adolescence are those who are worthy of emulation.

The superego: development and redevelopment

Superego development is characterized by competition, and it has as its task the acquisition of an appropriate blend of initiative and guilt. Freud described this period as the genital phase (thirty-six to seventy-two months). As the child becomes aware of gender as a boy or a girl, this awareness is expressed through the proper use of pronouns referring to gender. Erikson expanded the concept of the genital phase by ascribing to the superego development the task of acquiring an appropriate blend of initiative and guilt. Again, Freud referred to *angst* and defined it as pangs of conscience, which was in fact guilt; and guilt is the currency that is generated by the superego. Initiative represents the capacity to mobilize anger and invest it in a constructive and productive manner. It provides the foundation upon which competition rests. Hence, the capacity to initiate represents the freedom to be aggressive. Yet, it is held in check by the individual sensing and being aware of transgressions that may result from the exposition of anger and aggression and the incursion into the territory and rights of others. This awareness generates guilt (or guilt in anticipation); therefore, one does not do what is wrong, what is dictated by society as being wrong and what one knows instinctively is wrong. Yet when one has done so, being able to feel and acknowledge guilt feelings is as important to the superego functions as it is to undertake initiative.

Decision and selection characterize the redevelopment of the superego. The tasks are to incorporate appropriate mixtures of passivity and aggression, femininity and masculinity. The superego of childhood is "that which I must be." The superego of adolescence is "that which I choose to become," a mixture of fission and fusion.

Psychiatric disorders in adolescence

Psychiatric and related disorders of adolescence can be divided into two simple classifications: those which are associated with a defective or vulnerable component of the personality (i.e., ego, ego ideal, and superego), and those that are not. The former constitute the more serious disorders, as well as the more common. The latter, designated as the various adjustment reactions of adolescence, are generally transient and cause limited dysfunction. These adolescent disorders that are associated with defective and/or vulnerable personality components include the broad categories of psychosis, personality disorder, and psychoneurosis (or anxiety disorder).

Psychosis is a severe mental disorder in which a person's ability to think, respond emotionally, remember, communicate, interpret reality, and behave appropriately is sufficiently impaired so as to interfere with the capacity to meet the ordinary demands of life.

Individuals suffering from *personality disorders* display patterns of relating to the environment so fixed as to limit the likelihood of effective functioning or satisfactory interpersonal relationships. These disorders are deeply ingrained and form chronic habitual patterns of reaction that are maladaptive and often provoke the very counterreaction from the environment that the individual seeks to avoid. The diagnosis of personality disorder is not usually made in adolescence. One variant of a personality disorder in childhood or adolescence is the conduct disorder.

The chief characteristic of the *psychoneurotic disorders* is anxiety. The category of neurosis is so broad that it is no longer used as an official diagnostic term, although the new term *anxiety disorders* does not cover all the various disabilities that were once known as psychoneuroses. The anxiety of these disorders is expressed directly or controlled unconsciously and automatically by conversion or displacement into other symptoms or psychological mechanisms.

Usually manifesting itself during early adolescence, a psychosis can, in nearly all instances, be traced to an ego defect, personality disorders to an ego-ideal defect, and anxiety disorders to a superego defect. These defects arise, in turn, from stresses that impinged upon the personality and during that chronological period in which the relative component was being formed: ego — birth to twelve months; ego ideal — twelve to thirty-six months; superego — thirty-six to seventy-two months.

Mental mechanisms

These stresses represent a threat to the integrity of the developing personality component. To cope with such stresses, unconscious psychic processes are invoked to provide relief from anxiety and emotional conflict. These psychic processes are called mental mechanisms. Each component has available for its defense specific mental mechanisms:

COMPONENT	MENTAL MECHANISM
Ego	*Introjection:* Loved or hated external objects or persons are symbolically absorbed within the self. It is the opposite of: *Projection:* what is emotionally unacceptable in the self is unconsciously rejected and attributed or projected to others.
Ego Ideal	*Reaction Formulation:* The person adopts emotions, ideas, attitudes, and behaviors that are the opposite of impulses harbored either consciously or unconsciously. *Sublimation:* Instinctual drives that are unacceptable are converted into personally and socially acceptable channels. *Undoing:* Something unacceptable and already done is symbolically acted out in reverse, usually repetitiously, in the hope of relieving anxiety. This would include expiatory acts, compulsive ceremonies, and counting compulsions.
Superego	*Denial:* Emotional conflict is resolved and anxiety allayed by the disavowal of thoughts, feelings, wishes, needs, or external reality factors that are consciously intolerable. *Dissociation:* Emotional significance is separated from an idea, situation, or object. Dissociation may deter or postpone the experiencing of emotional impact, as, for example, in selective amnesia.

Although mental mechanisms are part of a normal mode of functioning, their overuse to protect the personality creates a dysphoria or unpleasant feeling. This dysphoria, preferable to a threat to the personality structure, is nevertheless unwelcome, and the individual still seeks a relative harmony free from the dysphoria.

This attempt at harmony is achieved by the development of what are called psychodynamics. When we speak of an individual's psychodynamics, we are speaking of something that does not appear on the surface, i.e., something which is not obvious. The study of psychodynamics assumes that one's behavior is determined by past experience, genetic endowment, and current reality, and it recognizes the role of unconscious motivation in human behavior. Psychodynamic theory is systematized knowledge of human behavior and its motivation, the study of which depends largely on the functional significance of emotion.

Through the psychodynamics acting upon the dysphoria, a tentative and relative balance can be achieved. As long as this relative balance remains unthreatened, the potential psychiatric disorder remains latent and covert. In terms of stages of development, this quiescent and covert condition corresponds generally to what is called the latency period, from age six to puberty. (This process is illustrated in the discussion of the process of depression.)

The balance or homeostasis ends when the stress associated with the respective component's chronological development during adolescence overwhelms the combined defense capability of mental mechanism and psychodynamics, and the latent disorder becomes manifest. Generally speaking, psychosis is manifested during early adolescence, personality disorders during middle adolescence, and anxiety disorders (or psychoneurosis) during late adolescence.

Psychoses

There are four major types of adolescent psychotic conditions: depressive disorder, schizophrenic disorder, schizoaffective disorder, and manic-depressive (bipolar) disorder.

Depressive disorder, which is probably the most common of the psychotic conditions of adolescence, is manifested by symptoms somewhat different from the classical melancholic picture of depression seen in adults. Depression is often called an affective disorder, a disorder of the emotions, while schizophrenia is called a thought disorder. To me, this is a misconception. All psychiatric disorders are disorders of affect and all involve perception and cognition.

Depressive disorders, in terms of their manifest symptoms in adolescence, have in common a withdrawal of emotion or affect from various activities, persons, and the environment by the victim of depression. The symptoms associated with this withdrawal (or to use the Freudian term *decathexis,* which means the removal of an emotional investment), are such things as boredom (a rare phenomenon in a normal adolescent), feelings of unreality, anorexia, depersonalization, and social isolation. Boredom is a withdrawal of interest, feelings, or affect in activities. Nothing has any appeal. These individuals cannot get the enthusiasm up to do anything. They who are bored are "all dressed-up with no place to go." These depressed individuals are aware of their potential to invest affect, but are unable to liberate it. This boredom is more technically described as *anhedonia,* the absence of pleasure from acts that are normally pleasurable.

Feelings of unreality are also a symptom of depression. Freud described such feelings as similar to seeing the world as a picture, flat, two-dimensional, and without life. It is as if the third dimension, namely, the feelings, are missing. Feelings of unreality are sometimes referred to as emotional anesthesia. These persons have no feeling for anything and are aware of that internally, as well as by the "flatness" of the world around them. Hamlet put it best when he said: "How weary, stale, flat, and unprofitable seem to me all the uses of this world" (act I, scene 2, 133–34).

Anorexia, the loss of appetite, is another manifestation of the decathexis of any feelings, so that food has no appeal. We must differentiate the anorexia of depression from the condition known as anorexia nervosa, which typically occurs in females from twelve to twenty-two. This disease is characterized by deliberate restriction of food intake (although appetite is still present in the early stages), a loss in excess of 25 percent of original body weight, and, in females, the absence of menstruation.

Depersonalization, another symptom of depression, occurs when the affect or feeling is drawn from one's body, so that one feels as if outside of it, observing the self. Again, the mechanism is the withdrawal of affect from its ordinary disposition.

Social isolation and withdrawal from friends, family, and self-imposed reclusive behavior are consequences of pain, dullness, or anesthesia which result from the above-mentioned symptoms: feelings of unreality, anorexia, or depersonalization.

The symptoms that are related to the affective component, but are more directly a consequence of the action of *introjection,* the mental mechanism that is basically responsible for depression, are melancholia, sadness, and a feeling of hopelessness or worthlessness. Introjection is the converse of projection: the loved or hated external objects are taken within the self symbolically. The ultimate effect of introjection and incarceration of affect within the self are suicidal ideas, gestures, and suicide attempts. Suicidal ideations are thoughts of suicide, while suicidal gestures are self-destructive acts that would not necessarily result in suicide. A suicide attempt is the consummation of the act, which, although it does not result in death, must be taken very seriously.

The sense of mattering

Adolescents frequently present a depressive illness in terms of bodily or somatic complaints. This is related to the psychodynamics most often associated with depression: namely, a sense of mattering. Healthy development of the ego confers upon the individual a sense of mattering intrinsically, i.e., of having intrinsic worth and value. But if development goes awry, an assault upon the ego poses a threat of having no value.

It is that ultimate threat against which the defense mechanism of introjection is directed. It is elaborated upon by the specific dynamics that arise from the circumstances of the child's environment. So that one matters, for example, for one's badness, one's unworthiness, is preferable to not mattering at all.

Once removed from mattering because of intrinsic badness, as being a bad person, is to "matter" because there is something bad or wrong with one's body. Hence, it is more palatable to believe there is something wrong or malfunctioning with one's bodily functions (that is, hypochondriasis) than to feel that one is a bad person. Pressing this a bit further, there occurs mattering because of one's bad behavior, which again is more removed from nuclear mattering because one is a bad person or because one has a malfunctioning body.

This kind of mattering because of bad or unsuccessful behavior leads to what are called the *behavioral correlates of depression,* those actions that are related to the depression or that express and release it. Just as children release depression or tension by hyperactivity, adolescents use action often impulsively. Adolescents who steal cars in the neighborhood or wealthy adolescents with a large allowance who continue to steal from their parents may be behaving in this way because of a depression. These actions are then interpreted as behavioral correlates of depression and in their prosecution and inevitable discovery, reaffirm the sense of mattering. A feeling of mattering because of bad behavior or because something is wrong with the body is more acceptable to the ego than a state of not mattering.

Underachievement — either social, academic, recreational or vocational — is another example of a behavioral correlate of depression. Underachievement presents an exposition of mattering because of one's failures or unworthiness.

Insomnia is also a symptom of depression. It usually takes the form of terminal insomnia (that is, waking up in the middle of the night and not being able to go back to sleep) as opposed to initial insomnia (not being able to fall asleep). This symptom is related to the threat posed to the ego's defense when the mind is more vulnerable, namely, during sleep, and when the defense mechanisms are less effective. Usually the anxiety of depression causes initial insomnia, but introjection results in terminal insomnia.

Delusions

The mechanisms and dynamics protecting the ego from nuclear assault constitute in themselves the depressive illness and symptoms. When these mechanisms are threatened from any stress and appear "shaky," delusions may then appear as part of the depressive illness. Delusions are fixed, false beliefs and, in most people's minds, are associated with schizophrenia. The reader should be cautioned that delusions may occur with depression. A delusion is merely the mind's affirmation of the dynamic, and it must be scrutinized to determine whether the material is depressive or schizophrenic, particularly if it is paranoid in nature.

For example, a depressive delusion might be: "I am a bad person. I know I am a bad person. I have done wrong." A delusion may be invoked if there is a weakening of the defense mechanism from a number of sources. The mind may then be brought into play to reinforce the perceptual quality of the dynamics in the form of a delusion. We remember the basic dynamic is that "I matter because I am bad," and then the various symptoms that arise from that attitude may no longer serve the purpose. Particularly in the course of therapy, there may be uncovering or other events of a stressful nature that may happen that threaten the defense mechanism's integrity. The mind may react by adding a further cognitive layer of defense, which will come out as a delusion. The person becomes convinced, knows that he or she is a bad person, and may even give illustrations of bad things done to validate this perception.

Hallucinations

In the event that the delusional system weakens, the perceptual mechanism responds by reinforcing the defense by auditory hallucinations: "I know that I did these things because I hear God telling me that I did them." The auditory reinforcement, perceptual reinforcement, and hallucinations associated with psychiatric illness are usually auditory, as opposed to visual, olfactory (sense of smell), gustatory (taste), or tactile (touch), which are usually due to organic causes. They represent the utmost effort by the mind to protect the defense against the potential uncovering of ego vulnerability. The hallucination must be heard in its context to differentiate between the depressive hallucination — "God tells me that I'm bad," or "my father tells me that I'm bad," or "I hear people saying that I'm bad" — from the paranoid, in which the delusion would be more projective, such as: "The world is a bad place and everybody hates me, but I don't deserve to be hated." The hallucination may be: "I hear voices plotting against me." The recognition of delusions and hallucinations as occurring in either schizophrenia or depression is a generally accepted fact among the profession, but most lay people tend to equate hallucinations and delusions with schizophrenia.

Vulnerability to depression in adolescence

Adolescence is a vulnerable period for depression. During the first part of adolescence (puberty to age fourteen or fifteen) adolescents undergo a grief reaction because of losing the parental relation enjoyed as children — innocence, even childhood itself. This leads to a withdrawal of emotional investment from parents and others and results in secondary narcissism. Accompanying this grief reaction, a depressive illness can easily be added, especially in an adolescent with an ego vulnerability. The blueprint is set. While normal adolescents move out of the grief reaction, depressed adolescents become mired in it. The normal grief or mourning grows into the severe depression of melancholia, instead of the equilibrium that might be expected after mourning.

Schizophrenic disorder in adolescents is not greatly different from the symptoms of schizophrenia in adults. However, unlike depression, which may occur for the first time in later life with no predispositional vulnerability, schizophrenia always starts in adolescence. When it appears later in life for the first time, so to speak, it either was unrecognized during adolescence or its cause must be assessed with great effort to rule out organic factors. Historically, there has been a change in the manifestation of psychotic illness in adolescence. What is now recognized as depression may at one time have been called schizophrenia. The four cardinal symptoms of schizophrenia, described by Eugen Bleuler in 1911, are:

1. Loose thought associations, where one idea or thought does not follow logically from its predecessor nor does it relate to its successor. This must not be just a single occurrence, but must recur with regularity over a fairly extensive period of time.

2. Autism is a state of complete withdrawal from interaction with others. (It can be found in depression.) Thinking bears a subjective character. If objective material enters into thinking, it is given subjective meaning. Autism generally implies that the material is derived from the subject him- or herself, appearing in the nature of daydreams, fantasies, delusions, and hallucinations. External reality gradually loses its significance, and persons are guided only by the inner workings of their being. This should not be confused with infantile autism, which appears during the first three years of life.

3. Ambivalence is a pathological state in which two mutually contradictory drives or emotions coexist and cancel each other out, rendering individuals incapable of action or decision. This state is much more severe and paralyzing than simply being of "two minds" about a subject.

4. Disturbance of affect or emotion is the fourth cardinal symptom of schizophrenia. The emotional expression may be inappropriate: individuals will laugh at a tragic subject or the emotion expressed does not match the content of speech. There may also be blunted or flattened emotion. With flattened affect, the voice may be monotonous or without expression. Sudden and unpredictable emotional changes, such as inexplicable bursts of anger, may occur.

In addition to these four cardinal symptoms, there are the so-called secondary symptoms — delusions and hallucinations — that may have the quality of a paranoid, persecutory element. There may be *ideas of reference* in which the individual receives special instructions, messages, or meaning from neutral and objective sources, such as a phonograph record, television program, or an advertisement or a billboard. These are related to ideas of alien control, for again individuals are governed in their actions by these messages or directions that are especially aimed at and directed toward them and no one else.

Garbled speech, another secondary symptom, is the extension of loose thought associations, to which the descriptive phrase "word salad" has been applied. Instead of the thoughts not hanging together, the words themselves do not make sentences. The further extension of this is the construction of nonsense words, neologisms, in which the letters do not even fit together into accepted words.

The vulnerability from which the schizophrenic condition arises lies in the ego, that part of the mind's apparatus that mediates between the person and reality. Stress, the feeling of not "mattering," or of having no value, lies at the heart of schizophrenia in the same fashion as this vulnerability lies at the heart of depression.

The defense provides individuals with a sense of mattering because of the "badness" of the world around them. The mechanism used is projection, and individuals' feelings are ascribed to the world. Through this mechanism, what is emotionally unacceptable in the self is unconsciously rejected and attributed or projected to others. Schizophrenia has a basic affective component, so that schizophrenic individuals with a projective mechanism at work to protect their ego vulnerability soon develop a dynamic, such as, "I matter because the world hates me," or "I matter because the world believes I am Jesus Christ." Those constructs then go on to cause these individuals to develop dynamics and a life-style that is based upon reaffirming that protection against the basic vulnerability of not mattering. They view the world as an alien place and tend to be more enforceably sequestered from the world in a protective sense, as opposed to depressed persons who feel "not belonging" and that it is their fault.

Introjection and projection

One can say simplistically that during infancy, when the ego vulnerability is in its inception, a "choice" is made between introjection and projection. When the principal stress causing the potential illness is from the environment (as opposed to the combination of neurophysiological factors and environmental factors) and when the affective quality of the environment is one of omissions, the mechanism "chosen" is introjection. When the affective quality of the environment is one of commission, the mechanism "chosen" is projection. For example, an overprotective environment which intruded upon the child would be an example of commission, as opposed to an environment which overlooked the child's needs, an omission. Overt rejection of the child would be commission, passive neglect an omission.

These conditions have early corollaries. In the condition of depression, a dramatic example would be anaclitic depression. Anaclitic literally means "leaning on" and refers to the complete dependence of the infant upon the mother or mother substitute for a sense of well-being. An anaclitic depression occurs during the first year of life as a result of a separation forced upon the child where the mother does not return (either being taken against her will or by death). The child regresses, does not eat, and may eventually die – this is a classical introjection: "I do not even deserve to eat." Autism is also an early corollary of schizophrenia. The child does not respond to being cuddled, withdraws from being held, and develops a world of its own making.

Schizoaffective disorder is an illness that is diagnosed when the clinician discovers a combination of schizophrenic, depressive, or manic symptoms and cannot make a differential diagnosis between affective disorder and schizophrenia. There is a mixture of the mental mechanisms of projection and introjection and the same type of ego vulnerability that requires their protection. From this comes a blending of dynamics, varying from "mattering" because of one's badness to believing that the world is an alien, untrustworthy, and persecutory place. Individuals may have a combination of symptoms from both principal conditions of depression and schizophrenia, in any kind of a mixture.

Fifteen years ago the terms *manic-depressive illness* or *bipolar disorder* were not mentioned because for many years it was believed that this illness did not appear during adolescence. Psychiatry now recognizes that manic-depressive illness may make its appearance even during early adolescence and may be preceded by hyperkinesis and hyperactivity. Its dynamics are similar to the dynamics of depression. Introjection is exclusively the mental mechanism. The manic stage of this condition is frequently mistakenly identified as schizophrenia. The clinical symptoms of the bipolar disorder include a cyclical swing from depression, which may last for many weeks, to a period of elation, i.e., the manic episode. The depressive phase may be characterized by all of the symptoms described above for depression. The manic eposide is characterized by the following: *Extremely high levels of energy* frequently associated with adolescents remaining awake for five, six, or seven days without apparent fatigue as a consequence. There may be *grandiose* thinking, which may be delusional. Speech is likewise energized and speeded up, and may be so rapid as to make it unintelligible. There may be a quality of logorrhea: these persons may talk continuously, filling the air with sounds. These types of speech patterns are part of the phenomenon called "flight of ideas," where there is a pressure of thoughts and need to articulate them. The term *hypomania* is a clinical syndrome that is similar to, but not as severe as, that described by the term *manic episode.*

The pre-bipolar condition may be identified in early adolescence as a continuum of the hyperkinetic situation that persisted through latency. This is not to say that hyperkinesis and hyperactivity in childhood will always lead to manic-depressive illness. The cyclical variations of bipolar illness may have a seasonal basis, with either the manic or depressive component becoming most florid in the spring or in the fall. The significance of alternation is that if one is dealing with a depressed adolescent, at least one year's experience with that adolescent should pass before ruling out bipolar illness. The cyclical phenomenon may also manifest itself as swings in mood from day to day and even in periods of vulnerability during a twenty-four-hour period. However, adolescents would need to have the associated symptoms, not just experience the vicissitudes of everyday life.

Psychotic illnesses in adolescents may be in such early stages that it is not possible to make a diagnosis. This is particularly true for young adolescents. However, one indication is a degree of dysfunction in all spheres: affective (e.g., emotional instability), cognitive (failure in school or underachievement), familial (can't get along with family), social (has no peer relations and has poor relations with teachers), and recreational. Usually if youngsters are faltering in all these areas, the global degree of dysfunction itself is justification for identifying someone as having a psychiatric disorder and, perhaps, an emerging psychosis.

A completely opposite condition, but also a precursor of psychotic illness in adolescence, may be found in the model teenager. Model teenagers have exhibited none of the normal adolescent emotional or psychological milestones. They have not matriculated into psychological adolescence. They are over-compliant, never rebellious, and are much more comfortable with adults than with peers. They are zealous in their studies, usually volunteer to take on responsibilities and chores at home, and enmesh themselves in extracurricular activities of the solitary kind. Yet the dynamic they reveal is a striving mightily to remain children and not letting go of childhood to become adults.

Personality disorders

Personality disorders include a wide range of difficulties in functioning effectively or in developing successful interpersonal relationships. They occur in adolescents, but it is generally acknowledged by the profession that many personality disorders cannot be diagnosed until the onset of late adolescence, before age seventeen or so. This observation is in keeping with the formulation of these disorders as arising from the ego ideal, the redevelopment of which takes place between ages fifteen and seventeen. The classification of personality disorders has undergone so many changes, additions, and deletions that it would be impossible and nonproductive to list them all.

A commonly employed mental mechanism in personality disorders is reaction formation, a mechanism in which the action or behavior is precisely the opposite of what the impulse or drive reflects. Reaction formation is perhaps best illustrated in the dynamics of the passive-aggressive personality disorder. An individual with this disorder, through inaction or passivity, is able to express hostility and aggression toward others. This behavior masks the aggression through total passivity.

The antisocial personality disorder is characterized by a history of continuous and chronic antisocial behavior in which the rights of others are violated. My colleague Dr. Edward Litin described the antisocial personality when he said, "Even though the door was wide open, he would crawl through the transom." Lying, stealing, fighting, truancy, and resisting authority are typically early signs in adolescence that there may be aggressive sexual behavior and substance abuse. An example of reaction formation at work here is the meretricious quality so commonly associated with the psychopath or "con-artist" who uses charm, physical attractiveness, and intelligence for totally illegal activities. This personality achieves success, but success built upon a house of cards. The appearance of success and competence is a reaction formation that covers up and disguises a pervasive shame, doubt, and lack of self-confidence.

It is important to make the distinction between the behaviors that result from psychotic illness and those from an antisocial personality disorder. The task of the ego-ideal stage of development is to form a proper blend of autonomy versus shame and doubt. Individuals with an antisocial personality disorder display on the surface a pervasive autonomy with no room for shame and doubt and may have no dysphoria or feelings of discomfort.

Learning disabilities

Adolescents labeled as antisocial or as juvenile delinquents might be suffering from learning disabilities, another problem of adolescence that may require both educational and psychiatric assistance. Learning disabilities in adolescents do not necessarily produce the more obvious signs and symptoms found in younger children (e.g., reversals or mirror reading). Manifestations are more subtle: short attention span, easy distraction, self-stimulating activities such as constant rocking, foot tapping, perpetual motion. The learning-disabled adolescent very often has a psychiatric problem that may be caused, in part, by a learning disability. Since learning disabilities result in difficulties with communications, the individual so disabled has had lifelong trouble making others understand why, although intelligent, he or she gets poor grades. He or she senses something is wrong, but may have no way of knowing the nature of the defect.

There are two possible psychiatric reactions to being misunderstood. One can react by giving up trying to be understood, surrendering, and withdrawing from the world—this reaction is called adolescent depression. Or one can substitute action or behavior for spoken language. This behavior often takes a negative or antisocial manifestation and is called juvenile delinquency. Instead of saying "I feel bad" or "I am really angry," the adolescent *acts* bad or releases anger in vandalism.

The combination of psychiatric and educational disabilities is very common, and the two conditions are frequently related. When pastors encounter adolescents who are either depressed or have been labeled as juvenile delinquents, information about their work in school and testing for learning disabilities will help to determine the direction for treatment.

Anxiety disorders and psychoneuroses

Guilt is the principal dysphoria that results in a host of psychoneurotic conditions from phobias to multiple personality. Psychiatrists now describe these conditions as "anxiety disorders" rather than neuroses. In my experience the incidence of such illness among adolescents is negligible. In general, adolescent anxiety disorders are either so obvious that adolescents must seek help, or they have little impact on adolescent functioning.

Regardless of the nature of the manifest illness, the affective component is tied to the past, so that as children grow, the affective life is not totally available to the present experience. For example, in a depression, the genesis or dysphoria of the depression is the consequence of needing protection that happened in infancy, at least fourteen years ago. Yet the depression colors everything in the present. Conversely, in an anxiety disorder, the affect is projected onto the future in anticipation of something about which the individual is anxious or fearful. This projection prevents individuals from living freely in the present.

Psychiatrists often treat this disorder by disconnecting the affect from the past or future and allowing it to be totally generated in response to the present. If one is immersed affectively in the present, in the minute, hour, or whatever, an experience becomes forever more a part of a person. That is how therapy works. The therapist's affect is for the patient and is generated by that encounter. The patient's affect is for the therapist and is generated conversely. The therapist's perception is of the patient, and the patient's perception is of the therapist. However, if in infancy, the individuals' affect did not yield a response, they had to be both subject and object. The affect remains only toward themselves and only tangentially toward others. Nor do these individuals allow others to perceive what they really feel toward them. In the early stages of therapy, patients impose upon therapists those feelings harbored toward therapists. But in the later stages of therapy, there occurs the liberation of affect which allows patients to live in the present.

The pastor and the disturbed adolescent

What can pastors do now that they have this knowledge about adolescent psychotic disorders when encountering an adolescent who suffers from these conditions that arise not in the present but from the past? How are these illnesses treated? Can they be cured? The successful treatment of psychotic illness among adolescents requires, in most instances, hospitalization, and usually a prolonged period of in-patient treatment in a psychiatric hospital or residential treatment center for adolescents.

Adolescents are malleable, and, as pointed out earlier, are undergoing a redevelopment of personality at this age. When they have an illness that is a consequence of a defect or vulnerability in the personality, it is possible to correct that vulnerability and successfully treat the cause of the illness during this stage. This is in contrast to adults, who, for the most part, if suffering from such a condition, are not so fortunate because their personality, almost by definition, is less malleable and does not lend itself to the successful interventions that are possible with adolescents. Treatment of adults, unfortunately, in many instances, is limited to treating the symptoms, palliating them, and helping them to live with the illness. Furthermore, in childhood and in latency, individuals are not yet ready for definitive treatment of the psychotic illness. Therefore, it is during adolescence that individuals are most responsive to treatment and their personality most available for corrective intervention. Depending on the location and availability of resources to the pastor, referral to the family physician would be the first step. If the family has no personal physician, then the local medical society can provide the names of practitioners of adolescent medicine or adolescent psychiatry in the area.

The pastor serves another role in helping parents understand the condition and, most importantly, to understand its potential optimistic prognosis if proper treatment is utilized. The treatment, however, takes a long time. It is also important that parents not feel guilty. Parents frequently blame themselves for the psychiatric problems of their children. Unfortunately, this blame and associated guilt have been all too often reinforced by earlier attitudes and by mental health professionals. In my experience parents have done their very best for their children. Although their unconscious attitudes and their own early environment that shaped them frequently constitute a factor instrumental in the development of the adolescent's personality vulnerability, parents seldom intentionally contribute to their children's problems.

Adolescent adjustment reaction

Although pastors may need to refer adolescents with a psychotic illness to other professionals, in most circumstances they can help those adolescents who are experiencing an adolescent adjustment reaction, a disorder that is not of a psychotic nature. Adolescent adjustment reactions vary from an exaggerated response to a healthy developmental process to transient pathological vulnerability. The exaggerated responses to adolescent development include: overdetermined opposition to authority, excessive risk-taking, and overzealous emerging in the group's norm or identity. Transient situational reactions include depressions in reaction (i.e., reactive depressions) to domiciliary moves, the loss of a pet, a break-up of puppy love, truancy, or running away. There might even be occasional shoplifting, drug use, "borrowing" the family car, or temporary slumps in grades. No underlying vulnerability to the personality can be seen, but there is a clearly recognizable stress, which brings on pathological reaction.

While the psychotic disorders of adolescence require intensive psychotherapy — and even psychiatric hospitalization — and while the anxiety or psychoneurotic disorders may require intense psychotherapy, adolescents and their families suffering through an adjustment reaction can survive outside the hospital if they receive psychotherapy, family therapy, or pastoral counseling.

Adolescence is a time of ambiguity, a new frontier. Its boundaries are vague, beginning with the onset of puberty and ending when relative self-dependence is achieved. Because the adolescent experience is inconsistent, fluid, indefinite, and imprecise, the adolescent needs and seeks consistent, definite, and precise guidelines from adults. The pastoral counselor may be called upon to aid the parents in providing this consistency. Adolescent protests are not aimed at undermining and defeating authority. Protests and challenges are really aimed at confirming the sincerity and genuineness of adults. While children accept the world and their parents as gospel, adolescents are wary of deception.

Consistent, precise, and definite limit-setting by adults is essential if adolescents are to negotiate this period successfully. Such setting of limits reduces the instability of adolescence and permits teenagers to devote attention and energies to more essential issues. If the authority is *credible,* adolescents can relax their testing. How do the pastor or the parents establish credibility with adolescents? We have spoken of consistency and definiteness, but listening, admitting mistakes, reversing bad decisions, and acknowledging imperfections are also critical components of adult credibility. Many parents have been so rigid in their limit-setting that admitting mistakes and revising bad decisions are precluded.

Two words essential to adult credibility are authority and discipline. A true authority is one who is the author of what he or she says, and does not need a rule book, childrearing manual, or other source as the basis of authority. A true authority is truly credible and believes in him- or herself. Adolescents need, seek, and want sincere authorities. A true ' authority (as his or her own author and editor) *can* acknowledge imperfections, be flexible, and correct mistakes. A true authority is not an authoritarian. An authoritarian fails to listen, is inflexible, never admits mistakes, needs to appear perfect, and in this effort may be inconsistent, indefinite, and imprecise. An authoritarian is never author of what he or she says, quoting and invoking rules and policies. An authoritarian does not believe in the self; he or she is never believable nor credible.

Over the years, discipline has become a victim of misguided disuse by contemporary adults. A *disciple* is a student, a follower of a believable teacher. The adolescents want, seek, and need to be disciples. The zealous participation of adolescents in contemporary religious cults is a dramatic illustration of these needs and the fact that these needs are no longer being met by other institutions in society, such as the family or the Church. To be a disciple, the adolescent must have adults who are worthy of imitation, whose discipline is then acceptable. Discipline is not punishment, retaliation, control, or suppression. Disciples are not ruled; they will follow a believable leader. Successful discipline occurs when the disciple surpasses the leader. If adults are true authorities, practice genuine discipline, and are sincere and believable, teenagers will be able to use their own energy to cope with the developmental tasks of adolescence.

REFERENCES

American Psychiatric Association. *Diagnostic and Statistical Manual of Mental Disorders,* 3rd ed. Washington: American Psychiatric Association, 1980.

Campbell, Robert J. *Psychiatric Dictionary,* 5th ed. New York: Oxford University Press, 1981.

Erikson, Erik. *Childhood and Society,* 2nd ed. New York: W. W. Norton & Co., 1963.

Mahler, Margaret S. *Psychological Birth of the Human Infant.* New York: Basic Books, 1975.

Spitz, René A. *First Year of Life: A Psychoanalytic Study of Normal and Deviant Behavior of Object Relations.* New York: International Universities Press, 1965.

Wilson, M. Robert, & Calistro, Paul. Adolescent Psychosis: A Holistic Syndrome, *Psychiatric Annals* 7 (5): 38–49, 1977.

5

The Young Adult

WALTER D. MINK

Young adulthood as a stage in human development is a relatively recent concept. Not surprisingly, the chronological definition of the beginning and the ending of the transition from pre-adult to adult status in American society is somewhat vague. Puberty signals adolescence rather than adulthood, as it once did, and such modern rites of passage as becoming a licensed driver, a legal drinker, a high school graduate, a voter, or a draft registrant do not confer adult status in an unambiguous way. At the same time, for many young people, completion of higher education, entry into a career, marriage, and parenthood have been extended beyond the early twenties, which formerly encompassed these major life events.

While entry into adult roles has become more diffusely defined in both routes and duration, it remains a transition of great symbolic significance for young people and the adults they join. The views of young adults about the opportunities or limitations of their future and the ways they test and relate to the prevailing values and expectations of adult society contribute to the character of a generation. The designation of each decade with a generational label, while inevitably inaccurate, is still instructive about the status of young adults in contemporary society and the ways in which succeeding generations are construed in popular commentary.

Dana Farnsworth, writing in 1969 in the first edition of this book, noted the troubled relationship between young adults and their elders at the time. Vivid portrayals of intergenerational conflict in the journalism and literature of the time remind us of the social consequences of the confrontation of an adult society with its youth. Yet a decade later, young adults are described as self-involved, security-oriented, conforming, and somewhat pessimistic about the future. Those who were seen as dedicated to changing the world appear to have been replaced by those who are concerned about surviving it. This dramatic contrast of the behavior of the young people of two decades suggests equally dramatic changes in values and motives. However, there may be greater underlying similarities than are apparent in the overt style of conduct. Farnsworth viewed the open conflict that he observed as an expression of disappointed desires to achieve the kind of relationship with parents and other adults which would support the development of an integrated sense of self. That need probably has not changed.

In viewing young adulthood and the problems attendant on its passage, it is important to recognize the interaction between the person and the social order and historical moment that are entered. The young adult is of an age that prescribes the significance of certain actions, choices, and events. A society at a particular time restricts or expands opportunities and rewards and authorizes or sanctions some activities and not others. Each individual also comes to the period of young adulthood with a personal history that influences the style of approach he or she takes to the significant activities of the age. Developmental psychologists and psychiatrists attempt to account for the constants and variables in developmental processes and the varying contexts in which they occur.

The first edition of this book was quite forward-looking in its emphasis on a life-span approach to the problems that mental health professionals observe in their practice. In the time since the publication of the first edition, a life-span perspective has become common in treatments of personality. The success of Gail Sheehy's *Passages* attests to the popular acceptance of individual life as a pattern of changes which can be recognized and managed. Young adulthood assumes special importance in the sequence of stages with their predictable problems to which people react and which they attempt to resolve in their development.

Developmental models: Childhood to adulthood

The idea of maturational stages of life has a long history. Examples of "life cycle" are found in ancient Hebrew, Greek, and Chinese writings. The famous "Seven Ages of Man" speech in Shakespeare's *As You Like It* is a widely quoted perspective on the span of life. The first systematic attempt to relate adult personality to a stage theory of development, however, had to wait until Sigmund Freud, with Jean Piaget and Erik

Erikson contributing substantially to Freud's model. In his theory of development, Freud emphasized the early years of life and considered the basic structures of adult personality to be established by age six or seven. Adulthood involves the establishment of productive work patterns and intimate relationships, but Freud did not elaborate an account of changes in adult experience as a function of age and significant life events associated with age.

Jean Piaget, the noted investigator of intellectual development in children, offers another proposal of developmental stages. Like Freud, he concerned himself with the progressions of childhood development with adult competence as the conclusion of the process. However, he pushed cognitive developmental stage models into adulthood, particularly in the area of moral reasoning.

Erik Erikson is generally acknowledged as the person who brought the idea of individual development through the entire life cycle to a wide audience. Erikson, a child psychoanalyst, begins with Freud's stages of child development, but in addition to the classic triad of oral, anal, and phallic stages (which Erikson calls by another set of terms), he extends development through five more stages, three of which are in the domain of adulthood. Erikson stresses the interaction of biological development and personal life history with the role and institutional structure of a society and its history at each of the stages of his sequences. A special feature of Erikson's theory is the idea that development proceeds by *critical* steps — critical in the sense of decision points that lead to progress, retreat, or irresolution in the elaboration of an integrated personality. The stages are defined in terms of polar outcomes of the resolution of the basic conflict of each stage. Erikson's ideas about the transition to adulthood through adolescence and young adulthood have been applied fruitfully by him and others to the interpretation of the experience of young people.

Developmental stage models have in common a relatively fixed pattern of sequences through which individuals pass as they develop from infancy to old age. Some theorists observe a universality to the pattern which they may interpret as reflecting biological determination, a common social recognition of age-determined roles and expectations, or a combination of the two. Some emphasize developmental tasks to be completed or conflicts to be resolved at each stage. Others, less dynamic, simply indicate the necessity of the prior stages to the achievement of subsequent stages. In all there is an ideal of progression to a level of greater integration, understanding, or competence than is possible at lower levels.

Developmental stage theories have their critics and many developmental psychologists prefer to be empirical in their study of the characteristics of different age groups and the social milieu in which they exist. In this chapter Erikson's model and those of two investigators — Daniel Levinson and Roger Gould — who were influenced by Erikson, will be used to help organize observations about characteristics of young adulthood rather than as explicit accounts of development necessities. It is important to note that these models have been developed primarily if not entirely as accounts of white American or European males. Whether or not women show identical or similar developmental sequences is a question that has not as yet been answered completely. Also, young people who are not white and who come from socio-educational backgrounds that are substandard are limited in self-perceptions, range of opportunities, and social roles expected of them.

Various writers propose somewhat different age periods for young adulthood ranging from a lower limit of seventeen to an upper limit of thirty. In this chapter, young adulthood will be considered to cover the span from eighteen — the average age of graduation from high school — to age twenty-five — the age when the majority of young adults have settled into reasonably stabilized patterns of adult life. Young adulthood seems to convey a relatively clear picture when defined in this way. When asked to describe "a young man" or "a young woman," middle-aged respondents chose the age range of eighteen to twenty-five. This appears to be a period when there is more stability and definition of social role than in early adolescence but without as yet full adoption of adult occupational, marital, or parental roles. This is "college age," a period of transition to, or perhaps postponement of, the complete assumption of the requirements of adulthood.

The transition to adulthood: Erikson

Erik Erikson proposes that the basic dilemma of young adulthood is to achieve intimacy and prevent isolation. In order to appreciate his emphasis on intimacy vs. isolation as the defining problem for the young adult, it is necessary to consider the preceding stage of late adolescence, which extends into the age span of many young adults. Erikson introduced the concept of *identity crisis* in his account of the challenge faced by adolescents. Identity refers to more than an answer to the plaintive question "Who am I?" To achieve identity is to commit oneself with faith and loyalty to those determining ideas and values that are incorporated as part of oneself and that are accepted in society. Adolescence is a time of testing limits in the roles that are assumed in the adult world and in its behavioral requirements. The negative outcome of the identity crisis is *identity diffusion* (or confusion) in which a sense of self merely mirrors a group or a situation rather than a consistent style of personal conduct.

Resolution of one stage does not have to occur before the transition to the next in Erikson's scheme, but failure of resolution influences the approach to the conflict in the succeeding stage. The achievement of intimacy depends on the adequacy with which the young person has formed an integrated sense of identity. Intimacy means much more than sexual intimacy and implies shared identity. It takes a person with a reasonably secure sense of identity to sacrifice it in an intimate relationship where "we" transcends "I." The isolated person cannot take chances with identity and may simulate intimacy while remaining impersonal. The inability to risk a sacrifice of identity may be strengthened by fear of the outcome of intimacy, including children and the care they require. Erikson presents a demanding definition of intimacy, but perhaps the high frequency of failures in American marriages indicates how difficult it is to achieve the strength of identity that permits the acceptance of the challenge of true intimacy.

The transition to adulthood: Levinson

Levinson emphasizes the ways in which individuals reflect the structure of society in their particular patterning of the world in their personal development. The basic developmental process in adulthood is the evolution of a *life structure,* the underlying design of a person's life at a given time. The evolution passes through a relatively orderly sequence of periods, which Levinson compares to *seasons,* marked by three major transitions, the first of which is an early-adult transition. Developmental tasks and life issues are specific to each period and give each a special character. Tasks can be performed adequately or poorly, reflecting the degree to which a life structure works in the world. Life structures are demonstrated in the important choices an individual makes and the consequences of those choices.

Daniel Levinson's stages are less a matter of moving from one level of integration to a higher one than one of progressing from one time set of changes to another. Adulthood begins with a transition from adolescence to early adulthood followed by the period of the first adult-life structure. Taken together they are defined as the *novice* phase of adulthood. Entering the adult world is a lengthy process, and Levinson states that it takes about fifteen years to emerge from adolescence into a period of "settling down."

The early adult transition poses two major tasks: to bring adolescence to a conclusion and to take a preliminary step into the adult world. The first is a process of termination, the second one of initiation. The major termination of adolescence is the establishment of independence from parents, but also includes separation from adolescent support groups and social norms. Separations are inevitably accompanied by a sense of loss or sadness and also by the anticipation, with mixed apprehension and hope, of a future.

Besides breaking away, the young adult must make critical explorations and choices. Examining earlier aspirations and dreams leads to a specification of a new "dream" with more clearly defined choices and goals. It is a problem for young adults to manage the tension between exploring alternatives and achieving stable structures. "Keeping options open" seems contradictory to "making something of one's life," and young people may appear to opt for one or the other. Work on one task may dominate another, but the non-dominant task is never absent. The outcome of the period of building a first adult-structure may be a relatively integrated pattern that includes entry into a vocation and selection of a marriage partner. This degree of satisfactory integration of compatible choices may not be the rule, however. As with the Eriksonian conflict of intimacy, some young people may avoid major choices and commitments and may consider their entrance into the adult world as incomplete, conflict-ridden, or lacking in direction.

The transition to adulthood: Gould

Roger Gould characterizes the major challenge of adulthood as the elimination of childhood consciousness and the achievement of adult consciousness. Childhood consciousness persists into adulthood as a set of false assumptions about what contributes to security and approval and the requirements for good conduct. Childhood consciousness, with its potential for hostility and fear, is overcome through understanding the ways in which it is expressed in adult life and how it interferes with development. Shifting from childhood consciousness proceeds stepwise and requires effort, and the attainment of adult consciousness is tested by the major challenges of adult life.

For Roger Gould, the young person at the threshold of young adulthood faces the important task of leaving the parental home and establishing a mode of independent living. The false assumption of childhood which must be abandoned is the belief that one always belongs to one's parents and their world and can always count on them for safety and rescue from danger.

The task of the emerging young adult is the completion of an independent adult identity. As Gould puts it, this stage requires the recognition that "I'm nobody's baby now." The individual must overcome the false assumption that doing things as one's parents would do them always brings success and reward and that parents will step in and make matters right when problems arise. Establishing an adult identity with its more open and sensitive adult consciousness permits the further exploration of the complexities of life and the self, leading to the recognition of human mortality.

The tasks of young adulthood: Making a commitment

The time of young adulthood as described by Erikson, Levinson, and Gould, as well as by others, is defined particularly by life events that occur during the period and by the tasks or challenges commonly faced by people of the age group. Landmark life events for young adults include completing their educational preparation, taking a first job with intentions to continue with it, marriage, taking on civic and community responsibilities, and joining established adult social groups.

These events suggest more than frequent occurrences, since they signify a group of accomplishments that are expected by young people and that they expect of themselves. The young adult who is not emancipated from dependence on parents or other adults, who has not become involved productively in the world of work or who has not established a prolonged relationship with a sexual partner, is likely to be viewed as immature, and these "problems" become reasons for concern.

The tasks usually associated with young adulthood have in common a theme of commitment. A commitment is both a choice and an affirmation. As a choice, commitment involves the discrimination of possibilities and the likely consequences of selecting some to pursue rather than others. As an affirmation, commitment includes feeling emotionally tied to activities, concerns, purposes, and persons who are perceived as part of one's self. In a very general way the commitments of the young adult are to values, to other persons, and to one's own possibilities as a person.

The making of value commitments by young adults is given a prominent place in the writings of Erik Erikson. The transition to young adulthood is a period of extremes of enthusiasm and idealism and polar opposites of rebellion, rejection, and refusal to commit oneself to anything. The extreme appeal of some religious and political movements can be interpreted in terms of the value sensitivity and vulnerability of young people. Allegiance may not be given easily, but when it is, it is often given wholeheartedly. Sometimes roles and attitudes are tried out whimsically or dramatically but usually with great seriousness. In some young people, the testing of acceptability may take the form of exploring what is unacceptable and sampling what is viewed as bad or dangerous. Finding one's place in a world of adult social values requires more than passive acceptance of what one has been taught.

In his studies of moral reasoning, Lawrence Kohlberg finds in young adults from eighteen to twenty-five a shift in values from a primary emphasis on reciprocity in interpersonal relations and the importance of meeting expectations (if one's own expectations are to be met) to an awareness of and commitment to the maintenance of a social order in which rules and roles are important. The ability to develop and accept an ethical policy is an important part of personal identity and requires a substantial opportunity to make choices. Kohlberg contends that the achievement of an ethical policy requires the clarification that comes through confronting values not in agreement with one's own.

The major areas of commitment

LOVE

The blending of love, sexuality, and caring in an enduring relationship is the major challenge of commitment in interpersonal relations for the young adult. As in the other commitments, there is testing and exploration of one's self and what is valued in other persons. The preoccupation many young people have with their attractiveness, their readiness to settle down, and how to express their sexual urges is often great and may come to dominate thoughts and fantasies. The establishment of deep, involving relationships is frequently fraught with doubt and conflict as well as great exhilaration and satisfaction. Of the three major areas of commitments—love, a life plan, and values—in young adults, falling in love is the one that is most difficult to characterize.

A LIFE PLAN

Committing oneself to a plan of achievement requires the melding of one's abilities and interests into a vocational aspiration. What is at stake in this area of commitment is the young adult's sense of competence and realistic expectation of success in what is undertaken. American society characteristically holds out a promise of great opportunities where success depends on hard work and a strong sense of responsibility. This shared dream is often hard to bring into congruence with actual access to career opportunities. The matching of interests and aptitudes to available opportunities, while maintaining a realistic self-confidence, can be a formidable task for young people. Not all who compete get ahead, and many young people resign themselves to accepting something less than they may have included initially in their fantasies of adult success. Christopher Jencks has shown that personal characteristics do contribute to economic success but so do family backgrounds and "luck." Being committed to one's own competence also requires a realistic appraisal of circumstances that permit its successful expression.

VALUES

The emphasis on commitment to long-term and reasonably stable values, relationships, and achievements seems to imply a stable world that presents a range of choices and permits progressive attainment of long-term goals, once decisions are made. A casual examination of the communication patterns, technological developments, and economic reorganizations during the second half of the century argues for increasing expectations of change—and fairly dramatic change. While establishing and maintaining long-term commitments will probably continue to be the task of young adults, the ability to anticipate and react productively to changing and often ambiguous conditions is an even greater challenge. Change—in one's vocation, most intimate relationship, or value orientation—is becoming a frequent characteristic of later reassessments of the commitment made as a young adult. The need to relate oneself to changing expectations and assessments of what is important may become a characteristic of adulthood for which future young adults will need to prepare themselves.

The self-perception of young adults

The views presented so far stress the conflicts, challenges, and tasks of young adulthood with their potential for problems and unsatisfying outcomes. Do young people view themselves and their lives in similar terms? In 1976 Joseph Veroff and associates conducted a replication of the survey that was published twenty years earlier as *Americans View Their Mental Health*. The young people of their survey span an age range that extends to age thirty. Compared with their counterparts of the earlier survey, these respondents were more willing to speak of their shortcomings and accepted aspects of themselves as less than the ideal they might like; but they also stressed a strong confidence in their ability to handle problems of life. The authors portrayed them as actively working out identity issues, quite aware of their strengths and weaknesses and particularly valuing their uniqueness. They viewed themselves as more socially skilled and psychologically sensitive than did the 1957 group.

They also expressed much more worry about their lives than did their counterparts in 1957. The authors suggest that this response reflects a reaction to a world where rules of social behavior are more ambiguous and futures less clearly delineated than in 1957. The sources of both happiness and unhappiness most frequently cited by young people are associated with finding one's station in life through work and with interpersonal relationships.

The paradox of young adults being both worried and optimistic may arise from the attention they give to discerning both the potential for accomplishment and the limitations that the future may hold. Generally, young people in the study viewed themselves as working with a good degree of confidence, but not without worries, on the tasks of establishing identities through self-examination and commitment to careers and relationships. They appeared to accept the developmental tasks of entrance into the adult world with an anxious but trusting expectation that they would complete them successfully.

Working out a sense of identity: The college years

Erik Erikson illustrates the ways in which societies and individuals provide for the accomplishment of the developmental tasks that are set for its youth. Usually there is some period of apprenticeship accompanied by what Erikson calls a moratorium, that is, a period of respite from adult social demands for the purpose of elaborating a sense of identity. Our society has come to recognize "a year off" as a way many young people informally grant themselves a moratorium. A more formal recognition of a moratorium period, however, exists in the college and university experience.

Over 50 percent of high school graduates now enter an institution of higher education. For those who complete the two or four years of a college curriculum, not only is the time extended before formal entrance into the world of adult work, but a milieu is provided in which the tasks of entering adulthood can be confronted and sometimes completed. While the student years cannot be considered typical experiences for young adults, they do provide illustrations of a variety of responses to developmental tasks in young adults. For many young people, it is during their experiences in college that they recognize and generally meet the challenges to commit themselves autonomously to their future.

The general education component of a college curriculum encourages inquiry and evaluation of knowledge and values. It is generally recognized that college graduates change in the direction of greater acceptance of diversity of attitudes and display more complex value structures themselves. William Perry has studied patterns of intellectual and ethical development in a college environment. He found systematic transitions from an absolutist position of good-bad polarities to an acceptance of uncertainty and diversity in value areas as legitimate and, finally, to personal commitments that inform and balance ethical decisions. For Perry and others, a truly liberal education should recognize and provide for both the intellectual and ethical development of students.

AUTONOMY

A major step of emancipation is taken by students who attend residential colleges or move away from home while attending school. Most young people expect increasing independence, but many are surprised to discover the degree of dependence on their families they experience when separated from them for the first time. In addition to managing separation, students must also adjust to living with strangers under intimate circumstances, which may increase the longing for the stability and support their homes provided.

Most colleges no longer operate in a surrogate parental fashion as they have in the past. Some students find themselves experiencing a degree of autonomy that is new to them in a context of new and diverse peer pressures. The exploration of freedom and different value orientations may become a testing of the limits of self-control. In these circumstances there may be excesses in the expression of autonomy, and some young people may find themselves unsupported by their previous values in a scene of conflicting demands. Others may become obsessive about the correctness and virtue of personal conduct. However, the testing of views and attitudes does provide a mechanism for ordering personal priorities and developing tolerance for the convictions of others.

SEXUALITY

While the climate of a college encourages intellectual concern with values and ethical behavior, there are more direct challenges to be met in the prevailing values of the student culture. This is most apparent in areas of sexual behavior and the use of alcohol and drugs. Although the "sexual revolution" on campuses has been exaggerated in the public view, college is nonetheless a place where sexual aspects of interpersonal relations achieve great importance. Many young people have already made their first venture into sexual activity by the time they reach college, but the general openness of college residential environments and the noninterfering stance of college administrators create situations where students are more directly required to make decisions about their own sexuality. Greater sexual expression does not necessarily mean greater promiscuity, since sexual relationships may involve students in commitments that in many ways are like the serious ones of marriage.

Greater acknowledgment among young people of homosexuality as a matter of personal preference may challenge some students as they explore their own sexuality. Most young people are vulnerable in the perception of their own sexuality. Whether through experimentation, reaction against concerns about heterosexual expression or sensitivity to preferences already noted in oneself, some students may involve themselves in homosexual relations that require them to come to terms with the significance of these relations for their understanding of themselves.

Whether involving sexual activity or not, interpersonal relations and their vicissitudes are of great significance to young adults, and students may find much of their time and concern taken up with the management of these relationships and their feelings about them. Separation from previous interpersonal support and negotiation of new relationships are often difficult, particularly when they involve the formation of a new supporting group. Students are often surprised at the significance and intensity of their interactions with those with whom they share living quarters or become involved romantically.

ALCOHOL AND DRUGS

Many young people reach the age for legal consumption of alcohol in college, and the social climate of most colleges and universities is conditioned by the role that drinking plays in it. Most students have had their first encounters with alcohol before entering college, but they have usually not had as easy access or as frequent opportunities to express their choice about drinking. With less accountability to adults about drinking behavior, some students may display problems of regulation and control that are submerged in the general student social environment.

Drug use of the kind that alarmed the public a decade ago is not common on campuses today. Initial experimentation with drugs is a phenomenon of a younger group today and most students understand the risks associated with promiscuous drug use. The reemergence of alcohol as the preferred social chemical has also changed the drug culture on campuses. However, fairly easy access to social drugs in college environments still puts at risk for dependent involvement with drugs those young people whose experiences and character make them vulnerable.

COMPETENCE AND CAREER CHOICE

While colleges provide a setting for the dramas of emancipation and establishing adult relationships and contribute their own social determinants to the ways in which students define themselves, it is in the domain of the assessment and confirmation of competence that institutions of higher education play their traditional roles. Whether the emphasis of the institution is on liberal, pre-professional, or vocational preparation, all students who persist face a requirement to make a commitment to a consistent and defined course of study. "What's your major?" is as frequently a part of personal identification as "What's your name?"

Many students arrive at college with some nominal career choice, since parents, teachers, and other adults encourage adolescents to make early decisions about what they want to be. For some the choice has been relatively easy. They know their interests and have been expressing them in high school. In making their provisional choices, others are influenced by currently popular or accessible areas or by the social prestige attached to the pursuit. Yet, for many, the early college years are a time for further exploration and discovery of talents and interests that can be directed into a career.

While colleges permit the exploration of educational options and the determination of focused interests, regular tests of performance and self-evaluation in comparison to others are part of the process. In times of restricted access both to higher education and to professional training and employment after graduation, evaluation of competence and educational accomplishment becomes a major career-determining influence. Students find themselves in the paradoxical situation of managing competitive strivings with the very persons with whom they are forming significant relationships.

A sense of confidence in one's abilities is hard won. Most entering students have not achieved the skill of assessing themselves realistically and with sustained faith in their ability to achieve. Fear of failure and fear of success complicate the ways in which students choose the areas for developing their abilities. Women students are particularly vulnerable to the traditional implicit designation of careers and disciplines as requiring skills and characteristics that men supposedly possess in greater abundance.

MOTIVATION

Motivational problems, including apathetic resignation from competition, may plague many students. The interplay of anxiety and depressive self-evaluation is common in student concerns about their competence, even among those who achieve well. The competitive requirements of some colleges or disciplines may place some students in moral dilemmas about cheating or plagiarism and encourage others to reduce tension in self-defeating or unproductive ways. Students find it difficult to be appropriately playful in a demanding achievement-oriented environment.

The idyllic view of college years must be tempered with the recognition that movement toward consistent commitments can be fraught with difficulties that may result in excesses of self-indulgence and impulsivity, poignant disappointments and defeats in interpersonal relations, and fragile self-confidence that is dependent on the evaluation of others for confirmation. Even for those who seem less unsettled by the college passage to adulthood, some may have avoided testing their commitments and accepted particular activities and courses of study as the path of least resistance.

The difficulties of college years should not be overemphasized, however. Most adults whom students meet in college are dedicated to encouraging the developmental progression to adult status. Peers are frequently more tolerant, accepting, and kind than the less mature companions of high school years. Broad educational opportunities often open new paths to accomplishment or stabilize developing competencies. The college milieu also is one in which questions of value can be explored and acted upon with greater acceptance and less risk than is the case at other ages. The problems that students have in college usually reflect the latent problems they bring with them, but the college experience may also support the amelioration and revision of earlier developmental inadequacies.

The college years of change require skills in the management of change. Students must negotiate such matters as time spent on studies and noncurricular activities, number and intensity of friendships, demonstration of altruistic concern for others, expression of sexual desires, control of impulses, and commitment to post-graduate plans. The ways in which they carry out these negotiations will have considerable effect on how they handle similar problems of balancing external requirements with a sense of internal consistency in their post-college years.

Psychiatric disorders of young adults

The psychiatric disorders of young adults do not differ in basic diagnostic features from the disorders of older adults. The characteristics of the era of young adulthood are unsettled and changeable enough that transient disturbances may produce behavior that would appear more pathological in other age groups. Therefore, some caution should be used in the application of diagnostic labels. The developmental tasks of early adulthood, however, are such that they may precipitate emotional crises for young people with more chronic problems. In counseling young adults, it is appropriate to be alert to indications of depression, anxiety, and schizophrenia.

DEPRESSION

Young adults are vulnerable to the circumstances that precipitate depressive episodes. Attempts to establish independence may arouse conflicts about dependence and feelings of loss of support. Investment in relationships may lead to disappointment and a sense of loss should the relationship falter. Attempts to achieve success in school or work may result in blows to self-esteem. Those who are inexperienced in handling the effects of disappointment and who have been sensitized by earlier experiences of loss and discouragement may show depressive symptoms beyond the expected response to distressing events. The sense of helplessness and hopelessness that occur in depression may be shown in the inability to study or perform other responsibilities, withdrawal from activities and relationships, and a pessimistic view about opportunities to be happy or successful. Most depressive episodes in young adults are relatively short-lived and self-limiting, but if a young person becomes more isolated, overly dependent, preoccupied with disappointment and hurt feelings, or expresses feelings that nothing will help, professional intervention should be considered. Suicide is always a possibility in the context of depression, and some young people can become excessively morose about the meaning and worth of life. Suicidal gestures may be made in an impulsive or dramatic way, but there is no clear basis for assessing whether suicidal gestures are "sincere" or not. Since suicide attempts are of such acute concern, it is appropriate to take expressions of suicidal thoughts seriously.

ANXIETY

Young adults have many worries, as might be expected from their concern about the future and the probabilities of success in their personal relations and their careers. Anxiety may appear as a free-floating sense of dread, as a specifically focused fear, or as obsessive preoccupations. Since a majority of young adults admit to frequent worries, the occurrence of anxious concerns is not by itself a cause for alarm. Of more concern are fears that limit social participation or the expression of abilities. Anxiety stemming from conflicts about independence, impulse control, or moral dilemmas may take the form of obsessive rumination about issues of right and wrong, past mistakes or embarrassment, potential misfortunes, or self-concept. Persistence of worried rumination or focused fear to the point of interference with other activities, particularly when the young person feels a loss of the ability to control repetitive thoughts or avoidant behaviors, signal the possibility that professional intervention should be considered.

SCHIZOPHRENIA

The expression of schizophrenia is sometimes subtle, sometimes flamboyant, and often may come to the clear attention of others during the years of young adulthood. It is in the very areas of moral commitment, interpersonal relations, and preparation for adult careers that the symptoms of schizophrenia may be manifested. Acute psychotic symptoms signal clearly that something is wrong. It is harder to interpret the gradual indications of failure to establish satisfying relations with others or the inability to perform successfully in school or work. Apathy, lack of motivation, unrealistic enthusiasms, withdrawal from social participation, disregard for dress or diet, excessive preoccupation — all may occur at one time or another in the life of young adults. If any combination persists and deflects the young person from achievement in the areas of developmental tasks, further evaluation is advisable.

The pastoral counselor and the young adult

The less severe but compelling problems that pastoral counselors are likely to see most frequently are those associated with the threshold experiences of young adults. Some young people may express distress about a particular concern such as freeing oneself from parental domination, coming to terms with sexuality, disturbances in a relationship with a lover or a close friend, or concerns about self-worth. Others may show problems in a number of areas simultaneously. Usually they are anxious, concerned, and sensitive. They may also be depressed, resentful, guilty, or apathetic. They are usually hoping for a sympathetic, friendly, older person who will be wise and supportive and who will not try to impose values or solutions on them. They may be involved in disturbed relations with another adult, which may make them wary or at least a bit skeptical.

The initial encounter obviously is one to be approached sensitively by the counselor.

Without minimizing the distresses of young adults, it is reassuring to note that as a group they are the most promising beneficiaries of counseling. Contemporary young people are more open, psychologically sensitive, and articulate than older persons or their counterparts of earlier generations. Their youth means that opportunities are more available to them, and they are less handicapped by rigid personality structures or a history of failure. They can entertain hope that they can resolve the issues that perplex them. It is that very hope that initiates the request for help. Those who already feel limited or defeated by life are not likely to assume that much can be done individually for them. This is the problem of many unemployed youth, particularly those who are thwarted by social attitudes toward their ethnic or socioeducational background.

Pastoral counselors are particularly sensitive to many of the concerns of young adults. Value conflicts provide an opportunity to explore the source of discomfort they have in assessing the ethical dimension of their experience. If the young person is approaching a commitment to another person and is anxious or ambivalent about it, the counselor's experience in premarital and marital counseling is useful. Since a frequent concern is one of personal confidence and value, the pastoral counselor is a proper person to help gain understanding of the meaning of human worth.

Young people may be very tentative in the ways they approach an older adult for assistance, yet they can be very astute in their assessment of that person as one in whom they can place trust and confidence. Theorists of young adult development emphasize the role that nonparental adults can serve as models, teachers, mentors, and guides during the transition to adulthood. Pastoral counselors have special opportunities to provide an example of what the adult world can offer in support and encouragement to those who are entering it.

REFERENCES

Colarusso, Calvin A., & Nemiroff, Robert A. *Adult Development.* New York: Plenum, 1981.

Erikson, Erik. *Identity: Youth and Crisis.* New York: W. W. Norton & Co., 1968.

Gould, Roger L. *Transformations: Growth and Change in Adult Life.* New York: Simon and Schuster, 1978.

Hultsch, David F., & Deutsch, Francine. Adult Development and Aging. New York: McGraw-Hill, 1981.

Huyck, Margaret H., & Hoyer, William J. *Adult Development and Aging.* Belmont, Calif.: Wadsworth, 1982.

Levinson, Daniel J. et al. *The Seasons of a Man's Life.* New York: Alfred A. Knopf, 1978.

Sheehy, Gail. *Passages: Predictable Crises of Adult Life.* New York: E. P. Dutton, 1974.

Veroff, Joseph; Donovan, Elisabeth; & Gulka, Richard A. *The Inner American.* New York: Basic Books, 1981.

6

Adults Have Troubles Too

FRANCIS J. BRACELAND

The troubles complained of by adults are as numerous as the birds of the air, and Dickens found them exceedingly gregarious in nature and "flying in flocks like birds apt to perch capriciously in strange places." Actually, troubles are the lot of all humans from infancy to old age, from birth to death. No stage of life can be singled out as a time of greater trouble than another, since each has its own special brand of difficulty. Though the spotlight of late has been monopolized by the bewildering array of the problems of adolescence, it is obvious to all that when we pass over the vague border into adulthood our difficulties are not over. We simply take on a new set of troubles. These troubles regularly are laid at the doorsteps of physicians and ministers.

One of our present-day difficulties lies in believing that we should not have troubles or, if we do, that there is some magic that will give us instantaneous relief or a psychiatrist available who will make them go away—preferably quickly. All nature and all history testify against this, for it is not written that our roads through life shall be especially smooth. Small and petty annoyances will always appear, and they seem to cause more trouble than serious problems.

It would be presumptuous for us to think that we could even mention, let alone describe here, the numerous troubles that assail adults, for our competence concerns emotional problems alone—and not even all of them. There is one thread that runs through all adult emotional problems, however, and that does merit our attention, for it involves misunderstandings with adolescents, older age-groups, family members, fellow workers, and friend and foe alike. The thread is communication, the tie-line that relates us to others. Once that line is impeded, cut, or broken off in anger, hurt, or obvious neglect, our chances of reaching agreement with others is materially lessened. The late President Kennedy on several occasions spoke of his regret at the breakdown of communications between nations, and frightening novels have been written about bombers losing radio contact with their bases with untoward results. If a slogan were needed, therefore, for our patients, our parishioners, or ourselves, it would be: "Keep your lines of communication open and, if necessary, your personal emergency telephone handy." It is necessary to keep one's "hot line" open with family, friends, and fellow workers, no matter how tense the situation or how seemingly great the provocation to disrupt communication may be.

Before beginning the discussion of our communication with others, it might help our understanding of the problems involved if we recalled that our troubles and emotional difficulties are due not only to our relations with other people or to external circumstances but also to the pressures and drives that arise within ourselves. They come from our past history and from the circumstances each individual has set for him- or herself. All of these are engraved upon the personality. So are the gratifications that result from past experiences and the deceptions a person may have perpetrated.

The complexity of the adult mental structure has been likened to a geological formation with the superposition of new strata over the passage of years. The earliest strata are, of course, the deepest and the most firmly molded; the latest are the deposits of more recent experience, hence more shifting and more subject to modification. Upthrusts from the depths occur from time to time, and tremors radiate throughout the whole person; sometimes these upthrusts are of volcanic proportions. In these instances one sees or hears about behavior and reactions that seem to be altogether foreign to the expected conduct of the individual.

The "adult" is hard to define

The person we call an adult is a composite of heredity, temperament, intelligence, and environment. He or she is not the mere addition of all of these things but a complicated product of their interactions. The overall picture of a healthy adult is that of a mature individual who is predominantly independent, has a good grasp of reality, is discriminating and adaptable, at ease with his or her conscience, and responsible for his or her own behavior, capable of both competing and cooperating with other adults with a minimum of anxiety and hostility.

The more mature the adult, the stronger and more stable the person is and the more resistant to regression. Regression is a mechanism by which we turn back in our action and behave as we did at an earlier emotional level. The more the child persists within us, the greater the tendency to childhood reactions and behavior. These childish reactions conflict with the adult's efforts to be mature, and with "adult" standards. These reactions have an enormous potential, and the more repressed they are, like steam under pressure, the more powreful they become and the more productive of inner tension.

It is this inner tension and anxiety that cause the bulk of our emotional difficulties. So widespread is this that we all have heard our present situation called the age of anxiety. Our problems are compounded by a lack of personal security and satisfaction and our difficulty in getting on with other people — the difficulty in communicating with others, which we will discuss in further detail, resulting in inadequate performance or with lack of satisfaction in work, recreation, social, or familial relations.

Walter Lippmann in his *Preface to Morals* said:

> . . . the critical question is whether childish habits and expectations are to persist or to be transformed. We grow older. But it is by no means certain that we shall grow up. The human character is a complicated thing and its elements do not necessarily march in step. It is possible to be a sage in some things and a child in others, to be at once precocious and retarded, to be shrewd and foolish, serene and irritable. For some parts of our personalities may well be more mature than others; not infrequently we participate in the enterprises of an adult with the mood and manners of a child.

The successful passage into maturity depends, therefore, on a breaking up and reconstructing of those habits that were appropriate only to our earliest experience. Lippmann also pointed out:

> When a childish disposition is carried over into an adult environment, the result is a radically false valuation of that environment. The symptons are fairly evident. . . . The childish pattern appears as a deep sense that life owes him something, that somehow it is the duty of the universe to look after him and to listen sharply when he speaks to it. . . . The childish pattern appears also as a disposition to believe that he may reach out for anything in sight and take it and that, having gotten it, nobody must ever under any circumstances take it away.

Console yourself

Before going further into the lives of adults, there is a bit of scaffolding which should be erected as background material for our discussion. First, the line between emotional health and emotional illness is hazy. It is probable that most of us at some time or other might stray a bit across the line due to worrisome problems (taking professional licensing examinations might be a good example), and all of us at times have "thick coming fancies" and extravagant ideas that resemble those evidenced by the emotionally ill. Therefore, as Lowell once observed, "console yourself . . . whatever you may be sure of be sure of this, that you are dreadfully like other people. Human nature has a much greater genius for sameness than originality." Second, neither Judaism nor Christianity ever held forth the possibilities of perfect happiness or constant good health on this earth. A person once asked Freud if his treatment would bring him happiness, and Freud answered that it would remove his symptoms; but for the rest he would have to remain with the suffering that is common to humanity. And third, if as adults we are to understand others, we must have some understanding of ourselves. Only those who respect and are at peace with themselves can be respectful of others and capable of relating to them in a comfortable fashion. An old Jewish proverb holds that "he who cannot be good to himself cannot be good to others." Erasmus in his *Praise of Folly* made a similar comment: "I ask you, will he who hates himself love anyone? Will he who does not get along with himself agree with another or will he who is disagreeable and irksome to himself bring pleasure to any? No one would say so unless he himself were more foolish than folly."

Furthermore our troubles and emotional difficulties are due not only to our relations with others or to external circumstances, but also to the pressures and drives that arise within ourselves. These come from our past history and from the circumstances each individual has set for him- or herself. All of them are engraved upon the personality; so too are the gratifications that result from past experiences and the deception he or she may have perpetrated.

Anxieties and fears

Why all this discussion of the adult mental structure? It is adults and their troubles that we are considering, and one of the serious troubles of adult life lies in becoming adult and reacting in adult fashion. The personality of an individual is always "becoming." The earlier layers of experience modify the later ones and in turn are modifed by them. The integration of the personality is not always continuous, nor is progress simultaneous everywhere. There are always irregularities; we advance in some areas and we seem to recede in others.

Let us assume now that we have safely traversed the uneven road to adulthood, and we are dealing with people who are raising families and doing the world's work. What problems do they worry about now? Have they changed in any way? Do they worry about nuclear warfare, rockets, and the possibilities of mass extinction? They may, at least some of them, but this concern is not admitted readily. Surveys made at different times indicate that the anxieties and fears of the populace change even though the "core" problems remain. Most of the surveys thus far indicate that people continue to worry about mundane things—things already mentioned—family problems, marital discord, economic status, jobs, automation, health, and the care of aged parents, rather than wars and rumors of wars.

Were a survey to be taken in the 1980s, it would indicate that people are quite concerned with economics, unemployment, high interest rates, and inability to find and pay for proper housing. As the children reach puberty, parents worry about their adolescents and drugs, alcohol, and a general looseness of morals. Most of all adults are uneasy about the senseless violence which is rampant: muggings, holdups, robbery, rape, and wanton killings. People feel unsafe in their own neighborhoods: few individuals feel free and secure enough to go out after dark. Newspaper, radio, and television accounts fill in the gory tales for people already fearful, thus adding to their distress.

We all are well aware of these findings of numerous surveys and polls, and may have to agree with Admiral Byrd that "the tolerable quality of a dangerous existence is the fact that the human mind cannot remain continuously sensitive to anything. Fright and pain are the most transitory of emotions, they are easily forgotten." To his comments, however, we add our own caution that there is frequently a remnant of anxiety which remains within us.

This situation, incidentally, forms the basis for some of the physical symptoms that people take to the family physician: they are the physical manifestations of fear, anxiety, and depressions, and in the aggregate they are spoken of as psychosomatic disorders. The implications of these symptoms are that we are whole individuals—mind and body, psyche and pneuma (or soul)—that something which affects us emotionally has some physical concomitants, and any serious physical illness of necessity affects us emotionally. (We will hear much more about psychosomatic disorders in the comprehensive medicine of the future.)

Stress

Admittedly, every adult experiences a series of worrisome problems to be solved. Some of them, which seem minor to others, loom large and serious to the one who has them. It has been said that it probably would astound us beyond measure to be let into our neighbor's mind and to find out how different the scenery appears from that perspective. Because we cannot enter into each other's minds, the transmission of thoughts, feelings, and attitudes from one mind to another is often unsuccessful. The balance between words and actions that transmit our thoughts and feelings adequately and those that do so only partially or not at all is an extremely delicate one, and there is always the possibility that the meaning and intention of our communication may be misunderstood or misinterpreted. Anyone who has ever had to write a directive or frame a law can attest to this; there is always someone who will find loopholes in it or even misinterpret it completely. Anyone who ever thought that he or she was making an intention clear and that his or her actions were altruistic and charitable, only to find oneself suspect and completely misunderstood, can attest to it more poignantly.

Jobs, emotional problems, and personal relationships

One may wonder why we consider jobs of men and women here. Why should psychiatrists interest themselves in work or in leisure? For a number of reasons:

—People do not become ill in a vacuum. They become ill in their daily surroundings, and because they spend half their waking hours at work, psychiatrists are interested, for work is the stage upon which a large portion of an individual's life is played.

—It is said that by far the greatest proportion of discharges from industry are due to personality problems rather than technical inaptitude. It is also estimated that the greatest cause of absenteeism after the common cold is some form of temporary emotional upset, even though it manifests itself in physical symptoms.

—Unrest and personality problems can render working conditions untenable.

—The conditions of a person's work are changing rapidly in this present culture and economy, and some individuals have difficulty in adapting to rapid change and fall by the wayside, hence the psychiatrists' interest.

A knowledgeable psychiatrist once observed that the unemployed person's most pressing need is to maintain his or her position in the home and with the family. If unemployment is protracted, "life deteriorates into sodden repetition of job seeking and lounging about the house. He or she no longer meets friends on the job and whatever limited camaraderie there was no longer exists. Therefore, work becomes a fundamental resource, a face to show to society, something to hold on to as long as possible."

It takes two to close the circuit

The point here is that many adult troubles come from misunderstandings and resultant coolness or quarrels with those who are our associates. Something has happened to the communications between us. Why, with all of the possibilities open to us, does this occur? Why do our messages so frequently miss their mark and fall so miserably short of our purpose? Why do we find it so difficult to reach mutual agreement or understanding with our fellow human beings? Part of the answer seems to lie in the close tie that exists between our ways of communicating and receiving messages and our ways of relating to other persons, both of which are extremely complex operations, consisting of an incalculable number of variations.

How do we communicate? On the face of it, the answer may seem to be obvious; but speech and writing, our main methods of communication, are not by any means our only ones. Many subtle signs and symbols reflect our personalities, feelings, attitudes, and beliefs, and they affect the meaning of our messages. Our real selves come through to others in gestures, sounds, movement, facial expressions, sometimes as an accompaniment to speech but quite often without our uttering a word. Our very manner or a slight gesticulation has a meaning of its own more widespread than the language of words. Some of our gestures may have only local or national meaning, but in general gesticulation provides us with a language which nature has given to everyone and which most people understand. In addition to the very obvious signs, however, there are shadings in tone or voice, variations in stress and speed of speech that further influence the impact of the message. Signs that at first seem fixed in content may have several meanings according to circumstances. For example, different forms of smile or laughter may indicate disappointment, cynicism, irony, malice, shame, despair, doubt, etc.

These variations may alter the true meaning of our communications in a multitude of ways. Moreover, they are altered further by the person who receives them; it takes two to close the circuit. Our messages do not fall on deaf ears nor unseeing eyes; they produce a definite response in the receiver, but this response may be altered in a multitude of ways. An offer to help someone in financial or other distress may be badly received and interpreted by the intended recipient as interfering, lording it over, or patronizing. One is never sure in offering assistance to a child or adult whether the offer will be received in the sense that it is offered. The receiver interprets the message in the light of extremely personal factors and makes a response conditioned by individual make-up, emotional state at the time of receiving the message, and the influence of the sum total of past experience. We can all recall having met people whom we liked or who liked us instinctively. We can also recall people who took violent dislike to us without our having said or done anything. These are examples of the reactions just mentioned; we have been invested with qualities or defects that we may not have at all, and we are judged by the other individual's make-up and past experience.

Messages — spoken, written, or implied — mean different things to different people. They arouse individual memories, conjure up dissimilar images, stir up a variety of emotions, and produce a wide range of unlike ideas, even when there is a common language and common interests and background between transmitter and receiver. We have all heard someone say: "Yes, it's true, that's what he says, but I have my own opinion." Clearly, then, communication that is subject to so many variables is bound to be subject also to many distortions. Each individual operates within his or her own frame of reference and finds only such meaning in communications as experience permits.

Loneliness and our need for people

There is fairly concrete evidence that communication is a social function, and that human beings are social animals we can have no doubt, since our every experience proves it. People depend upon relationships with others for their very existence, feeling secure only when they belong to someone or some group large or small. Experiments have shown that humans need this contact with other human beings in order to maintain their equilibrium. We could discourse at length upon various aspects of loneliness as we talk about communication, but much of what we might say would be foreign to our thesis. Generally, the best treatment for loneliness, though it sounds like a contradiction, resides within ourselves and proceeds from the self-possession that directs our way of life. One cannot profit from a personality designed by somebody else and neither can one come to grips with loneliness through solutions drawn up by strangers, even if they are experts. A lonely person cannot wait for friends to come to the rescue. Friendship begins with our reaching toward others. Those who wait to be rescued from loneliness, it is said, experience even more anguish than those who take the problem in hand and move out to people despite the risks.

There is a loneliness in old age, too, which while it is not of major concern to young adults, they should know about. There are more than seven million elderly below the poverty line, many of them in hovels, afraid to go out lest they be mugged and their few miserable possessions stolen.

The presence of other human beings is vital to our existence from birth onward — we need one another and must get along together or examine the reasons why our communications with others fail. Our nonverbal communications are extremely important, and knowledge of this phenomenon helps to understand the problem. The history and record of the manner in which these phenomena start in infancy and how they grow make for a fascinating story that is too far afield to record here. We learn, for instance, that beginning in infancy the way the mother carries, feeds, and tends to the child; her warmth, her softness, and her manner mean everything to the child when words mean nothing. This is the beginning of so-called nonverbal communication.

The details of the development of communication skills in childhood and in various stages of growth are fascinating but need not be discussed here. We see that human beings are bound to their fellow humans from their very beginning and that adults face life with the knowledge, the standards, and the values derived from their family relationships. The signs and symbols with which they communicate at each level grow out of their early background and become more complex as adulthood is reached. If they have adapted well during the various stages of growth, their methods of communication will be adequate and they will have acquired their own personal stamp. If not, the wise guidance of a psychotherapist can be a corrective experience in which individuals can learn to understand what is going on within themselves and their relations to others, and they will be better able to communicate in areas where communication earlier was difficult.

Physicians and ministers can help

The Greek dramatist Aeschylus (525–456 B.C.) noted that "words are physicians of a mind diseased," and certainly this is evident in psychotherapy today — words from the patient, not the physician. Thus, in a warm, giving relationship the therapist, whether psychiatrist, family doctor, or minister, helps to heal the wounds inflicted by people who had never learned to communicate in a healthy way. In this atmosphere of acceptance, the patient or parishioner can recognize his or her thoughts, redefine values, and gain a new outlook on the self and its problems.

Just as communication between patient and therapist helps to restore mental health, so communication in other settings helps to maintain it. A great part of the success we achieve in living depends on how well we are able to establish bases for mutual understanding with the people we encounter. Mature individuals, who have succeeded in integrating themselves into a larger world, keep in touch with that world at all levels of activity. Their contact with other human beings helps them to transcend the harsh realities that often confront them. They are going to be buffeted by troubles — all of us are — but in communication with others they find reassurance and a sense of security. They satisfy basic needs for prestige and the respect of others at work, at play, or in social activity.

People can sense in each of us sincerity and interest, attention and a willingness to listen and to see their side of the story — their hopes, their desires, their fears. They can detect the hireling, too, no matter what his or her profession or business; people are particularly adept at this. They may be fooled once but rarely a second time. You have often heard the statement: "I don't know what it is — he has always been nice to me and never did anything to me — but I just don't like him." This approach has more justification than the statement one girl made: "I don't like her and I'll find a reason for it yet."

Defining differences

It looks now as though we have come around full circle, back to the make-up of the individuals as the essential factor in all communication, and at least to some idea of the troubles in our interpersonal relations. We have long since passed the stage when we were dependent upon receiving communication through our skin, but we still say occasionally that "he or she gets under my skin," either as a record of like or dislike of a person. Effective communication, therefore, overcomes obstacles and prejudices. It implies feeling for others and consideration of other points of view, even those in disagreement. This kind of communication can lead to constructive action; it permits people to define their differences and reach agreements. Hasn't it ever struck you as strange that people, who will bravely disregard all danger and sacrifice their lives for their fellows on the battlefield, will make such little effort to communicate with or live with their fellow human beings in peace and understanding in their own cities? "To be understood is a pleasure; to reach an agreement is expedient and pleasant; to be understood and reach agreement is deeply gratifying." To be able to communicate with others has many other good results: it guards us against intolerable loneliness, engenders vitality, and gives us hope and courage for the tasks that lie ahead.

Patient-parishioner and counselor relations

The art of medicine is to see people, not as problems to be solved, but as sensitive human beings to be helped. Sometimes we even have to help people who do not want to be helped or who believe they don't. That is why the physician talks of the importance of doctor-patient relationships. This is no mumbo jumbo, as detractors have sometimes stated; it is the essence of medical practice. It is in this relationship that cure takes place. It requires warmth, kindliness, and understanding, and though the doctor must be scientific, scientific knowledge is not enough for dealing with people. People still have high regard and affection for their personal physicians and ministers, but medicine in the aggregate and religion in general both seem somehow to have failed in their communications with lay people—failed to impart the most attractive and useful elements of their images to the public. This is extremely unfortunate, for humans who are poised, often precariously, between this world and the next, are in need of all the help that physicians and ministers can give them.

We have learned in other chapters of this book that the words which are to be used to assuage people's ills and troubles are to be used sparingly. Persons with emotional problems who visit physicians and ministers need understanding, kindness, interest, and assurance of a willingness to be of assistance within the bounds of reason. If one listens carefully enough, the source of the trouble becomes apparent. The callers only rarely need advice; they more often need a sympathetic ear. There are nuances to their problems that only they know, and a therapist who is too facile with ready advice may entirely miss the real cause of the trouble. Words, like medications, must be used with great care.

The troubles lie within ourselves

S. I. Hayakawa, the semanticist, speaks of the words we use as essential instruments of humanity and observes that depending on our unconscious attitudes toward the words we hear and utter, we may use them either as weapons with which to start arguments and verbal free-for-alls or as instruments with which to increase our wisdom, our sense of fellowship with other human beings, and our enjoyment of life. I subscribe heartily to this idea. Starting arguments and verbal free-for-alls is a potent cause of many adult troubles. Sometimes we do not even have to argue—our unconscious attitudes seem to betray our anger and hostility —then we wonder why everybody doesn't love us.

William James thought there was a plane below all formulas and all enmities due to formulas where people could meet each other moving about and recognize each other as members of the same family inhabiting the same depth. I believe this is true, and from what we have learned about people, I believe that the surface conditions that interfere with communication with our brothers and sisters often lie within ourselves.

Down through the ages people from all walks of life have arrived at the same conclusion: the possibilities of tragedy—maybe the reason for much of our trouble—lie within ourselves. Maybe even our trouble in communication, resulting in cutting our tie-lines with family or friends, rests with ourselves. This is a difficult admission to make, but if we can make it, we can set about to erect the poles and restring the wires to those with whom we have quarreled. Maybe we can even approximate that dynamic security that rests within ourselves and then, like children who have assured themselves of the love and security of their own families, start out to communicate with the rest of the world.

In the meantime, with our lines restrung, we will keep them operating, and even, if necessary, reach for our own personal emergency telephone. The days are gone when, like the disappointed father or the tragedian in the play, we can tell people never to darken our door again. They are likely to believe us and do just that, and we will be the chief losers.

REFERENCES

Byrd, Richard E. *Alone.* New York: G. P. Putnam, 1938.

Ginsburg, Sol W. *Psychiatrist's View on Social Issues.* New York: Columbia University Press, 1963.

Lippmann, Walter. *Preface to Morals.* New York: Macmillan, 1913.

Lowell, James Russel. On a certain condescension in foreigners. In *Oxford Book of American Essays,* 166–93.

7

Midlife: Problems and Potential

FRANCIS J. BRACELAND

U ntil a few decades ago writings, popular and scientific, about middle age and its problems were scarce. Attention was focused upon the young with an occasional side-glance at the elderly and their health and housing problems. Contemporary culture still reserves many of its accolades for the vigor and freshness of youth and bestows on old age a kindly disinterest and sometimes its pity. The past is prologue to the present and the present to old age, and everyone approaches old age at the rate of sixty minutes per hour. Those who are in middle life are particularly aware of this, and there is no doubt that for some the time is a menace of sinister proportions, not only because of the specter of waning physical powers but also because of what that fact portends. Yet in another time, H. Allen's exhortation in *Anthony Adverse:* "Grow up as soon as possible for the only time that one really lives is from thirty to sixty,"[1] was received as wise advice. "The young," he said, "were slaves to their dreams and the old servants of regrets."

Phobias about middle age plague both men and women, although earlier it was thought to be most marked in women. The psychiatrist Edmund Bergler wrote an important book on people's middle-aged revolt against time, biology, and their own inner make-up. In it he discussed those hitherto conforming and even successful individuals who began to feel a sense of failure in achieving their heart's desire and, with time running out, became preoccupied with making up for lost time. They stand in marked contrast to a group of people (described by G. Stanley Hall) who spend their youth in preparing misery for their old age and then spend their old age in repairing misconduct of youth.

Indeed, middle age today was considered old age at the turn of the century. Life expectancy for the male was then forty-seven years, and only 4 percent of the population was over sixty-five. The 1980 census, however, reported the survival rate of males to be seventy-two years. J. Siegel and C. Taeuber, in the February 1982 *The Gerontologist,* wrote:

> The early results of the census show that there were about 25.5 million people over age 65 years in the United States on April 1, 1980. These constitute 11% of the total population and include about 15 million women and 10 million men. Another 22 million fall into the 55- to 64-year age range so that one-fifth of the population is 55 years old or over.

Several factors are responsible for increased longevity, but there is no need to detail them here. It is the fact of longevity and the larger number of the elderly that are important to our discussion. Today's middle-age men and women are the first middle-age group to encounter two "generation gaps"—one between themselves and adolescents and the other between themselves and the elderly.

No hard and fast boundaries define the start or ending of middle age. Bernice Neugarten (1968), an authority on the subject, noted that middle age has only recently been distinguished from young adulthood, and even now the young-old are being distinguished from the old-old. In fact, chronological ages are not dependable markings because of the differences among groups and cultures of what "middle age" means. Generally, the limits are set arbitrarily between forty to forty-five and sixty-five to seventy years of age. Actually, these numbers are only for convenience and do not follow slavishly upon any laws of nature.

Middle age thus delineated is a segment of the life cycle and potentially a period of great accomplishment. It is sometimes called the fulcrum upon which the younger and older ages pivot. Medically, it is the most interesting stage of life, and for many it is a period of great fulfillment— one that is alive and active, one in which the individual has real opportunity to acquire knowledge and wisdom. Ordinarily, the person in midlife is less harassed by the libidinous drives of the young and the enfeeblement of the elderly. It is a time for mature consideration and progressive achievement; yet it can also be a time of life to bear heavy responsibility. Often those in midlife are called upon to raise the young and support elderly family and relatives emotionally, physically, and even economically. Roadblocks will occur as they do in all ages, but, in general, a person is much better emotionally and physically and has wider experience—all of which allow for making wise decisions.

Confronting middle age

When men and women approach middle age, they may show first a concern for their bodies. Shakespeare in *As You Like It* (act II, scene 7) described men in middle life "in fair round belly with good capon lined"; we still mark the waistline as one of the first onslaughts of middle age. Yet, it is also a time when people seriously start taking stock of themselves. While most of us will never go through the trauma of the American hostages in Iran, Lawrence Kennedy's reflection on his experience puts into sharp focus what men and women in middle age potentially face: "When you have been through a death threatening experience," Kennedy said, "you are suddenly confronted with your real self. Most of us go through life chasing after a person who never really existed — our idea of ourselves." Kennedy then recalled the advice given to the group of returning hostages by a psychiatrist who treated them en route home: "Don't try to chase after an idealized self. Come to terms with the person you really are." Sean Sammon, a psychiatrist and a monk, observed that Kennedy's comments summarize well the developmental tasks that confront midlife men and women — accepting one's own eventual mortality and beginning the journey away from early adulthood and its experimental quality and toward the inward focus of the middle years (Sammon, 1982, p. 15).

Normal pressures accompany every period of life; each age has its characteristic emotional aspects. Ordinarily there is no marked impairment of ability in men or women in middle life, although some physical slowing is normal and should be expected. The individual may become aware that age is having some effect, but the situation differs for each person and times may even vary in the same individual. There may even be some compensatory gains that make up for the fractional losses. By this time, most men and women have established a way of life for themselves and hold a job or follow a way of life that is more or less appropriate for their tastes and abilities. If they do not, an element of discontent exacerbates the problems they normally encounter in facing the tasks of middle age.

QUESTIONING COMMITMENTS

The age thirty has an important part to play in our transition to the middle years. In describing the "age of thirty" transition, Daniel Levinson (1978) points out that the end of this transition is the end of the preparatory phase of early adulthood. Most men and women have completed the allotted time for exploring and getting established in the adult world. It is time to enter the "settling down" period that marks the culmination of early adulthood and produces final fruits (and thorns) of the period. The shift from the "age of thirty" transition to "settling down" is one of the crucial steps in adult development. This transitional period is set as beginning at thirty-two or thirty-three years of age and usually ending at forty or forty-one. Often a vague sense of uneasiness and depression accompanies this period. People ask, what is missing from my life and what parts of it must I change or give up in order to be fulfilled? Men and women often wonder whether they had committed themselves too soon to work or marriage. It is a time when one wonders again—have I chosen the right job? Have I attained my proper niche? Am I being appreciated or would I do better somewhere else? Both men and women harbor doubts of being properly appreciated at home and may even turn to an outside romantic interest. How often have we heard about the husband who became attracted to some lovely young lady, usually twenty-three or twenty-four, whom he encountered in his work and who thinks he is wonderful and even said he looks distinguished? For some, the middle years are even designated the dangerous years. Marriage problems may increase in intensity, and the question of separation or divorce is tossed about. The incidence of divorce is said to be greater between the ages of forty and forty-five than at any other time, except for the first two years of marriage. Oscar Wilde cogently described these dilemmas: "The gods have two ways of dealing harshly with us—the first is to deny us our dreams—the second is to grant them" (cited in Sammon, 1982, p. 19). Apparently, though, neither way is without its problems.

CONSEQUENCES OF YOUTH

Various studies of the middle aged indicate that despite the difficulties middle-aged persons encounter, they ordinarily exhibit mastery of their daily situations and for the most part demonstrate noteworthy qualities of resiliency. As part of growth, we become aware that as changes take place within us, inevitably there will be emotional and biological development keeping pace with the passage of time. Psychologically, physiologically, and emotionally, change is part of growing older, a phase which requires a medley of skills to meet the challenges. We may notice in middle age what we will find dramatically evident of old age, that our personal habits and tendencies have become sharpened, sometimes even to the point of caricature. Unfortunately, not everyone mellows with age. Sometimes when people remark that "he hasn't changed a bit," it is not intended as a compliment.

To a degree, all of us have shaped our own destiny, and it becomes more apparent in middle life. This shaping results from many things. It depends not only on a person's constitution, temperament, and endowment but also upon education, training, belief, and a whole welter of external forces. All of these things are involved in an individual's internal life and have much to do with values, ways of looking at him- or herself and at others. Other influences have to do with expectations, convictions, and prejudices and even the occasionally delusional thinking that may creep in unbidden. One's philosophy of life is quite important at this stage of life. In other words, both what we have done with the years and what the years have done to us are major determinants in how we handle our ease or unease in middle life.

BETWEEN PAST AND FUTURE

Crises will arise, of course; in the minds of some individuals they occupy themselves with what the future holds for them and their family. These concerns may bring with them a train of symptoms about which the physician hears. Much of the anxiety that arises is due to a restiveness. Suddenly everything in life seems turned around and topsy-turvy. Some individuals get depressed, and the consulting physician would do well to advise them against any drastic change, such as in business or marriage, until the anxious and depressive symptoms clear up.

In this interregnum between youth and old age, a great variety of morbid symptoms surfaces. Sammon (1968) places the next period of life-evaluation and changes at about age forty. "Early adulthood," he says, "is dying but the era of the middle adulthood has not yet arrived. The period between these two events, the midlife transition, is important in the life of every man and woman." The middle aged begin to become more aware of their own finiteness. Parents and friends may die; they note changes in themselves; and they sometimes lose zest for what they are doing.

Beyond this trying time of early middle age is the middle period, which goes on well into the sixties. The orientation in life shifts from past to future. One thinks now not of how long he or she has lived, but how many years are left. For some, it is a traumatic time. Some youthful dreams have to be given up; things have changed; some old friends, perhaps some family, have "dropped out"; new faces appear at the workplace or neighborhood. The question arises: what have I done with my dreams — what do I do now? In this period, the questions asked come thick and fast. Yet, for others it can be a most loving and most satisfactory and creative time. They are less tyrannized by ambition. Instinctual drives are not as strong as they were, but they are still there. This is not the last chance to change or to grow. Levinson (1978) says we can continue to work on our developmental tasks even through later transitional periods. He writes, "As long as life continues no period marks the end of the opportunities or the burden of further development."

Symptoms of midlife change that are referable to bodily systems may appear; these usually result from tension and anxiety. The patient, however, may interpret them as signs of serious physical disease and seek medical help. In the examination of the patient for these physical complaints, the family physician has an opportunity to be of service, not only to the patient but to the family as well. He or she can either treat the emotional symptoms or refer the patient to someone who will. The physician who knows the patient best, and the one whom the middle-aged or elderly patient trusts most, is the physician best suited to help in these circumstances.

DEPRESSION

More likely these tensions and anxieties, if left unchecked, can lead to neurotic illness in the form of mild or moderate depression. Symptoms may be vague, manifold, or ill-defined; they include fatigue, loss of interest in work, family, and friends, or widespread aches and pains. There may be irritability, heightened anger, and resultant feelings of insecurity. Sometimes the only symptoms of depression are peevishness, complaining, restlessness, and a tendency to useless overactivity; but often they are disturbing to family members, who see only the unrest and do not understand what underlies it. The sufferer casts a pall upon the household and the family suffers; the children make themselves scarce, and the spouse frequently becomes upset as well. There are few people to whom to appeal, unless the individual has some relationship with a minister, family physician, or close friends. But it is likely that in the withdrawal from society, the person has estranged him- or herself from all of them and would consider any efforts of theirs to help as interference.

SEXUAL ANXIETY

Certain physiological problems related to these emotional changes — like insomnia and sexual dysfunction — may become more apparent and even frequent, and these add to frustration and depression. Insomnia often accompanies times of stress; it can be the result of anger, guilt, overwork, or disappointment. Among the middle aged, early morning awakening is fairly common and may suggest some form of depression. The temptation to take various sleep-inducing drugs increases, but these medications may only complicate the condition and add to the depression. Though sexual relations in men and women continue into old age, the middle aged may notice a falling off of sexual desire and perhaps less than satisfactory performance. Such diminishing of sexual desire and performance becomes particularly worrisome for the male who equates his sexual ability with his masculinity. Generally, he should not get depressed about it, for much of the impotence of men in this age group is psychologically caused. Neugarten (1968) believes that the diminution of the male prowess (and the female responsiveness) results from repeated attempts at sex and from psychologic rather than biologic factors. She points to the boredom and the repeated attempts at sex, complicated by a preoccupation with thoughts of career or family pressures, by mental and physical fatigue, or by health concerns, particularly in the male.

DANGER OF DESPAIR

The emotional symptoms that arise in this period are often exaggerations of the individual's normal personality and a replaying of characteristics that were developed at a much earlier age. When these symptoms become severe and progress to the point where there is a break with reality, the individual is said to have a psychosis. Among women, because of the more apparent physical changes brought about by menopause, these emotional strains may be sharp; but they rarely lead to psychosis. Men do not experience a "menopause." The changes they undergo may be less striking, but certainly are noticeable.

If, however, such an emotional upset does take place, but is experienced as a gradual process, then very likely the individual has been able to accept the regressive changes that accompany the aging process. Yet in other individuals these emotional upsets can be very threatening and lead the individual to isolation. If at this time the person loses someone or something dear, he or she may worry and become depressed. The person may conclude that life is over. Physiologically, this may not be so; but psychologically, if his or her life was maintained by a strong emotional investment in the lost person or thing, then life may indeed be thought of as empty. In other situations, such as in a job, a person may experience the feeling of failure as something overwhelming. Old conflicts may revive; physical strength may decrease; the will to "continue the battle" may be lost. No matter what the precipitating cause, the resulting emotions may be those of depression and even despair. If the person blames others for his or her troubles, ideas of persecution are liable to eventuate into full-blown delusions. The individual directs inward upon the self the attention formerly taken up by a number of external interests, and this inward preoccupation may result in a hypochondria that disturbs the individual and those around him or her. If the person renounces friends and usual pleasures, such action only complicates matters.

The foregoing paragraphs offered general comments on the problems both men and women can expect to face in the middle years. The following sections suggest some of the more particular problems of women and men in middle age, the middle aged and the care of elderly family members or relatives, retirement, and the psychiatrist's and the minister's response to the middle aged.

Women in middle age

Not until 1950 did the United States census figures show definitely that most women as a group outlive men, although this idea had wide circulation in prior years. Since 1970, figures indicate that there are about 109 women to every 100 men in the population. Several factors help explain the change. Women have a biological advantage in outliving men, as many recent studies have shown. Cultural and social circumstances may also be favorable to women; for example, in middle age, women have fewer of the pressures and less of the tedious and limiting work of being a mother or homemaker. Medical advances, too, have increased women's chances of survival; fewer women now die in childbirth.

With this recognition that women live longer than men, there has been an independent and growing change in the attitudes toward women and their roles in American society. The "raising of consciousness" effected by the women's movement has allowed women to seek fulfillment in the professions and job market, in addition to choosing to be a mother and homemaker. On the whole, compared to even a generation ago, women enjoy more opportunities and have more options in choosing a lifestyle. If she is married, it is not surprising to find her husband engaging more in the care and raising of the children and in the housework (such behavior is not yet the norm, but it is a far cry from the day when the woman was confined to the house). Indeed, the greater number of women in the work force has altered traditional ideas about women and their abilities. Many can be found in responsible positions in business and industry; even such male bastions as airline pilots and astronauts are open to females. Women, even older women, are going back to college or furthering their education. More women than before work as lawyers and doctors. Thus, the picture for middle-aged women has changed markedly since World War II.

Yet despite these changes, women still must face the problems of transition into middle age. Professional women are finding that they are not exempt from the problems of the workplace that middle-aged men experience. Women like men have to deal with the workings of politics and favoritism, even in large corporations. They will see that rewards do not always go to the most capable, and that jealousy, backbiting, and at times even a touch of scandal present stressful situations of another sort. Those who have married, with a family and a successful home life, may find it easier to deal with these problems in middle age. Some young women, on the other hand, decide to make a place for themselves in business first and then raise a family later. However, gynecological studies show that women have much better chance of successful pregnancy before age thirty. In view of this, some women may decide to start a family first and then enter the ranks of the employed.

For a long time, the transition into middle age in women—the climacteric—was regarded as hazardous and depressive for all women. Up to a surprisingly recent time, the distress and symptoms of menopause which women showed were thought to be signs of involutional melancholia. That is, the woman grew depressed because of the loss of her role as mother at menopause. Earlier clinicians who thought this "melancholia" to be very real and distressing, conjectured that as much as 25 percent of the diagnosed involutional female population destroyed itself through suicide. It was blamed on "glandular changes," an idea that no longer holds credence in the profession. Other reasons for the depression included "waning of sexual attractiveness," "the empty-nest syndrome," and "husband's preoccupation in making a living."

To be sure, women regard the climacteric as a turning point in their reproductive lives and are aware that various endocrinologic changes are taking place within them. However, they no longer need to think of this change as a hazard. There may be some discomfort, generally not enough to require medical attention. There are, of course, some women who do mind the changes and some who do require medical help because of discomfort of hormonal change. But because of research in the aging process and of the middle aged and elderly, we are now better prepared to help women deal with this period more effectively.

Most women generally have a healthy concept of themselves and value their dignity in the scheme of things. If a woman had been brought up to cherish the idea and ideal of her own self-worth and guard her own prerogatives, she will continue to do so in middle age. But just as the male has his own set of fears and concerns about middle life, so too does the female. (Gaskill's discussion in this volume is helpful.) Some may feel that life at middle age has already poured out all it has to offer, and their personal importance is diminished. In these instances, there can be doubts about her self-worth, fear of old age, a decrease of responsibility now that the family is grown, and an increase in getting tired more often. They notice that the skin loses its youthful elasticity and that mucous flows less freely. Sexuality wanes, although today that change is nowhere near the dread it used to be. When it does occur, some other psychologically stressful situation usually triggers it, such as a strained family situation, boredom, or emotional exhaustion. Most women can handle these problems reasonably well, but those unable to cope may experience depressive symptoms. These symptoms, when associated with self-blame or missed opportunities, can definitely lead to anxiety and depression.

At this time, too, a woman may show increased concern about her partner's health, and the unwelcome prospect of a life alone may intrude into her thinking (the same is true for the husband who sees his wife's health beginning to fail). Widowhood requires a whole rearrangement of a woman's life, no matter whether such change is expected. (What is said here about the widow also pertains to the widower.) Becoming a single person again changes her whole social life considerably and presents her with a whole new social constellation. If she is attractive, women friends who feel insecure about their marriage may feel threatened by her new-found availability. In other social situations where couples tend to be the rule, she may be left out because she is single. The friends of her married life may not prove to be friends in her widowhood.

In some women the impact of a spouse's death lasts longer than is generally supposed. Somatic symptoms may accompany her grief, and these somatic problems may become significant. The recovery to normal life takes time; she (like the widower) needs to work through her grief. Efforts to cheer her up at this time may not always prove helpful. The young middle-aged widow may have a particularly difficult time in living through the mourning process. She still needs to raise the children, while trying to find her new identity. The way to help the bereaved is not to try to argue them out of their efforts at denial or escape from grief, but rather to encourage them to describe their feelings; otherwise, such feelings may develop into real emotional problems. One should be careful, however, of interfering or prying into her feelings and hesitations. Such close and personal counseling is better given by an intimate friend or a professional person.

Men in middle age

In addition to the noticeable physiological change, men in middle age also encounter psychological stress of a kind not experienced in earlier life. Stressful situations, particularly in the workplace, make adjustment during this transitional period difficult. These stresses may influence or be influenced by his home, family, and marital relationship and by his doubts about his self-image and masculinity as bodily changes take place. Illness, business reversals, rebuffs, disappointments with friends, failures of promotion, loss of face in business or in the community — any of these problems may threaten a man in middle life much more than they would have at an earlier time. He thinks that the years are moving too rapidly and jeopardizing his chance for correcting the reversals. Mild depression is not unusual under these circumstances. In the somberness of that depression, a man in middle life may fall into a period of self-analysis that may increase the depressive mood. He examines himself through the dark glasses of discouragement and perhaps acknowledges that he must settle for much less than what he once thought were essential objectives. Worse yet, he may find that he has achieved all his goals, yet only to realize that they are devoid of emotional satisfaction.

Much of this depression (and anxiety) may be related to his job. A man in middle age may become depressed after having been promoted to the top position in his business or profession. Finding himself alone at this dizzying height and afraid of losing his status and prestige, he becomes depressed and anxious. The very successful man of fifty may have accumulated along with his wealth so many obligations, offices, and memberships that he cannot get off the mad merry-go-round, even when he needs time off for the sake of his health. The moderately successful man, under the pressure of passing time, may drive himself (or his wife or confreres will pressure him) toward greater and greater accomplishments, only to place himself under greater strain and anxiety. Such a man, say psychiatrists, may develop anxieties about a son — or a symbolic son in the person of a young man — who threatens to displace him at home or in business. This kind of man has never resolved certain conflicts with his own parents and is therefore vulnerable in his role as an elder; even his relationships with business rivals and family members become sources of stress. The man of mediocre accomplishment is equally pressed. Fearing that his time is running out or his manhood is at stake, he may find it more necessary than ever to go out and prove, at least to his wife and family, that he is somebody important. His limited abilities may conspire against him; yet failure at this point is particularly bitter. He may also reach outside of his family for affirmation of his self-worth and estrange himself from what should be one of his greatest sources of satisfaction.

Situations at work may be especially difficult to bear, even though unpleasantness is encountered in all walks and at all times of life. These middle-aged men are scared, insecure, fearful that they will be slighted or that someone will get ahead of them—responses that are quite natural during this unpredictable time of life. Their behavior, however, may plague others and evoke hostility; they may make general nuisances of themselves. If permitted, they can even cause midlife crises for fellow workers.

Such anxious middle-aged men can be placed in different grades, from the benign to the malignant. The quiet ones, who believe everyone is against them but keep mainly to themselves, cause little trouble. In fact, many people in the workplace harbor a whole system of delusions, but they keep quiet and are of little trouble and don't bother anyone. It is the hostile ones who cause the trouble. They blame employers for discriminating against them for some unknown reason. Though often brilliant workers, these individuals sow dissension wherever they go. Their guard is always up—someone is always doing something to them—and their capacity for causing trouble is enormous. Figuratively, they get their teeth into something and will not let go. The basic reason underlying much of their reaction, sometimes unknown to themselves, is a desire to gain control. They think that once in control, all will be well for a while (maybe!). Yet, whoever these men are they should be treated with understanding, kindness, and patience. Of course, there may come a time when one needs to treat them with benign neglect and forebearance and to pay little attention to them. To be sure, their self-doubt and fears can become overwhelming to others at times.

In this trying phase of life, men (and women) will often increase their consumption of alcohol. In fact, it is often the first evidence of trouble in middle age. The stress they are experiencing makes excessive drinking easy and dangerous; one should not overlook such behavior too quickly. Alcoholism is a major problem nationally, and it is most widespread among men between ages thirty-three and fifty-five. It symptomizes underlying trouble. It reaches indiscriminately into the ranks of professional men just as it does into other groups. Most victims of alcoholism are anything but lazy. Many are talented and wonderful people when sober. Only recently, however, have we come to regard alcoholism as an illness that can be treated, instead of considering it evidence of moral weakness. We deal with it openly among professional men, in part because we know the havoc "industry's billion-dollar hangover" can inflict. Yet consequences reach beyond industry and professional life. The disease can break up a home as easily as it can lead to a loss of a job. The cure for alcoholism must come from the individual, who realizes that he needs help rather than denying his illness.

(Alcoholism among women is not a problem to be ignored. There are many cases of housewives who, bored during the day or incapable of handling the stress of raising children, will drink excessively. In addition, with more women entering the professions and competing with men for the top executive positions, they too are not wholly exempt from the strains that can lead to alcoholism.)

Elderly parents and relatives

Because people are living longer — the 1980 census tallies three times as many persons over age eighty-five and twice as many in the seventy-five to eighty-four age group than in 1970 — middle-aged men and women face the likelihood of caring for elderly parents and relatives. To be sure, the middle aged have always looked after the elderly, but never has it been so widespread in America. So, the middle aged must become aware of and sensitive to the plight of the elderly, if the relationship between them is to be meaningful and harmonious. Some families are fortunate to have several adults caring for the elderly. Yet how many times have we heard of bickering among these adults who try to shun their responsibility toward older parents or relatives. Such petty argument only exacerbates an already difficult situation.

The care of elderly parents and relatives involves specific medical, housing, and economic aspects. But it is a situation also entwined with deep emotions: anxiety, guilt, confusion, pleasant and unpleasant memories. Isolated parents, especially if their partner has died, are especially troubled. For example, husbands who have been so long dependent upon their wives have a particularly hard time. Fiercely independent and proud, some will not venture to ask for any help, let alone welfare aid. Middle-aged offspring of such elderly parents may experience confusion and even denial of the aging process before them. Instead of showing patience, care, and real demonstrations of love, many such individuals consider elderly parents and relatives to be hindrances and interruptions in their own busy lives.

Barely a decade ago it was customary to hand the elderly over to "rest homes," where a professional staff could look after them like dependents. Their children would make occasional visits, more from a sense of duty than from real concern. Fortunately, the new sensitivity in gerontology, especially as pioneered by Elizabeth Kubler-Ross and the hospice movement, has reminded the middle aged that the elderly are still entitled to their dignity and a fullness of life. It is encouraged that the elderly be kept at home, among familiar surroundings and the people who are dear to them. Such an arrangement does impose some real burdens upon the middle aged. To be sure, these responsibilities can lead to more stress, in addition to the ones they have to cope with in their own transitional period. There are no simple answers. Some public services, such as "Meals on Wheels," "Mother's Helpers," and other programs, can ease some of the work. But nothing can take the place of companionship and personal care in affirming these elderly at this last phase of life.

Thoughts of retirement

Only a couple years ago people looked forward to retiring at age sixty-five. The mandatory retirement age is now seventy. Whether it comes at sixty-five or seventy, retirement marks an entry into a new phase of life. Some anticipate it as a time to relax and to do things, like traveling, that they never did because of work. But retirement can also be a painful time. After the initial novelty of not having to work wears off, some retirees will get fidgety because they have run out of things to do: they get bored. They no longer have the support of the workplace to keep them busy. So, all the strengths and weaknesses in the personality—the same strengths and weaknesses that were there before retirement—percolate to the surface. And very few of these traits disappear in old age.

If the retiree faces this period without an agenda or a positive attitude, loneliness—and its accompanying anxieties—can creep in and cause real problems for the individual. Loneliness often lurks under the unspoken fear of oncoming old age. One often hears the plaintive statement that a person feels lonely; it is probable that everyone has experienced this feeling at one time or another. It is a strange and paradoxical phenomenon. While the monk alone in his cell is not lonely, the individual in the midst of a crowd is often wretchedly so. Our aloneness sometimes is coupled with feelings of emptiness, and both, in the last analysis, represent a form of basic anxiety.

Admiral Richard Byrd (1938) on one occasion wrote a note in his diary that expresses dramatically the sensations of loneliness that can assail individuals in all age groups: "Something I don't know what, is getting me down. This would not seem important if I could put my finger on the trouble, but I can't find a single thing to account for the mood. Yet, it has been here and tonight for the first time I must admit that the problem of keeping my mind on even keel is a serious one." And then, soon after, he wrote that he was conscious only of the solitude of his own forlornness, and added: "This morning I had to admit to myself that I was lonely. Try as I may, I find I can't take my loneliness casually. It is too big. But I must not dwell upon it; otherwise I am undone."

Though women and men in middle life rarely experience loneliness so intensely, the admiral's thoughts are worth pondering, for they indicate that sometimes the vague unrest which all of us experience may be due to an unrecognized and unwelcome form of existential loneliness. It is said that its conquest can be accomplished by all who are willing to find and destroy two underlying obstacles: self-love and hostility. Both make it impossible to communicate properly with people in the environment and render it difficult for us to see or feel a real relationship with others.

This brings us to a brief consideration of the necessity of keeping our lines of communication with friends and family open. Sometimes there is a temptation to cut them because of fancied hurt or slight or even a real disappointment. This is an extremely important matter, for it has to do with one's relationship with adolescents, family members, older age-groups, fellow workers, and friend and foe alike. Communication is the thread that relates us to others, and once it is impeded or broken off in anger, hurt, or obvious neglect, our chances of reaching agreement or continuing relationships with others is impeded.

The minister's role

It is assumed that the minister who is called upon to deal with the problems in question has some knowledge of counseling techniques and of both the good that can be accomplished in the counseling role and the dangers that accompany it. Therefore, a few comments about the pitfalls of treating distressed people in the middle age group conclude this essay.

Depressed people are at times potentially suicidal, and the risk of suicide is increased in the middle and older age groups. Failures seem to be especially poignant, and the possibility of recouping losses or rearranging one's life seems almost negligible. Many of the problems that arise in middle life are not beyond help, but if the person involved believes them to be, the situation is just as serious as if they were truly beyond all assistance. Therefore, if the person is brought to the minister by a family member—he or she will rarely seek help alone—the minister must determine whether the situation is beyond his or her competence.

One cannot assume that because the patient is religious, he or she is automatically protected against suicide; a person who becomes sick, hopeless, or depressed enough is no longer capable of acting according to earlier beliefs. If there is any question of suicide, or if the counselor thinks there is any possibility of it, expert opinion should be sought even if family or patient protests. Current professional opinion holds that depressive illnesses are treatable and that some forms of therapy seem to be particularly efficacious. In the past, these patients in the middle age group were sick for periods of eight months to three years, and only 50 percent of them were destined to recover; illnesses in the involutional period were wretched and worrisome to all concerned. Patients in these age groups seemed to suffer more than those in other categories. Now, fortunately, approximately 90 percent of them recover with appropriate therapy and, if hospitalized, can usually return to their families within a period of six weeks to two months.

Our population is increasing, and more people now live long enough to acquire the illnesses of middle life. Undoubtedly some of these distressed people will consult the family doctor or the minister, for these professionals are the first line of defense against mental disorder. The way in which they handle the problem will determine the individual's future. Surveys indicate that 42 percent of the people who seek outside help with their problems first consult a minister. Working within his or her own province, the minister can provide relief for many individuals whose sufferings are caused by difficult life-situations and problems with work, school, marriage, or personality adjustment. Intelligent counseling often helps to clear up these so-called environmental difficulties. The minister qualified to give such help has an understanding of the motivations, actions, and reactions of others that is based on a solid foundation of self-understanding and a genuine desire to help. He or she also knows when to refer someone for professional psychiatric care.

While the minister is deciding whether an individual is to be taken into counseling or referred elsewhere, the general rules of good counseling hold. A relationship must be established; this is the basis for all helping situations. The minister must listen carefully, giving necessary time and displaying interest, patience, and a willingness to help. Tolerance and acceptance are necessary; condemnation, moralizing, criticizing, and blaming are to be avoided, for any of these negative attitudes is bound to put an end to the relationship. The counselor's attitude should be one of quiet confidence that avoids a promise of quick or miraculous solutions to problems. The realistic benefits of counseling, and its limitations, should be set forth as honestly and as objectively as possible.

Depressed individuals frequently maintain attitudes of hopelessness and self-condemnation; often these reach delusional proportions. Attempting to argue these individuals out of delusional ideas is a useless venture, no matter how silly or obviously wrong they may be. These ideas are not amenable to reason; they are emotional in nature and are beyond rationality. Such efforts only result in the counselor's feeling exhausted and hopeless.

Centuries ago Cicero wrote that people who have no resources in themselves for securing a good and happy life find every age burdensome. To this we may add: It is the failure to recognize or to deal satisfactorily with our emotional problems that is the cause of symptoms in middle life, rather than defects in our hormones or glandular secretions; it is our unfortunate neurotic accretions, rather than our internal secretions. This is a good thing to know, for it indicates the proper method of attack on these problems and the possibilities of their solution.

Ralph Barton Perry, in his *Plea for an Age Movement,* suggests that life is a continuum of awakening to the attainment of greater heights of human excellence. And he offers us the following valuable philosophy:

> Whether a man shall live toward the past or toward the future, is for him to decide; and he can change his mind as often or as late as he likes. Time extends in both directions, and neither is ever closed. Let us, therefore, consider every anniversary as the opening of a new chapter, rather than as the closing of an old, and our many years gone by as an accumulated capital to invest in the years to come.

REFERENCES

Byrd, Richard E. *Alone.* New York: G. F. Putnam, 1938.

Levinson, Daniel et al. *Seasons of a Man's Life.* New York: Alfred A. Knopf, 1978.

Neugarten, Bernice. *Middle Age and Aging.* Chicago: The University of Chicago Press, 1968.

Perry, Ralph Barton. *Plea for an Age Movement.* New York: Vanguard Press, 1942.

Sammon, Sean. *Human Development* 3(1):15, 1982.

8

Emotional Problems of Aging

FRANCIS J. BRACELAND

It is vanity to desire a long life without caring whether
it be a good life or not.

—Thomas à Kempis

W ere a text needed for a dissertation on longevity, one would do
well to consider an observation from the *Gateway to Great Books:*

Amid the uncertainties of life, this much is certain—whoever lives long
enough will grow old. Whoever grows old will first grow older, and whoever
lives to sixty or seventy will be old much longer than he is young. What
follows from this succession of obvious certainties is the common sense conclusion that we should prepare ourselves for all of life and not just the part
that passes fastest.

What is implied also is, if we are to attain longevity, we must first go
through the process of aging and remain for a considerable period in the
senescent state. *Senescence* is a gentle term; no other word in English so
aptly designates the normal process of aging. Unlike the term *senile,* it is
not pejorative and yet it marks the passage of time. "Senile" and
"senility" have such a ring of finality to them, often unjustifiably. We are
better off without using these terms except on few occasions.

Who are the elderly? We make a mistake when we think of the elderly
as a homogeneous group, for they are not. Some are rich and some are
poor; some are sick and some are well; and most of them fall somewhere

in between. Psychological and social pressures weigh heavily upon them, as they struggle vainly to retain roles beyond their competence and are denied them for various reasons. Sources of gratification evaporate, yet personality needs are as strong as ever; they flow through channels cut long before. The rigidity traditionally associated with old age is, in part, an expression of the need to maintain a world that used to be — a world in which self-esteem, satisfaction, and relative mastery of the environment occurred at least some of the time. Inflexibility and a rigid life-routine are sometimes adopted as defenses against this existential anxiety.

Writers have rarely been kind to the elderly. Sir Walter Scott "saw old men counting their youthful follies o'er till memory lends her light no more." I prefer the modern writers, like Henri Nouwen who sees old age as the gradual fulfillment of the life cycle, in which receiving matures in giving and living makes dying worthwhile:

> Aging does not need to be hidden or denied, but can be understood, affirmed and experienced as a process of growth in which the mystery of life is slowly revealed to us. Without the elderly we might forget that we are aging. The elderly are our prophets — they remind us that what we see so clearly in them is a process we all share.

Why do people get old?

There are numerous theories concerned with the process of aging, and wherever there are numerous theories it means no one really knows. Ewald Busse discussed the subject at length at a 1982 meeting of the American College of Psychiatry and reviewed those theories he thought to be worthy of continuing attention. There are too many to detail here. We can mention only a few. There is the exhaustion theory in which an organism is thought to have only a fixed store of energy which runs down. There is a theory of the accumulation of deleterious material. There is a theory of aging consisting of a deliberate biologic programming, which he thought a possibility. Then there is also a theory that when a cell divides some of the cells are committed to senescence. He spoke also of psychologic theories (several of them quite involved) and social theories such as the disengagement theory. Immunologic theories also have come under consideration. Of particular interest, he said, is the relationship between the onset of acquired disease, the influence of social stresses, and the importance of life-styles.

In discussing the neuropathology of the elderly brain, Busse mentioned several findings of interest. One of the earliest which continues to hold significance is the gradual loss of neurons, with accumulating evidence that this loss is not evenly distributed throughout the brain. In addition, the body's immune system may falter. Two age-related lesions most frequently assumed to be major causes of senile dementia are neurofibrillary changes and senile plaques. Also a fairly new important observation is the sevenfold increase in aluminum in the brains of patients with Alzheimer's Disease. One cannot tell as yet whether this large amount of aluminum is a primary contributing factor or whether it accumulates as a secondary phenomenon. It is even speculated that large amounts of antacids used for gastric distress might be in some way dangerous because they often contain aluminum hydroxide. At present all of this is in the stage of conjecture.

Regardless of what the cause of aging is thought to be, several things are certain. At some point in life the tissues and energy reserves cease to expand; a maximal development is reached, and then a gradual decline. Somewhere between the point of maximal expansion and the final end point, there is a period that denotes the onset of old age. This period is poorly marked and uncertain, and often it is determined by the observer, by the measuring rod used, or by the purpose of the evaluation. Thus the deciding factor may be the degree of tissue degeneration, the industrial usefulness, or even the psychological or sociofamilial attitudes operative in the culture, rather than the exact chronologic age of the person.

Other certain essential functions of human beings are shaped by external events, and certain phases of senescence can be provoked and hastened by social forces; by loss of security, material or emotional; by isolation; or by feelings of uselessness. Only too frequently elderly persons find themselves exiled from the satisfactions of earlier years to a gray sort of no-man's land, alone, misunderstood, and misunderstanding. In few branches of medicine are the biological, social, psychological, and pathological factors seen to be so sensitively attuned as they are in the emotional and the mental disorders of old age. Although physicians and ministers have had little to do with the social or economic segments of the problem, medicine as a discipline has had much to do with the adding of years to human life.

Physiologically there occurs a gradual impairment of homeostatic capacities in older individuals, along with degenerative tissue changes. Emotional pressures in themselves play a part in the breakdown of homeostasis, for emotions, as well as toxins, can become psychonoxious. Old age is a time of unusual emotional stress. One by one the props of individual security vanish. The body image is distorted; the whole physical machine begins to sputter. The satisfactions of work and independence are missing now, and the individual feels lost in a seemingly purposeless, hectic world. Companions of a lifetime are removed from the scene, and the imminence of one's own exit may incite fear, rebellion, or even despair.

Dealing with old age

Though many elderly persons seem to carry on as though nothing has happened and seem not to feel the pressures of age, yet psychological and social pressures of necessity weigh heavily upon them as they struggle to retain roles not always within their competence. Some are denied them simply because they are old.

Centuries ago Hippocrates wrote that it was change, especially great change, that was responsible for disease. Since then other sages have confirmed that marked change in the culture and environment demands new adaptive measures, and disease often is a consequence of failure of adaptation. It is hardly necessary to recall that the elderly do not take kindly to rapid change or to new situations, and with their vital supports weakened by age and by rapid changes in the present culture, large numbers of them are cast adrift in their own forlornness. Growing old today presents one of the most difficult tasks in human development. Human nature sometimes seems to rebel against what appears to be a dethronement of people in aging. Some never accept it; they fight it and eventually some succumb to bitterness and hang on as grouchy citizens. Today's changes are deep and all-pervasive and proceeding more rapidly than ever before. It is as if a whole new culture is forming. Much of what the older age group believed in, held dear, and was sustained by has been challenged and altered.

Frustration, disappointment, insecurity, organic impairment — all such factors give rise to anxiety and each reinforces the others. Unless the personality retains sufficient integration to cope with the difficulties of aging and enough compensations are available to make up for the inevitable losses, morbid behavior may evidence itself. Shorn of prestige, bereft of old landmarks to adaptation, aging individuals may be prone to distort the environment in which they live. The environment does not take kindly to this. Intolerance begets intolerance, and the social climate may actually become as hostile as individuals have imagined it to be. As their problems increase, so do their incapacities. Evidences of senile change then begin to show themselves.

It has been noted that the roles in which older people have most to contribute, if they have negotiated the previous phases of their life cycle successfully, stand at the top of the social development scale. They are roles that meet the broadest problems of adjustment and orientation and in which wisdom should be a premium. Elders have contributions to make, not only in intellectual circles but also in areas requiring the rapidly dwindling skills of equanimity, grace, and manners.

Rejection

As far as this present culture is concerned, old people are no longer in the stream of things; it is youth and the potentialities of the future that monopolize people's attention. Older citizens are often actually impelled to draw into themselves, and this, unfortunately, often tends to fix attention upon one's physical health and to slip easily into psychosomatic disorders. Unconsciously there is hope that through symptoms and suffering they will receive the sympathy and attention that otherwise would not be accorded them. Even elementary attention and psychotherapy are of help here, providing they accompany real human interest. Other patients in this group react rather badly; they are those of a more introverted nature, for this lends itself more easily to isolation. The denouement of this type of reaction is a ferocious narcissism that might easily lead to a break of all ties with reality. Thus, the elderly may find themselves in a group poorly understood and resented, although this attitude is usually hidden beneath a superficial veneer of solicitude for the group's welfare. They are often pitied, but without real sympathy and feeling, by the younger age groups.

The fear of being unable to take care of oneself and of becoming a burden to others is a phobia ever present in the minds of many people because, as a consequence of it, they hazard social rejection and consequent loss of their own self-respect. Unfortunately, some rejection of the elderly is due to an unconscious fear that old age will be the eventual lot of the rejector — this also lies behind some of the rejection of the mentally ill. Some of the social rejection has an esthetic basis, for age sometimes brings with it a loss of social graces and carelessness in various spheres. Some of this is anything but lovely, and the hostility that these characteristics engender is not always disguised. The consequent reaction only serves to drive the individual more and more into self-centered, irritable, and restless modes of behavior.

The attitudes of society are even magnified in the specific family situation, where the resentment is enhanced by propinquity and is reinforced by feelings of guilt. Very real and practical problems confront the children who are sheltering these aged people, but the ramifications of these relationships are too involved to explore in detail here. The way in which the grandparent is shoved about is common knowledge, as is the way the children take turns as sitters and keep a watchful eye on each other. One knows, too, of bitter quarrels between husband and wife, and how marriages are threatened and sometimes broken by the continued presence of an aged parent. There is no secret, either, about the emotional disharmony that may be rekindled on the basis of ancient conflicts between the aged parent and the son or daughter who is now providing the home. Long-smoldering resentment over happenings far in the past may goad the children into domineering and hostile attitudes, with consequent quarrels, tears, and hurt feelings.

Parents relinquish unwillingly positions of dominance once held in the family, and this frequently incites clashes of opinion. At the same time aged parents have the universal need for love and acceptance, and when they become aware of familial rejection, they respond with a reaction pattern designed to reestablish inner security. This may take the form of temper tantrums or other attention-seeking behavior, or in other cases the aged person may adopt aggressive behavior to make sure that he or she is not overlooked. These efforts failing, depression, illness, discouragement, or complete isolation are all that are left. Suicidal gestures, or even successful suicide, may be next.

Encouraging signs

Before dealing with a number of the psychological problems — from simple rejection to serious psychoses — that the elderly may experience, it should be noted that the aging process, or growing old, is not as bleak as some would like to believe. There are many evidences that society as a whole is becoming much more sensitive to the elderly. For example, the new interest in the problem of aging is one advance, along with the general acceptance that aging in itself is not a disease process and not all mental or emotional symptoms that individuals evidence in the later years denote senility. We find that most of the emotional illnesses encountered are not irreversible. Many of the symptoms, were they evidenced by members of the younger age groups, would be carefully traced down and treated, while among older individuals they are often "shucked off" and dismissed as being due to "their age." The fact that depression and acute confusional states in addition to acute brain syndrome all are treatable and reversible is missed unless the patient falls into sophisticated medical hands.

In addition, a basic issue such as the part aging rather than disease plays in effecting intellectual change has become increasingly open to question. As a result, one should always consider functional or acute organic processes as causes of intellectual changes, particularly those of recent onset. The work of E. Busse and his group several decades ago was one of our first encouraging reports. Eisdorfer, one of his colleagues, put it succinctly when he reported: "We studied a sample of people between the ages of sixty and sixty-nine and we fully expected that their intelligence would drop off after ten years. But with one notable exception their intelligence after ten years was undiminished." It is apparent, therefore, that while aging is associated with various losses, older people can indeed learn. One must admit, however, that many would be hesitant about putting their learning abilities to test in Madison Square Garden.

As to memory, that bête noire of aging, there is encouraging news there too. Some observers conclude that, contrary to the prevailing stereotype, the inevitable decline of memory with age as a clinical symptom is a complex phenomenon in older persons in which complaint must be differentiated from performance. Complaints, they say, can occur with or without an actual deficit in memory. Impairment on memory tests was, as would be expected, strongly associated with evidence of organic brain dysfunction. In some instances persons who complained about memory actually functioned better than those who did not complain.

Nor should mild depression hinder the enjoyment of living. Many of the cognitive symptoms exhibited by the elderly are due to varying degrees of depression. There now is a whole host of antidepressants available to the physician, which could prove to be a boon to individuals, especially if the drugs are accompanied by skillful psychotherapeutic efforts. (It is my belief, however, that drugs should be used sparingly and monitored frequently.)

There are many other advances being made in the treatment of the emotional and psychological problems of the aged. Many of them reflect the sensitivity that the elderly are human beings who also need attention, care, and love. The more we are aware of the range of illnesses unique to the elderly, the better we can respond to them. Thus, it is useful to explore how the elderly react to rejection, retirement, the aging process, illnesses, and psychoses.

Jobs and retirement

The aged find that the modern economic and industrial technological schemes have no place for them. With the exception of some skilled trades and professions, it is extremely difficult for a worker over the age of forty to find a new job. Thus, many men and women are often discarded vocationally and rendered economically impotent and unproductive by factors beyond their control. There are other important implications in having a job, aside from the financial security it affords. The individual is given prestige in his or her own eyes and a feeling of social approval. There is a feeling of having a place in the busy work-a-day world, and sometimes this affirmation is even more important than financial return. The loss of this ability to contribute and earn respect demeans an individual in his or her own estimation.

There is a great deal of pressure in labor and in industry to get rid of the older worker, and now retirement is one of the poignant facts of life. Numerous plans are in operation — some of them intricate — to soften the blow. Psychologically it is still a blow, no matter how well prepared one is for it. Separation, anxiety at first, and depression later are frequent concomitants to the cutting off of an individual from a job that was considered his or her own, no matter how much he or she may have complained about it. Some adapt to retirement willingly; more do so unwillingly; and some not at all. The first group is blessed; the middle group constitutes the irritable and the difficult; and the third group contributes to the ranks of the depressed.

Retired persons gradually bereft of the companionship of old friends and coworkers characteristically become lonesome, complaining, and self-centered and may make excessive demands on children, physicians, and ministers. This is well recognized and the efforts of prophylaxis — mental hygiene if you will — are important and should have been begun beforehand. One should retire to something, for a retired person retains all of one's attributes, foibles, joys, and sorrows. No one can pass from an all-consuming way of life to one of inactivity without emotional repercussions.

The manifest illnesses

Except in isolated instances, it is improbable that the common stresses of aging will in themselves precipitate abnormal emotional reactions in individuals who previously have shown satisfactory and stable personality patterns. Rather, people who develop psychiatric problems in later life are usually those who had difficulties of adjustment earlier. Statistical information is lacking on the incidence of neurotic or psychotic phenomena in the second and third decades in patients who develop severe reactions later on. Nevertheless, careful investigation reveals that the actual emotional breakdown has been preceded not uncommonly over a period of years by changes in the personality. These changes

usually are in the nature of accentuation of certain personality characteristics. For instance, careful examination of the history of an individual
with a senile paranoid reaction may show a pre-morbid personality in
which the suspiciousness and tendency to blame others for troubles have
been evident long before there was any sign of the onset of a psychosis.
The beginning indications of the paranoid make-up are extreme sensitivity with false interpretation of events, exaggeration of minor offenses
to the degree that they are considered deliberate insults, complaints, false
evaluation of the individual's assets, and a poor capacity for adaptation.
There is a tendency to blame others for causing disappointments and
failures, and even minor stresses may intensify the basic insecurity of
these individuals, so that primitive defenses are called forth. It is only
when there is a certain amount of systematization of these false interpretations and occurrence of outright false accusations against others
that the presence of a psychiatric disorder is suspected. Occasionally, the
initial symptom directing attention to the condition is an aggressive out-
burst that appears completely inappropriate to the existing situation.

As is apparent in the neuroses and psychoses of earlier life, the particular clinical syndromes that appear may be correlated with the types of
personality patterns of the individuals in question. Thus, agitated depressions occur in the obsessive, rigid, inelastic individuals who have trouble
adapting to changing conditions. Manic reactions occur in persons who
have severe mood swings; paranoid individuals become delusional.
Needless to say, among all of them there is considerable overlapping due
to varied shades of accentuation in personality make-up, just as there is
in youth. The importance of cerebral impairment in this picture lies, not
in the specific personality changes arising from specific lesions, but in the
reduction of the individual's capacity to adapt and to deal with stresses.

Strangely, the diagnostic picture may appear differently in a different
light. Some patients with early cerebral damage may simply become
more adaptable, and their general improvement is marked by a lessening
of hostility and aggression, with an increased acceptance of dependency
needs. True enough, as they become more tractable, there occur minor
defects in judgment, increased insomnia, and a train of lesser symptoms.
But the overall effect is that they can be cared for at home rather than
banished to large hospitals.

Etiologic factors

Diagnosis of emotional disorders in the elderly is difficult in the early
stages because older people are more liable to somatic illness, not only
because of lowered resistance but also because of acceleration of progres-

sive biological changes that are part of the normal aging process. Neurologic changes produce decline in the cognitive functions almost universally and, indeed, as indicated by intelligence tests, this decline (which may start as early as the thirties) progresses slowly until the late fifties and then accelerates. Tests for organic deterioration provide a measure of the individual's loss of abilities. The functions examined by the various tests include memory, learning, comprehension, judgment, the ability to make inferences and to elaborate, and the speed and accuracy of performance. In the older person, in addition to actual impairment of abilities, there is a diminution of perception and of execution that militate against achieving scores once within his or her power.

By their thirties most individuals have established a way of life in which they are settled and a type of work in which they gain increasing experience, so that they are equipped to deal with most situations of a stressful nature that they are likely to meet. In adult life most people function within ranges that enable the achievement of normal adjustment, and they are hopefully pursuing the attainment of the aims and goals that were set up as representing security, gratification, and satisfaction during their adolescence. With the early fifties, however, comes the reckoning, and this is extremely important. With the realization of advancing age, the questions that were so troublesome in adolescence have to be answered: Have those objectives that had previously seemed desirable been attained, and are they indeed as attractive as they then appeared? These questions may be posed consciously or unconsciously—in the realm of work, in the realm of the home, and in the realm of the community.

As individuals move into the seventh decade, they are faced with further manifestations of biological change and perhaps with radical alterations in social and economic status. Such problems as increasing competition with younger rivals, threats to economic independence, enforced retirement with fundamental changes in routine, and lack of anything to replace lifelong patterns are intensified. Further threats are the changing values of the times, a decrease in authority and prestige, the loss of friends by death—and thus a narrowing circle of companions and peers, increasing loneliness and isolation, a growing feeling of uselessness, and fears of invalidism and of dependency on others. Aware of the loss of physical capacity and with a growing realization of inadequacy in mental performance, individuals are called upon to deal with these factors of major significance at a time when their biological structure is becoming less efficient and less able to deal with change.

The part played by malnutrition and lack of essential vitamins in the production of senile conditions, particularly in the delirious states, is still unsettled. Treatment with large doses of vitamins, as recommended by some investigators, has not uniformly achieved the results desired. Nevertheless, many old people have over prolonged periods allowed their diet to become monotonous and inadequate, and the resulting malnourishment may render them more liable to acute disturbances. This is especially true when the individual is exposed to additional stress. Thus, acute delirious conditions sometimes occur in old people following the fracture of a large bone and subsequent immobilization.

Defense against, and symptoms of, illness

It is known that among the early signs of senescence are lapses of memory. Not only may there be failure to recall recent events, new acquaintances, etc., but sometimes the initial symptom recognized by the patient is the inability to recall the name of someone with whom he or she is relatively familiar. Great care must be taken, however, to differentiate a pathological memory loss from the lapses of memory which are due to defects of attention—the lot of most of us at various times. These latter lapses result since the name or event was never actually registered or was registered only marginally because attention was directed elsewhere.

Mistakes in judgment and a certain carelessness in detail are common in early senescence, and there may be less acute appreciation of the problem or the topics under discussion. Individuals may be aware of an increasing tendency for conversation to wander, with a trend toward circumlocution. It is said that as we get older, our bodies get shorter and our anecdotes get longer. Whether or not individuals are aware of these failings may have some effect on their status. Such failings are noticed by others, whose reaction in turn may lead to responses of a defensive nature. The threat to the security of self-esteem may be met by either a conservative or an aggressive reaction; that is, persons may withdraw from all situations that are likely to make difficulties obvious, or they may seek out occasions in order to try themselves out. Successful handling of the problem proves to them, at least, that the defects are nonexistent.

Some of the manifestations of the effort to maintain the status quo may be a narrowing of interests, a staunch adherence to methods and patterns long familiar, a rigidity of outlook, and suspiciousness of change. There is, consequently, an overevaluation of the past and an increasing depreciation of the present. Daily activities become more and more restricted and more routine. Further, there may be accentuation of the characteristic modes of reaction, so that any threat to the life system will produce a response greater than that merited by the stimulus: irritability, loss of temper, hasty statements that may be regretted, rash decisions, and insomnia. All of these increase and provoke still greater insecurity, so that more overt anxiety may be engendered.

The basis of the aggressive type of defense is essentially a denial of loss. With consciousness of the decline in one or more spheres of power—whether in competition with young rivals at work, in sexual activity, or in any area where gratification is sought—an attempt is made by the elderly to prove to themselves and to others that they are as able as ever. Tasks requiring physical strength, endurance, or superior performance may be undertaken by individuals in competition with members of the family or colleagues at work. Even if this aggressiveness does not achieve conscious and overt expression, however, it may result in anxiety manifested in somatic or mental symptoms. Likewise, the sexual drives, giving rise to fantasies, conflicts, and unacceptable sexual activity, may produce guilt and anxiety, all the more so because the culture in which we live tends to deprecate even normal sexual activity in elderly persons.

Somatization of anxiety, i.e., the reflection of anxiety in physical symptoms, may occur in any of the physiological systems, with complaints of palpitation, breathlessness, tremors of the head and extremities, loss of appetite, indigestion, aerophagy (gulping air and belching), constipation or diarrhea, headaches, frequency of urination, insomnia, etc. The mental symptoms may include such complaints as loss of power of concentration, feelings of tension and nervousness, or feelings of impending danger. Not only may there be lack of desire to leave the home or to undertake normal activities, but there may also be actual fears of going into streets, of crowds, of subways, etc. These phobias are thought to represent the inadequate resolution of conflicts in which sexual or aggressive drives are unsatisfactorily repressed, and the object or situation represents occasions in which there may be temptation to gratify these drives—the person who fears to leave the house may actually fear going to some "forbidden" place.

Illnesses a little more serious

In the conditions mentioned so far, the individual is still relating to the environment, but if there is loss of opportunity for gratification or if there are feelings of aimlessness and lack of purpose, the aged person may completely withdraw and focus attention on the self, thus engendering hypochondriacal symptoms. Whereas in anxiety states there are somatic accompaniments of anxiety, in hypochondriasis no evidence can be found upon medical examination to justify the intense preoccupation with bodily function. The most common focus is on the gastrointestinal tract, with emphasis on eating, digestion, and bowel function. It has been suggested that the factor responsible for this is not only the impairment of the physiological functions involved but also a regressive psychological defense by which gratification is sought on the infantile level. However, any system may be the center of hypochondriacal symptoms, and the medical practitioner may be called upon to deal with complaints of disorders of the excretory, cardiovascular, respiratory, or musculoskeletal systems. There may be complaints of general fatigue, representing loss of adequate motivation and of interest in external objects. Characteristic of these conditions is the self-concern, the egocentric preoccupation of the patient and, with due allowance for the age of the individual, an absence of sufficient evidence of physical disease to account for the symptoms.

Hypochondriasis in pure form, without evidence of marked alteration in mood, is frequently encountered; but simple neurotic depression and severe psychotic melancholia also occur just as frequently in the older age group, and the differentiation can be extremely difficult. Therefore, when the opinion has been reached that the source of the physical complaints is not physical in origin, special attention must be directed to the possible presence of depression. Dissatisfied with the life they envisage before them, deprived of their self-esteem, and consciously or unconsciously holding themselves responsible for their failure, aging persons are liable to develop conditions in which self-destructive tendencies are prominent.

In general, patients are aware of being sad, but one must nevertheless be alert for those occasions when no complaints of depression are made and when careful inquiries are necessary to elicit its presence. Such conditions, if allowed to progress, may develop all the signs of psychotic depression with hypochondriacal delusions, marked anxiety and agitation, delusions of degradation in the spheres of health, wealth, and worth, and intense feelings of guilt as a result of which self-destruction becomes a sacrifical expiation.

A special clinical picture during later life which appears to be confined to individuals in the higher executive class is the development of depressive reactions in those who, judged by the normal worldly standards, have recently attained success, such as promotion in their occupations, and in whom one would expect to find contentment and satisfaction. The psychodynamics of these depressions include such factors as heightened fears of inadequacy attendant upon increased responsibility, feelings of being out alone with no one to depend upon, and consequent mixed feelings about the position achieved. Such personalities have long been driven to seek the success that symbolizes for them the final resolution of insecurity, only to find the search has been in vain. This presents an area for research in the field of industrial psychiatry in terms of recognition of the types of personality best suited for the very highest level of executive direction and of those that perform most efficiently in less exalted positions.

The psychoses and therapy

The most serious of the emotional illnesses facing the elderly are the psychoses. The considerable variation in the relative incidence of arteriosclerotic and senile conditions, as revealed by the figures from different hospitals, illustrates the difficulty of present-day classifications. As an etiological factor, it is probable that arteriosclerosis has been too greatly emphasized. Classically, these illnesses present a fairly well-defined clinical picture commencing as early as the fifth decade. There is a history of headaches, twitching, dizziness, prickly sensations, or other somatic symptoms accompanied by the general feelings of ill health. However, until a major episode — epileptic, fainting, or convulsive — ensues, there are few essentially psychiatric symptoms.

In some institutions the diagnosis of arteriosclerotic dementia is not made unless there is focal evidence of cerebral damage. Subsequent to the attack, some improvement is noted; however, more episodes follow, after each of which the level of improvement attained is less than that prior to the attack. Dating from the attack, there may appear any of the functional features indicated earlier — anxiety states, hypochondriasis, depressive reactions, confused episodes, paranoid outbursts, fluctuations of mood, etc. Physicians are quite familiar with the irritability, anxiety, or depression experienced by hitherto very active individuals when, following illness or operation involving parts of the body other than the head, they become dependent on others for all their needs. Functional symptoms in such patients arise as the reactions to the impairment of function, to the threat of life, and to the fears of dependency that physical illness entails.

The roles of the minister and the physician in the care of the elderly with emotional problems are well delineated. Ministers are well acquainted with their role as "physicians of the soul." They were bringing comfort and solace to the aged and their families for generations before psychiatry got into the act. It is they whom the family will call upon for almost everything except obvious medical matters. It would be fatuous for a clinician to discuss the minister's role with him or her. It might be helpful, however, to outline what possibilities for therapy are open to the physician and how on occasions the minister can help. Both roles are essential, each in its place. If the efforts of physician and minister can be coordinated, it will benefit the patient.

The evaluation of the incipient signs of psychopathological processes in later life is rendered difficult because of the intimate relationship of organic and psychogenic symptoms. Clear-cut affective conditions— depression, anxiety, elation, apathy—present no abstruse problems in diagnosis when they constitute the central complaint; but somatic symptoms, which bulk so largely, require that the physician be constantly vigilant. The first step, of course, is a thorough physical investigation, including all pertinent laboratory studies, in order to convince the physician of the absence of gross organic pathology. Such information must be conveyed to the patient in such a manner that he or she will feel that complaints have not been lightly disregarded. The importance of the effects of the emotions on the body should be made plain; the tendency of the patient to focus attention on the abnormal bodily function should be explained, and emphasis should be placed on treatment directed toward correcting the underlying emotional disorder.

Thus prepared, most patients are ready to undertake examination of their emotional problems and to participate in dealing with them. The recommended plan of therapy should lay emphasis on revealing the psychological background of the present situation, with reassurance, explanation, and suggestion of the main methods of dealing with it. A full history is necessary, and information provided by members of the family or others closely associated with the patient is of inestimable value in the rapid evaluation of personality changes and of the significance of particular symptoms in terms of the drives and self-esteem of the patient. Encouragement of goals that will offer gratification and reexamination of aims that are likely to lead to frustration are notable aspects of reeducation. The abandonment of ambitions that can no longer be achieved must be accompanied by the acceptance of lower standards and by the participation in activities wherein the use of the individual's assets will be rewarded.

Deep investigation of personal conflicts involving instinctual drives is not indicated for this age group. In other words, the zealous therapist must constantly remember that by the time we have attained late middle life, most of us have had many things happen to us which have been carefully laid away, either satisfactorily or unsatisfactorily, and to dredge them up now and add them to our present cares might result in serious consequences. In fact, on many occasions the patient's wish to ventilate old difficulties must be tactfully diverted lest there result undesirable aftereffects, such as guilt or anxiety.

In addition to dealing with the psychodynamic aspects of the illness, there are innumerable subsidiary forms of therapy helpful for the elderly patient. The use of medications in small doses to alleviate anxiety is certainly indicated, though prolonged or excessive prescription has to be avoided — no need to remind physicians that older persons are liable to develop adverse reactions to the cumulative effect of medications and that much smaller doses of sedatives and other drugs usually suffice.

Manipulation of the environment may take a prominent place in the treatment of those patients in whom domestic, social, or economic factors have been of major significance. The provision of suitable living arrangements, explanation to the family of the difficulties of the aging and suggestions as to how to cope with the patient, the preparation of adequate and attractive meals, measures to improve the general health — all contribute to the welfare of the person under treatment.

There is no need here to go into the actual therapy utilized in hospitals in the care of senile and arteriosclerotic patients. If there is a depressive overlay to the symptoms, it usually can be lightened by drugs or somatic treatment. If the organic changes are well advanced, however, there can be only routine hospital care as good or as poor as that provided in the particular institution in question. Good nursing care is a necessity whether in the home or the hospital, but in these days of personpower shortages even that is sparse. All in all, the situation is not a happy one, and those patients who are badly regressed and nearly helpless mercifully do not linger long.

Growing old gracefully

Growing old need not be as dreadful or frightening as these few foregoing sections make it out to be. Certainly, illness — both physical and emotional — may occur, just as it does at other times of life. Much of the fear of facing this period of life, however, can be alleviated by simply being aware of this change in life and in preparing for it. The New York Legislative Committee upon looking at the common mistakes in growing old identified ten such failings. I have taken the liberty of recasting them in a more positive way, so that we might think of them as ways of easing into growing old:

- There should be a willingness to slow down and leave off a high-pressure way of life.
- There should be a willingness and effort made to serve others.

— There should be an orientation toward the future, not the past.

— There should be preparations made for retirement.

— There should be an acceptance of and rapport with the younger generation.

— There should be outside interests.

— There should be cultivated an independence of spirit.

— There should be an adjustment to the change in income level.

— There should be an openness to learning new things.

— There should be a readiness to face reality as it is.

We hear over and over again of how important it is to be in touch with others. The old fixed rules of mental health still hold, especially those connected with keeping the lines of communication open with family and friends. In order to be meaningful the communication must be within the frame of reference that the times require. This is not always easy for the elderly for their interest is frequently in the past, as we have already mentioned, and when one remembers that people in their eighties have seen such changes as in transportation from horse to cars to Concordes, and in communication from telegraph to present-day communication by satellite.

Another maxim of the aging period is well settled and should be accepted; namely, that there is no necessary parallel between chronologic and psychologic age. The saying that one is as old as one thinks and feels is not simply a flippant remark. Pathologists have demonstrated at autopsies that the brains of some people who had been labeled senile actually showed few serious pathologic changes, and on the other hand some of those who occupied important positions until death showed evidences of severe brain pathology. The trouble with many individuals who exhibit senile behavior may be that they have "quit" — have "given up." They have failed for some reason, recognized (or unrecognized) even by themselves, to stay in the mainstream of daily life. To lose interest in life at any time ages one mentally and physically. Monotony induces depression or fixes depression already present. To sit and stare in space or lost in memories means rusting away. Such people may be sound physically, but they are not flexible enough to grow old gracefully, which is a process that involves mental readjustments. To salvage them we must fill their times, revive their interest in life, and encourage them to use their hands and brains.

It is obvious, then, if our belief in the dignity of the human person is to be anything but a catch-word, that we are going to have to find some workable solution to the present-day wastage of human resources. Social planning for the utilization of aging individuals anxious to be occupied is laudable for them, but to others it may seem artificial. Could people be like Cato—who at eighty-four wrote treatises, studied a new language, and every evening reviewed the events of the day so that he might keep his memory in order—there would be no trouble. It would be as Cato stated: "The man living the midst of such studies keeps his mind in full stretch like a bow and never allows it to go into old age by becoming slack."

The methods of prevention and the management of the emotional problems of the elderly are neither as difficult nor as futile as was, and in some instances still is, sometimes believed. Psychiatrists have changed their opinions considerably over the years and now look at these elderly individuals as people who have problems and who have chosen special personal ways of meeting them. These responses may sometimes be pathologic and obviously misguided, but they probably were chosen to avert a disaster in coping with life.

How, then, can one face the crises of aging in a positive fashion? First by accepting aging as something positive, not simply something to be endured. One must accept it as a new phase and new style of life and seek to discover the values and the precious opportunities available to make it worthwhile and fulfilling. The alternatives to a positive approach are unhappy ones.

Growing old gracefully thus necessitates a change of venue—the pressures, the push, the striving for recognition and advancement which formerly occupied the earlier period can now be viewed with a philosophical detachment and a new perspective on life, on love, and on the real meaning of existence. This brings with it a deeper insight and a true knowledge of the value of all things without the biases that earlier drove the person on. Young people can approach the older person without resentment, since the latter have exchanged their throne of power for the seat of wisdom. They have discovered their own true value and can be appreciated by those of lesser life experience. This wisdom cannot be learned from books, nor can it be acquired in schools or universities. Only a lifelong process of gradual growth and maturing can bring this wisdom of the heart. The wise patience and calm of a mature person can be an encouragement, guide, and stimulant for others. Coping with loneliness can be done only by becoming our true selves and living with a genuine love and compassion for others.

Growing old in a positive way can be like crossing a desert into a promised land. Aging makes a person aware of how unstable and transient are so many things in life. Wealth and external achievements, beauty, and health are fleeting and perishable. However, experiencing instability is one thing; developing a new awareness of what is lasting and eternal is another, and this brings with it new meaning and hope.

The person who has kept mentally active, curious, and thirsty for knowledge has the best chance of enjoying and being creative in later years. It is difficult to think of Justices Holmes and Brandeis as having been old men, for they were so dynamic mentally. The older person who can become interested in the arts, literature, or crafts need never feel lonely or unoccupied. The person who reads and can cogitate or who works with the hands and creates will never find the world tedious.

Old people also need evidence of real family life. They need a modicum of attention and a reasonably generous dose of being listened to. Efforts to keep them in contact with contemporary affairs are helpful; efforts to keep their lines of communications open are essential. Affection is better than drugs. They need to know that they are still regarded as being in the land of the living. They should be prevented from indulging in even self-rejection, which can threaten the person who experiences segregation and desolation. Nouwen correctly observes that this self-rejection strips the elderly of their feeling of self-worth. This loss of self-worth, he says, becomes most visible in those whose whole identity is tied to their past lives. "There can hardly be a more alienating feeling than that which believes I am who I was."

Occasionally we find real pleasure in old persons, even in their looks, for it is, as Nouwen noted, "The person shining through." We appreciate the person and wonder how he or she did it and whether or not we can do it. If we really want to know, writes Nouwen, we should not turn to scientific treatises but rather to philosophy and seek as much help from the ancients as from the moderns to appreciate the experience of a human life and its richness. Indeed, more than thirty years ago M. Gitelson made a statement, which might well guide us in caring for the old, the retired, and the disaffected:

> Knowing that the old ones are really insecure and anxious, the physician will lend them his own strength, not with a pat on the back and a wordy reassurance, but by the living fact of his willingness to stand by and help in every way. There should be no talk about inferiority feelings, no talk about compensatory devices, no talk about anxiety — no jargon of any sort is necessary. One must simply understand how the old person feels and conduct oneself with due consideration for the validity of these feelings.

To this, we may add what Nouwen offers, that "aging is not a reason for despair but a basis for hope, not a slow decaying but a gradual maturing, not a fate to be undergone but a chance to be embraced."

REFERENCES

Busse, E., Barnes, R., Silverman, A. *et al.* Studies of the process of aging; the strengths and weaknesses of psychic teaching in the aged. *American Journal of Psychiatry* III, 896–901, 1955.

Butler, Robert N. *Why Survive?* New York: Harper & Row, 1975.

Fox, Nancy Littell. *How to Put Joy into Geriatric Care.* Bend, Oregon: Geriatric Press, 1981.

Gitelson, M. The Emotional Problems of Elderly People. *Geriatrics* 3, 135–50, 1948.

Mace, Nancy L., & Rabins, Peter V. *The 36-Hour Day.* Baltimore: Johns Hopkins University Press, 1981.

Moss, Frank E., & Halamandaris, Val J. *Too Old Too Sick Too Bad.* Rockville, Maryland: Aspen Systems, 1977.

Nouwen, Henry J., & Gaffney, W. *Aging: The Fulfillment of Life.* Garden City, New York: Doubleday & Co., 1974.

Rathbone-McCuan, Eloise, & Hashimi, Joan. *Isolated Elders.* Rockville, Maryland: Aspen Systems, 1982.

PART THREE

Common Pastoral Problems

1

Crisis Intervention

HOWARD P. ROME

The word *crisis* is derived from the Greek *krinein,* meaning "to decide." It is synonymous with turning point, climax, juncture, point of change, judgment. Therefore, crisis decisions always involve theories of action rather than theories of knowledge. The character of the crisis is derived from the relationships explicit in the situation. Its orientation is founded upon a schema of serviceability. Any explanation is an effort to use the forces of socialization as a strategy. Crises are the crucibles out of which many innovations emerge; new models of action often receive their initial direction from attempts to cope with emergencies.

When a need is perceived, it is associated with an undifferentiated image of activity focused on object gratification. Anxiety arises from ungratified needs and overwhelms the psychic process of denial. Thus the birth of crisis reaction is inherent in the phenomenon of object loss. Franz Werfel has written, "Love is nothing more than the capacity for passionately developing the picture of a human being in our inner dark room." The tendency to find one's own moods in things outside the self has been designated the "pathetic fallacy." Hence the dialectical contention, or more precisely the characteriological struggle, is between what Freud termed "the consciousness of inner identity" and finding one's thoughts and one's identity pictured in outside events.

Erikson (1968) has posited eight developmental stages which, in his own words, are "derived from the various stages of the psychosexual

265

development that were described by Freud as well as from the child stages of physical, motor, and cognitive development." If these experiences are handled expeditiously, the outcome for the person is continued maturation and enhanced development. If, on the other hand, the stress inherent in the crisis is not handled adequately, earlier and heretofore latent psychological conflicts may be exacerbated and play a determining role in shaping the form of the new conflict, giving rise to the characteristic repetitive series of symptoms that psychological theory holds to be a characteristic of all neuroses. It follows that persons undergoing a crisis are amenable to corrective influences when skilled intervention of cogent and relatively brief duration is applied. The iron, it may be said, is hot at the time of crisis.

Developmental crises

There are critical transition points in every change of place, state, social position, and age. These exist in all cultures everywhere, ancient and contemporary, primitive, peasant, and urban.

Birth is the first crucial transition the individual makes as a living being. Birth is not only a biological experience but a social crisis as well and is attended by rites, magic, ceremonies, observances, and taboos. Next in sequence are name-giving and baptism, the formal ceremonies whereby a nominal identity is conferred upon the individual and the rite of initiation into a Christian sect or denomination is performed. (Adoption is an acculturation process, a legal ceremony that simulates the biological process of birth, by which a designated social authority grants to an individual all the privileges usually associated with birth rights.) Confirmation is another rite in the chain of developmental crises by which the recipient is admitted to full communion after successfully completing a prescribed course of instruction. Marriage follows next in the life and status of the individual. The ceremony attendant upon marriage is laden with symbolic overtones designed to secure certain privileges and is a guarantee of rights for the newly established family. And, of course, death is the last great transition ceremony, critical for the family as well as the individual. Inasmuch as time's arrow flies in but one direction, all these are points of no return. Because they are universal experiences, they are termed developmental, maturational, or situational crises — standard transition points in the life cycle of the individual and the family.

Crises of this category, inasmuch as they are inevitable, depend heavily on social mores and social custom for working out the least disruptive resolution and mobilizing the most support. In other words, these are the socially institutionalized ways of intervening in times of crises. They are known in anthropological circles as *rites of passage:* formalized ways that are socially approved for the customary transitions throughout the development-maturational cycle. As Dr. Kluckhohn states:

> There is a "philosophy" behind the way of life of every individual and of every relatively homogeneous group at any given point in their histories. This gives, with varying degrees of explicitness or implicitness, some sense of coherence or unity to living both in cognitive and affective dimensions. Each personality gives to this "philosophy" an idiosyncratic coloring, and creative individuals will markedly reshape it. However, the main outlines of the fundamental values, existential assumptions, and basic abstractions have only exceptionally been created out of the stuff of unique biological heredity and peculiar life experience. The underlying principles arise out of, or are limited by, the givens of biological human nature and the universalities of social interaction. The specific formulation is ordinarily a cultural product. In the immediate sense, it is from the lifeways which constitute the designs for living of their community or tribe or region or socio-economic class or nation or civilization that most individuals derive their "mental-feeling outlook" (Kluckhohn, 1958).

Our secularized culture by and large is characterized by more casual arrangements of the rites of passage. Anticipatory socialization, that experience which conditions in advance the behavior required for the assumption of new roles, tends to be left to the discretion of the individuals directly involved. The social prescriptions for expected behavior in these new roles are consequently highly variable and, insofar as the community as a whole is concerned, relatively unstructured. These universally critical transitions in an otherwise "normal" family frequently provoke disruption in the persons directly involved and, to a lesser degree, in the family-as-a-system (Parsons & Fox, 1952).

The family-as-a-system is a coping mechanism of paramount importance in experiencing and resolving these developmental crises. Frequently one sees evidence of this in the form of the crisis itself becoming a rallying point of a new-found family solidarity. This is particularly striking when the members of a family are faced with the characteristic turbulence of one of these developmental crises such as illness.

Before I treat a patient. . . .
I need to know a good deal more about him,
Than the patient himself can always tell me.
Indeed, it is often the case that my patients
Are only pieces of a total situation

Which I have to explore. The single patient
Who is ill by himself, is rather the exception (Eliot, 1950, p. 114).

These are cultural configurations, the moral principles that comprise the social philosophy of a society. As such, they delineate the ethos of a culture, since they motivate the behavior that furnishes meaning to relationships and supply the moral sentiments by which family members are influenced.

In our present-day society, it is taken for granted that one primary function of the family is to prepare its members for their anticipated daily quota of frustrations. The normative belief is the confident expectation that each member is entitled to and will get the needed support, reassurance, and encouragement. It is customary to allow the opportunity for regression that a respite within the family affords from the cultural compulsion to be habitually independent and self-sufficient. One speaks of this as a welcome opportunity to "let one's hair down." Being "in the bosom of the family" has the obvious connotations of regression to a childlike status, being in a warm and comfortable mothering situation, being home. Admittedly this is an indulgence, but it is a socially endorsed and legitimate indulgence permitted in a crisis if it is temporary and does not exploit the succor afforded by the family's empathy.

Western culture has moved away from the fixed and structured customs that less sophisticated cultures prescribe and follow compulsively in order to facilitate passage from one developmental epoch to another. Consequently, it devolves upon the individuals and the family to compensate for the deficit. Since their preparation is for the most part *ad hoc* and improvised rather than ritualized, it is likely to be fraught with tension and anxiety. This is another price paid for secularization; developmental crises, generally speaking, are more personal and hence liable to more traumatic experiences than they were in earlier times.

Each of Erikson's developmental stages is a crisis in the sense of connoting a turning point rather than a threat of catastrophe. If all goes well, the infant acquires trust, proceeds to autonomy, and then continues to initiative. The schoolchild develops a wish to make things, a sense of industry. Adolescence presents the identity crisis, which, if successfully mastered, leads to the experience of intimacy. The adult concerned with bringing up the young enters the stage of generativity. As old age arrives, integrity may finally be achieved. Each of these stages has its negative counterpart: mistrust, shame, guilt, inferiority, identity confusion, isolation, and despair. These are the ontogenetic homologues of what has been described previously from the viewpoint of transition stages in the socialization process (Erikson, 1968).

Coincidental crises

This category of climactic and potentially disruptive events is in a temporal sense coincidental, in that critical events occur at random times in the lives of most persons. While they are always expected, they are unpredictable and therefore constitute the hazards of everyday life that have to be endured and hopefully overcome by the best available adaptive means. They include accidental injuries, including fatal accidents; life-threatening experiences, such as the risks of war; natural disasters, earthquakes, floods, tornadoes, etc.; major and minor physical and mental illness; the psychological trauma of surgery; suicide; those stresses that are incidental to a loss of income and retirement; status and geographic relocation (employment and economic changes, immigration), etc.

These crises are provoked by all incidents whose magnitude approaches catastrophic proportions for the individual. A forewarning of the imminence or the fear of death is a typical example. While the average person knows that death is an ever-present liability and that life is contingent, this knowledge is for the most part intellectual, meaning that it is treated as merely another impersonal, objective sense datum. Death is what happens to other people; "It won't happen to me—at least not for some time to come" is the rationalization that protects the average person from the necessity of contemplating his or her own nonexistence. It is personal inasmuch as it is the culture's counterphobic way of disposing of a fearsome inevitability (Feifel, 1959).

There are lesser but symbolically related aspects of this same phenomenon. They may be induced by a sudden change that results in a radical dislocation of the individual's life-style and the customary adjustment. Examples include such events as an enforced immigration, as was true of many Germans in the years immediately prior to World War II; a narrow escape from an accident; the experience of an illness that is associated with the high probability of a fatal outcome; or an injury with crippling residuals, such as amputation or blindness or brain damage. These are examples of coincidental crises—life-disrupting events that radically change what was anticipated. Most people expect a "normal" life to consist of a series of not-especially-disturbing events, but actual statistical reality indicates the likelihood of quite another state of affairs.

When they are viewed collectively, such catastrophes have certain psychodynamic traits in common. There is anxiety, both psychic and that which is reflected in somatic-tension states. These are portrayed in the typical life-style of the individual. In turn, a life-style also implies the response of coping mechanisms that have as their general objective a stabilizing effect. Coping techniques act to effect release from paralyzing anxiety or escape from the temporary halt induced by the dilemma, achieving these by making an unequivocal decision among a variety of alternatives.

Since ministers are frequently the resource appealed to in a crisis, it is important for them to understand the structure of crisis and the process of intervention.

In an assessment of the crisis, it is necessary to determine whether the more troublesome symptoms come from the catastrophe itself or are the consequences of an improvident way of dealing with it. For instance, the injudicious resort to addictive narcotics or to alcohol is an example of a dysfunctional way of coping with the necessity of deciding among a number of equally hard choices. These improvident solutions invariably generate further crises.

Eric Berne (1964, pp. 73–81) has epitomized these crises as "life games." He says that in its full flower the game *Alcoholic* is a five-handed game, although the roles may be condensed so that it starts and terminates as a two-handed one. These are the dramatis personae of this crisis situation:

  — the Alcoholic, the one who is "it";
  — the chief supporting role is that of the Persecutor, usually played by a member of the opposite sex, usually the spouse;
  — the third role is that of the Rescuer, usually played by the family doctor or a substitute;
  — the fourth role is that of the Patsy or Dummy, the one who aids, abets and sympathizes;
  — the fifth role is that of the Connection, the direct source of supply.

In the initial stages of *Alcoholic,* says Berne, the wife may play all three of the supporting roles. At midnight she is the Patsy, allowing herself to be exploited; in the morning the Persecutor, berating her husband for the evil of his ways; and in the evening the Rescuer, pleading for a change in his ways. The payoff comes from the hangover, in which indulgence in self-castigation is the true name of the game. Crisis intervention in this kind of life-game depends on what role is assigned and what role is taken, and the congruence between the roles.

Alcoholic is the paradigm of many related crises in which drugs play both a major and a minor role. The widespread abuse of hallucinogens, amphetamines, tranquilizers, and sedatives is said to reflect an ideological as well as a generational struggle that is worldwide in scope, psychedelic in form, and anti-traditional in character. It seeks to reverse Marx's dictum and say "opium is the religion of these 'new' people" (Bottomore,

1968, pp. 82–105). Then, too, the spirit of the time—the *Zeitgeist*—lends a distinct flavor to the different capacities and tolerances for individual and collective stress. People adapt to the commotion of turbulent change in different ways as well as at different rates of accommodation.

Obviously, there are many background factors responsible for this variation. Perhaps the most compelling are earlier socialization experiences. Social conditioning and biological factors inherent in one's genetic endowment constitute both the necessary and the sufficient elements involved in the formation of the individual's buffer system, coping mechanisms, resistance or vulnerability to the stress of change. These adaptive ways are not always equally effective, inasmuch as they do not function at the same degree of efficiency for everyone or for the same person at different times.

Social criticism explicit in social change is the ideological crisis of our time. Between the radical right and the radical left our traditionalist society is being sundered on a scale that is universal in its pervasiveness (Lerner, 1958).

Christopher Lasch says that the rise of the new radicalism in the United States coincides with the emergence of the intellectual as a distinctive social type (Lasch, 1965). He defines the intellectual broadly as a person for whom thinking fulfills both the function of work and of play; more specifically, as a person whose relationship to society is defined principally by a presumed capacity to comment upon it with greater detachment than those more directly caught up in the practical business of production and power.

Mass society has a tendency to break down into its component parts, each having its own autonomous culture and maintaining only the most tenuous connections with the general life of the society, which as a consequence has almost ceased to exist. The most obvious victims of this process are adolescents. This is Lasch's definition of the "new radical": one who promotes a melange of efforts to liberate the socially and radically disenfranchised by means of political action; one who is engaged in a fevered pursuit of experience for experience's sake, who conceives of life as an experiment, who identifies with the outcasts of society, who has a "feeling of beleaguered hostility" toward the rest of society.

OUTLINE FOR THE MANAGEMENT OF AN ACUTE CRISIS

1. Since by definition the affect in a crisis situation is intense, the situation manifestly calls for help from a resource person who, it is hoped, will play the role of Rescuer.

2. Determine if the crisis is within your sphere of competence. If so, does it require you to control, to render first aid, to summon someone who is more expert, to be a source of referral, to render obstetrical service? In short, apprise yourself of what needs to be done *immediately* and set about doing it or setting in motion the actions that will get it done.

   2.1 Be prepared by being familiar with local resources. Know the physicians who will respond to emergency calls and have their telephone numbers readily available. Similarly, know the ambulance service and the procedure for arranging for an emergency admission to the nearest hospital. In preparation for crises, visit the local police department or the sheriff's office, and learn under what circumstances they can and will be of assistance. Have at your disposal a notebook with the names, addresses, and telephone numbers of social agencies, Alcoholics Anonymous, suicide prevention center, etc., so that with the least commotion and the greatest dispatch you are able to arrange for a definitive referral.

3. The call for help may or may not express a consensus.

   3.1 If it does, you may assume that there is tacit agreement to defer to the Rescuer — at least for the duration of the acute emergency. The group is prepared to accept as a leader one who can organize, direct, manage. As a consequence, deference is paid to the Rescuer.

   3.2 If there is no consensus, then in addition to all else, the control aspects of the situation are in question. In effect the Rescuer is asked, "Who asked you to butt in?"

   3.3 The critical situation realigns, polarized along lines that question the role of the Rescuer and by implication his or her competence, authority, and partiality.

   3.4 This secondary impasse has to be resolved before dealing with the primary crisis.

      3.41 Assure the parties concerned of your neutral role.

      3.42 Verify this by giving the specific details of your identity, qualifications, and the reasons why you answered the call for help.

      3.43 Offer to leave with the provision that the neutral role of Rescuer will be taken by someone agreeable to all concerned.

4. If, when you have judged the crisis to be less of an emergency than life or death and have determined that it is within your sphere of competence, elicit the following information:

4.1 Where has this happened? The answer to this question will automatically set limits upon your activities. It will also determine, in part, whether you are solely responsible *at this time*. For example, your responsibility is vastly different if you are called to a police station, a local tavern, a hospital, a home, or on the street. The circumstances of a crisis in any one of these situations define what you are required to do.

4.2 When has this crisis occurred? Your response is shaped according to the time when you first encounter what is judged to be a crisis. It is different at 10 A.M. and at 4 A.M.; New Year's Eve is different from an ordinary weekday afternoon, etc.

4.3 How many persons are immediately or remotely involved? Are they all present? The role of the Rescuer hinges on obtaining as many versions of what the crisis is about as there are participants. This is not to say that the crucial issue is necessarily related to the "facts" of the situation, but rather to that perception of the "facts" as they are seen by the persons involved.

4.4 It is important to ascertain who, if any, of the dramatis personae was responsible for initiating the cry for assistance. Patently, this person is amenable to help. It also follows that the caller's role in the crisis situation gives you cues. If a man called you, you are "his man" and will be expected to be partisan to his cause until you specifically avow your neutrality.

Thus, if you are summoned by a wife who has been beaten, a husband who has just discovered he has been made a cuckold, a daughter who has been ordered never to darken the parents' door again, an officer of the law, or a nosy neighbor who wants to titillate his scoptophilia, quite obviously the roles you are expected to play vary considerably.

5. You must first determine the *sequence* needed to terminate the crisis as quickly and as expeditiously as possible.

5.1 The clues and cues for this are given if you view the crisis as a live-action, real-time sociogram. This observation will structure the problem insofar as you can deduce it from what is said, who has said it, in what order they speak, and the emotions they manifest. You are also able to glean from the drama clues as to the power structure of this *ad hoc* group. Try to formulate answers to such questions as: Is this a revival of an old melodrama played repetitiously by the same cast? Or is this drama quite new, at least for these participants who have not had previous occasion to learn their parts? Who are the principal actors? Who plays the supporting roles? Who are the spectators? Who are the claqueurs? Who is it that wants to bring you up-to-date by volunteering to give a précis of the drama's previous acts? Is what you have been told a bowdlerized or an unexpurgated version?

5.2 Armed with this additional information and beginning to crystalize your formulation of the crisis, you have to reassert your neutral stance by a firm insistence that everyone will benefit from a de-escalation of the crisis.

5.3 Your role is that of an *authority;* not an *authoritarian.* You strive to be a catalyst, "a person whose talk, enthusiasm, or energy causes others to be more friendly, enthusiastic, or energetic."

5.4 At this time your goal should be to manage the acute situation only, and arrange for a follow-up in the form of a referral, a later appointment with you, whatever seems to follow next in sequence.

5.5 You take over completely *only* if the emergency of the crisis warrants.

6. In all crises the expectation incumbent upon the Rescuer is *Do something!* Sometimes, it is well to remember, to *do nothing* is actually the *something* that is needed. Your presence in the role of a neutral provides an opportunity for discharge of the accumulated tensions.

7. Remember that authority is most authoritative when it is not exercised. Use your authority as a moderator to arrange an orderly sequence of history-telling.

7.1 Arrange for the most obviously agitated, visibly disturbed historian to be first.

7.2 By thus acting to remove first the most disruptive element in the crisis, you demonstrate control and establish your authority. This is the beginning of the restructuring of order out of chaos which is the essence of all crisis intervention.

8. While you may be uncertain as to the outcome, it is incumbent upon the Rescuer to act *as if* he or she were sure: to portray the calm reasonableness that Dickens said was an "emblem to humanity of the rest and silence into which the storm called Life must hush at last."

8.1 To accomplish this, you must use as levers as many of the ordinary social conventions as possible to re-establish habitual behavior. People are creatures of habit, literally programmed by social indoctrination to follow cues in a conditioned-reflex, automatic response. Therefore, if you smoke, ask for a match and an ashtray. Or request a glass of water or a cup of coffee. Ask if you may sit down; pick a seat near the most disturbed person. Sit back in the seat, look the picture of relaxation, at ease, comfortable, not worried. If time permits (this can be determined by whether the original call required that you respond immediately, within minutes, or at your earliest convenience), be dressed and look as you ordinarily do.

8.2 Proceed to the site of the crisis under your own power. This avoids the necessity of being dependent upon anyone else for transportation and avoids what might be interpreted as partiality.

9. Limit the situation, by whatever means at your disposal, to those immediately concerned. This is in the interest of essential privacy. Ask the spectators to leave the room. If they are members of the family suggest that they might amuse or pacify the children, take the dog for a walk, see about making coffee, etc. Displacement activity in the throes of a crisis is salutary.

10. Look for signs that indicate the "pecking order" of the group, in order to utilize normal social controls.

10.1 Look for clues as to coalitions, allegiances, and cliques which may be potentially divisive.

10.2 Act as if you have all the time in the world so that no one feels abused, overlooked, deprived, or subordinated.

11. In regard to *action,* you have one of three alternative decisions to make.

11.1 Is there a need to act, and if so, what action is necessary?

11.2 Does the action on your part have to be taken now; if not, when?

11.3 Do you need more time or data on which to base your answer to 11.1 and 11.2?

12. If action is required, try to contrive the circumstances so that it is least disruptive. Action taken in heat and/or haste is likely to be in error.

12.1 If you decide to act, act decisively. Once the decision is made, you must see that there is no vacillation.

13. If you decide to make a referral, do not prematurely commit yourself or your consultant to a specific course of action. To do so vitiates the need for the consultation. Make sure you have laid the appropriate groundwork, such as determining that a hospital bed is

available, that Dr. Smith will be free tomorrow at eleven o'clock, etc.

14. When properly handled, crises have an inherent potential for leading the participants to a heightened maturity. Give the participants the opportunity to start this working-out process so that they will feel entitled to the success.

15. The reward of the Rescuer is personal satisfaction. But do not expect to be rewarded on every occasion. You can't win them all. However, you can do your best and this will moderate the guilt you will feel at having failed — sometimes.

REFERENCES

Berne, Eric. *Games People Play: The Psychology of Human Relationships.* New York: Grove Press, 1964.

Bottomore, T. B. *Critics of Society: Radical Thought in North America.* New York: Pantheon Books, 1968.

Eliot, T. S. *The Cocktail Party: A Comedy.* New York: Harcourt, Brace, & World, 1950.

Erikson, Erik H. *Identity: Youth and Crisis.* New York: W. W. Norton & Co., 1968.

Feifel, Herman. Attitudes toward death in some normal and mentally ill populations. In Herman Feifel, (ed.), *The Meaning of Death.* New York: McGraw-Hill, 1959.

Kluckhohn, Florence R. Family dynamics: variations in the basic values of family systems. *Social Casework* 39, 63–72, 1958.

Lasch, Christopher. *The New Radicalism in America, 1889–1963: The Intellectual as a Social Type.* New York: Alfred A. Knopf, 1965.

Lerner, Daniel. *The Passing of Traditional Society: Modernizing the Middle East.* New York: The Free Press of Glencoe, 1958.

Parsons, Talcott, & Fox, Renee C. Illness, therapy and the modern American family. *Journal of Social Issues* 8, 31–44, 1952.

Wertel, Franz. *Estrangement.* New York: Viking Press, 1937.

Care of the Critically Ill and the Dying

NATHAN SCHNAPER

H ow many of us have heard those worrisome words: "So-and-so is critically ill, even dying." *Critically ill* and *dying* are not synonymous, however. Except for a sudden death, critical illness, no matter how brief, usually precedes dying. Only on looking back can we really see the terms *dying patient* or *terminal illness*. Doctors tend to use these terms in rather precise ways. Critically ill patients are those individuals who are in a life-threatening crisis (including those who have suffered serious and severe medical, surgical, or physical trauma). The outcome of this crucial period to the patient is uncertain and dangerous.

This chapter presents some general principles about the understanding and care of the critically and terminally ill. It will also discuss the concerns of the severely physically traumatized and the care of patients with cancer, and it will offer comments on the grief process. Although this chapter's orientation is basically medical, this approach provides an overview that offers insights and understanding for the clergy.

The critically ill patient

The critically ill undergo tremendous psychological stress. The illness or trauma disrupts psychological as well as physical functioning, and these patients face a great deal of uncertainty. Those who tend them need to be aware of the acute manifestations of this heightened anxiety. Because severe illness or trauma disrupts ordinary functioning and operations, conscious controls are threatened or diminished, thus allowing greater leeway for unconscious reactions and fears to come to the fore. Those working with critically ill and dying patients and their families shoud be aware of certain mental mechanisms and defenses and of the *unconscious* that are likely to be accentuated in coping with illness and its consequences.

Secrets are things we can tell others; fantasies are thoughts we tell only ourselves; and our unconscious are thoughts we cannot even ourselves be aware of. The unconscious workings of the mind are revealed in dreams, slips of the tongue, mental symptoms, and hypnosis. Our unconscious retains all our impulses, memories, and emotions associated with experiences. It is timeless, with little regard for reality, and therefore condones contrary wishes without doubts or negation. The more painful or disgusting an experience is, the more likely it will be repressed into the subconscious. It is a powerful source of energy that determines one's psychic behavior and arbitrarily compels an individual to react impulsively or repetitiously in certain situations and, at times, in an irrational way.

In the care of the critically ill, the helpers and family members will have to deal with the unconscious of the patient as well as their own. Reactions will include transference and specific defense reactions. A patient may use a variety of defense mechanisms to cope with anxieties. Frequently, one will see denial, displacement, projection, rationalization, and regression—all as ways of dealing with (or denying) the present condition.

The helpers

Because critically ill patients find themselves in special circumstances and under unique pressures, ordinary coping mechanisms may be unavailable or ineffective. The available defenses then become overutilized and distorted. Since helpers have their own personalities, with preferences and limitations, and their own defensive structures just as the patient, they need to be sensitive to possible conflict within themselves that might make treatment of the patient less than objective. Whether they are medical or paramedical personnel or ministers, helpers derive partial motivation for their chosen professions from a need to be all powerful, i.e., to "run" peoples' lives. This proclivity in no way denigrates these helpers or their work. Usually their need is sublimated, and as a result, society benefits. Where such need is not completely sublimated, the stress of experiencing the failure of one's power to "cure" can provoke anxiety. In such instances, defenses familiar to helpers come into play: they too can use rationalization, suppress awareness of the patient, or deny the patient's right to complain. Most serious (and dangerous) is anger. If the patient rejects medical or religious intervention, such helpers may sense a threat to omnipotence in what seems to be a deliberate act of the patient. They themselves become angry and rejecting of the patient. Anger and rejection, overt or covert, are never useful responses to the critically ill.

Other helpers, although not troubled with problems of omnipotence, are bothered by closeness. Struggling with illness, the patient draws the helper from a peripheral position into a relationship of central significance. The patient becomes more dependent, such that the shift in relationship constitutes a threat to the helpers' need to be observers from a distance. For instance, helpers can reject suggestions for referral to consultants, hospital, or nursing home, or they may employ other techniques of avoidance.

Some helpers need to be loved, a need that is closely related to the desire to be omnipotent. They fear the patient's anxiety, frustration, and demands. They find it difficult to be realistic. Any lack of sympathy from others, no matter how firmly the reaction is based on reality, makes them feel hostile to the patient. This type of helper cannot offer the patient a brief, simple explanation; even a brief "It's God's will" becomes a three-paragraph lecture. Overelaboration and overexplaining signal their own anxiety (Schnaper, 1964, p. 34).

Most of the time, the relationship between patients and helpers is more important than procedures. Such a relationship considers the personality of helpers. They should not try to act a role, but utilize their personality as an instrument. If their usual mode and style is authoritative, they should be thus with patients. Given this honesty, patients can experience the helpers as sincere persons (Schnaper, 1961, p. 486).

Critically ill patients and their families find themselves under stress from the illness itself and its danger. In view of this stress, the health care (helping) procedures themselves and environment can not only be life-saving but also confusing, disorienting, and distressing.

The intensive-care unit

Critically ill patients and the intensive-care unit share a very special reciprocal relationship. A picture of an ICU comes to mind immediately when one learns that an individual is critically ill: a patient in an ICU is *ipso facto* critically ill or "dying."

There are many and varied types of ICUs. They include medical, surgical, coronary care, stroke, neurological, pediatric, burn, and others. To patients and family members, these units are frightening. Most ICUs are windowless and impersonal, with highly mechanized monitoring systems, and overloaded with auditory and visual stimuli, much like a "science fiction bunker" (Hay & Oken, 1972). The psychological symptoms of patients in this environment run the gamut of depression, delirium, hallucinations, delusions, neurosis, and psychosis. Aggressive in its therapeutic efforts, the ICU's team and equipment are housed in an area of the hospital adjacent to its particular service, and its patients are usually in-hospital transfers with established diagnoses. Treatment may demand at a moment's notice a variety of resuscitative, changing diagnostic, and therapeutic measures for survival.

Severe multiple trauma

A well-established trauma center is an ICU "plus." In contrast to the general ICU, it is self-contained with its own operating and admission rooms, physicians (including neurosurgeons, infectious disease specialists, etc.), nurses, anesthesiologist, and other support staff, including psychiatrists, social workers, housekeeping personnel, etc. The patients in this center usually have severe multiple injuries involving two or more systems and/or life-threatening illnesses that result from overwhelming infections, suicide attempts, drownings, poisonings, ruptured aortic aneurysms, gastrointestinal hemorrhages, etc. Most patients, particularly those involved in highway crashes, arrive by helicopter. Physiologic shock and varying levels of consciousness (or more often, unconsciousness) are the rule.

The life-saving approach is multidisciplinary and appears to be organized chaos. Patients' clothes are cut away, while lines, tubes, and catheters are placed in veins, arteries, and orifices, including tracheal intubation. Surgical techniques as well as medications, physical aids, laboratory procedures, Xrays, and electronic monitoring are instantaneous. Once patients are stabilized, they are transferred to a critical-care recovery unit, where intensive therapy continues.

The patients

The emotional responses of the patients in the trauma center include psychotic, neurotic, and behavioral reactions to real or fantasied threats of their illness or injuries. Their experience is mainly one of stress. Even minor surgery can constitute a severe psychological threat to patients. Any effort to understand these emotional responses must be predicated on an understanding of the fact that persons facing trauma bring to the encounter individual personalities, which provide a defense against the illness or injury and the factors that caused it (Schnaper, 1969a).

Any threat (e.g., illness, surgery, or narcosis) marshalls coping mechanisms. The specific problems threatening the traumatized patient include the following (Schnaper, 1975):

HELPLESSNESS

In any illness people become dependent on someone else for healing and comfort. The defense of regression follows dependence. Caretakers are viewed as protecting or parental figures. The more severe the physical injury, the more intense the patients feel the abandonment and separation from family. The degree of regression is proportionate to the severity of the injury and intensifies patients' magical expectations of their helpers.

HUMILIATION

Injury and hospitalization also engender desperate feelings of indignity in reaction to hospital procedures, e.g., the bedpan, catheters, and taking of blood samples. Severely traumatized patients are necessarily exposed to these procedures in the admission area and throughout their hospitalization. If they are unconscious when admitted, they experience this humiliation retrospectively when they awaken. If they are semiconscious when admitted, they may see their clothing being cut off and the other procedures as assault and battery, especially if they had been drinking alcohol.

BODY IMAGE

Body image is the conscious and unconscious concept of the physical appearance patients have of their bodies. It can also include their car and clothing or the perception of the environment, all of which contribute to a sense of identity. It includes emotional attachment to a particular body organ; e.g., a woman may object strongly to the surgical removal of a breast. In severely traumatized patients, the threat of mutilation of the body is often an overwhelming strain.

MENTAL SYMPTOMS

Traumatized patients may experience an altered state of consciousness due to either physical or emotional causes. Examples of physical causes are open-heart surgery, metastatic carcinoma, and massive asphyxia with resultant cerebral hypoxia. Emotional causes usually result from a defensive dissociation between themselves and the injury to avoid an emotionally painful situation.

A patient behavior frequently observed when they are awakening or still semiconscious is masturbation. The fondling of genitals while basically sexual, is infantile, a regressive, self-comforting, and self-reassuring response. Very few patients are aware of their actions in this regard.

Families find themselves in sudden crisis, in acute shock, totally unprepared, and burdened with overwhelming anxiety. As they obtain more information about the patient's physical status, they undergo phases: high anxiety and confusion, denial, anger at their relatives, remorse, grief, and then reconciliation and recovery. Active intervention by a psychosocial professional is mandatory.

Psychiatric patterns among trauma patients

Often patients admitted to the trauma center suffer from head or spinal-cord injury and usually have had severe injuries involving multiple organs, bones, and body physiology.

OPEN-HEART SURGERY

Although patients who have had open-heart surgery are not usually seen in trauma centers, a brief comment about them can serve as counterpoint to the trauma patients. Many articles (Rome, 1969; Braceland, 1974) report that although cardiology patients have advance notice and are more prepared than trauma patients for emotional trauma, they often face postoperative emotional difficulties. Some have "hidden" psychoses, but more generally they experience a temporary delirium.

Postcardiotomy organic brain syndrome (delirium after open heart surgery) is a case of an altered state of consciousness with a physiologic and psychologic etiology. Such patients bring to surgery a mild, perhaps undetectable deficit in brain oxygenation (ischemia) caused by illness. Such factors as more than eight hours of anesthesia, more than four hours of bypass time, hypoxia, microembolic phenomena, blood transfusions, the ICU atmosphere, sensory deprivation, and possible preoperative psychiatric disturbance may well contribute to patients' emotional state after the operation.

HEAD AND SPINAL-CORD INJURIES

These approximate multiple trauma. Most of the writings have been oriented toward the posttraumatic syndrome or posttraumatic neurosis

(Ruesch & Bowman, 1945). Because head and spinal-cord injuries often result in permanent emotional or physical disability, rehabilitation should be sought in these cases (Mueller, 1962).

Head injuries usually produce subjective symptoms. The usual pattern comprises headaches, fatigue, vasomotor debility, dizziness, poor concentration, irritability, personality changes, and vague somatic complaints. Experts disagree on the source of these symptoms (see Weinstein & Lyerly, 1968; Braceland, 1974; Miller, 1961).

In my experience the real culprit of posttrauma problems is *time*. If rehabilitation of the patient with posttraumatic syndrome is undertaken within the first six months, patients usually do well. If it is undertaken after two years, the rehabilitation potential falls to near zero. During this prolonged interval, patients grow dependent on spouse or family for financial and emotional support. The male patient has the added problem of role reversal, and no amount of money can motivate him to "get up the nerve" to face the outside world. A similar pattern prevails in active individuals who have retired from work, particularly those who have not planned for retirement.

Posttrauma care of patients with spinal cord injuries can only be considered in the context of physical and emotional rehabilitation. Second cervical-spine transections are the most serious because the patient cannot survive without life-support systems. These injuries generate the most debate in the polemical area of euthanasia.

PARAPLEGICS

According to Miller (1961), the emotional problems of paraplegic patients stem from the role reversal from independent to dependent. They initially react with depression, despair, bitterness, and grief. How well patients adjust depends on their personality assets or liabilities. Some preoccupy themselves with frustration, autistic thinking, and dependency as they relate to their physical limitations. Others are motivated to set new goals and accomplish social, economic, and vocational objectives, in seeking a new role in life.

The body image problems of paraplegics are different from those of amputees. The latter experience phantom-limb sensations. Paraplegics' efforts at denial of limb loss are difficult because they can "see" their extremities. They also have to adjust to other physical disabilities: root pain can be severe, bladder and bowel control may require many surgical procedures, and sexual capability can be an overriding concern; however, the latter can be alleviated by physical and plastic aids and ingenuity.

SEVERELY TRAUMATIZED PATIENTS

The individuals are usually victims of automobile accidents, shootings, stabbings, falls, etc., and are generally in shock, unconscious, and near death upon arrival at the trauma center. Unlike cardiotomy patients, they are unprepared for the experience because of its suddenness.

The core experience for trauma patients is unconsciousness. After three to fifteen days in this state, and after regaining consciousness, they attempt to fill the void retrospectively. Of sixty-eight patients interviewed after gaining consciousness at the Maryland Institute for Emergency Medical Services (MIEMS), forty-three were amnesic, eight were initially amnesic but subsequently recalled their experiences, and seventeen recalled the experience without difficulty. The latter two groups used fantasies and distortions in their recall (Schnaper, 1975b).

Many traumatized patients are amnesic, but some, if given enough time and fed bits of information by relatives, begin to remember and report "dreams" they had while in the unit. An almost universal theme of these fantasies is imprisonment. This idea is understandable because of their confinement to bed and attachment to many tubes and lines. Patients' reasons for being incarcerated are highly individualistic and predicated on their particular psychological development. Of twenty-five patients interviewed at the MIEMS, twenty-two recalled feeling that they were being held prisoner — fourteen of these patients remembered feeling that they tried to escape.

Interwoven and perhaps interrelated, with the fantasies of imprisonment is a very real death-like experience. At times, patients will hold a conviction that they are dead; at other times, they doubt as to whether they are dead or alive. Some patients report both experiences. Others, feeling the uncertainty, encounter and observe death. Of twenty-five patients interviewed, eighteen recalled feeling they were dead. Fifteen patients said that the feeling of death was "just nothing," and three were not sure whether they were dead or alive. None of the twenty-five patients expressed feelings about dying. The eighteen who reported a death-like experience referred only to the state of death, not the state of *dying*.

One can readily identify with such patients. They are incarcerated in a featureless cubicle and have no contact with the normal world. There are no windows, pictures, or flowers — just masked, hatted, uniformed wardens who usually hurt them. If they are conscious, the patients are deprived of sleep by twenty-four-hour monitoring, the hiss of a respirator; and background noises. Even their transfer by helicopter contributes to the patients' sense of physical disorientation. Disorientation and depression occur frequently in the unit. Staff members should be alert to these later symptoms and respond appropriately and quickly. Providing such personal items as photographs and tape recorders, as well as verbal reassurance, can comfort and orient the patient.

Delirium vs. psychosis; ICU vs. trauma center

Two pertinent issues merit discussion. One is the differentiation of postoperative delirium from postoperative psychosis, and the other is the difference between the typical ICU patient and the typical trauma-center patient.

Classical delirium demands an investigation of organic causes. Functional psychosis requires watchful waiting and proper supportive measures. Psychosis is usually resolved in forty-eight to seventy-two hours and can be established by ruling out organicity and by finding out if the patient has had a history of predisposition to psychosis. Disorientation and visual hallucinations suggest a metabolic disturbance and/or toxicity.

Both psychosis and delirium may be evident in the ICU and the trauma center; patients in these types of facilities differ. Patients in the ICU, as a rule, have had time to adjust to the idea of hospitalization. Trauma patients, because of the unexpectedness of their situation, had no idea that such a thing would happen. The trauma-center patients are usually unconscious when they are admitted, and that unconsciousness may be prolonged; they waken to total confusion. Not only are trauma patients unprepared for the hospitalization, but they must account retrospectively for the void in their consciousness. One of the twenty-two patients at the MIEMS who recalled feeling imprisoned felt that he was being held because he had killed a school bus full of children with his heavy truck (his injury occurred when he was crushed between the body and the cab of his truck while parked) and because he believed that he had urinated in bed. He observed his death by seeing his name on a tombstone. Another patient, a widow who had been injured when she drove her car over an embankment, dreamed that she was being held to be sold into white slavery.

The crucial dynamic in both cardiotomy patients and traumatized patients is a system of defenses. The cardiotomy patients have had the opportunity to mobilize their defenses; the trauma patients have not. With the return of awareness, trauma patients' defenses are intensely mobilized as they seek an explanation for the void in their consciousness. Although this is usually a homeostatic effort, it evokes painful images of death and fantasies of "badness" as reasons for incarceration. These unrestrained beliefs are the products of severe psychological regression accompanying the injury. Emotionally, these patients are children in a punitive situation that they feel they deserve. My belief is that all of the anecdotes about life after death/life can be explained phenomenologically as altered states of consciousness.

The trauma center staff

The staff forms the "heart and soul" of the ICU and the trauma center. Collins and Ballinger (1969) stated that "people, more than anything else, determine its value." In a trauma center there are many emotional compensations for the staff in their affectively intense and critical caretaking. They carry great responsibilities and can thereby gratify their omnipotent fantasies. They also encounter great stress, frequently compounded by fatigue. In addition, there are different transference and countertransference attitudes among the physicians, nurses, and ancillary personnel.

PHYSICIANS

The recent emphasis on the study of the total person and the recent increase in specialization have had a curious impact on patients. As a byproduct of this situation, patients are cared for by scientists rather than family doctors (Schnaper, 1969). The trauma team aims at combining various medical and surgical specialities to treat the patients' multiple injuries and their psyches – to treat the total person.

For physicians the sense of omnipotence is a double-edged sword. It spurs them to work long hours, far beyond the call of duty. Saving patients' lives is paramount. When physicians succeed, they radiate charm and good humor. On the other hand, when their omnipotence fails, they can be irritable or, after a long, hard battle to save a patient, shed tears for themselves as well as the patient. There are some physicians who experience a patient's death as an attack on their training, competence, person, and the integrity of their fantasies of being godlike (Schnaper, 1961). Hay & Oken (1972) reported the reaction of physicians in an ICU when a patient was failing. They became very authoritative with the nurses, demanding that they be waited on. Also, they either disappeared or tried all sorts of vain heroic measures.

The emotional tensions of the trauma center predispose physicians to peaks and lows in their relationships with their co-workers. Dedication to the task of saving lives, however, supersedes transient human frailities. The test of the physician rests in the number and quality of the lives saved.

NURSES

In the trauma center nurses are an integral part of the decision-making process and are involved in the crucial aspects of patient care. They may be required to act without hesitation, often on the basis of their knowledge and experience alone. Diagnosis becomes an important part of their job if they are to initiate treatment with the split-second timing necessary to save a life. Emphasis is on coordination, planning, and patient assessment so that crises can be avoided. Their responsibilities can be overwhelming or gratifying, irritating or satisfying.

For the nurse the ICU and trauma unit are inherently stressful environments: the machines (they must also be mechanics), the constant stimuli, and the overload of patients, some of whom are bloody, incontinent, and/or dying. Coping requires some degree of defensive detachment. The routine can be repetitive, and patients' relatives are always around. The nursing administrative staff is not always aware of the demands made on nurses in the trauma unit.

Unlike other ICU physicians and nurses, those in a trauma center must wait until patients regain consciousness to establish a relationship with them. Physicians, as well as nurses, must develop skill in communicating with tracheostomized patients, who cannot talk and who may be delirious. They must anticipate, sense, and read the patients' eyes, gestures, and body language. At all times they must also be available to reassure patients' families, either in person or by telephone.

MINISTERS

Although patients are either unconscious or awake and uncommunicative, ministers have a role here. The staff as well as alert patients observing their presence on the unit feel a sense of reassurance. They see someone who manifests caring in an unobtrusive calm manner. The resultant peacefulness is pervasive. The family of the patient is usually in dire need of reassurance and stabilization while the patient is confined to this frightening theater of operations. Ministers can be of great assistance to the family members as they attempt to cope with the trauma.

Care of the traumatized patients begins with preventing complications if possible. In the case of cardiotomy patients or other alert patients destined for an ICU, psychological explanation and preparation are imperative. Transfer from the ICU as soon as medically wise is essential. Efforts in "softening" the ICU atmosphere and having a psychiatrist as a member of the staff are recommended.

The presence of multiple trauma requires immediate and aggressive therapy. When time is essential, one cannot be mindful of the humiliation patients might feel because clothes are being cut away. One cannot do psychotherapy on dead persons. Once patients are stabilized, there is time to be aware of them as persons who feel threatened and have mobilized defenses. This is not to imply, however, that the trauma team should neglect a *humane* concern for patients.

Some suggestions have emanated from patients' experiences and were reported during interviews. When patients are unconscious (or seem to be, as with a stroke), they need to be spoken to, called by name, touched, and handled as gently as possible. Obviously, prognostications at the bedside are avoided. Patients who start to detail "crazy ideas" need reassurance, verbal support, and appropriate medication. While some staff members may feel uncomfortable viewing patients fondling their genitals, no effort should be made to interfere. Those patients who do recall masturbating describe the accompanying feeling as nonerotic, but one of "feeling safe," a "security blanket."

The patient with cancer

Not all extreme cases are found in the ICU or trauma unit. Although there are many life-threatening diseases (e.g., renal, cardiac, neurologic, pulmonary, etc.), the cancer patient can serve as a model for discussing the emotional problems that accompany a life-threatening illness. Despite the pessimistic view of cancer, it need not be hopeless or desperate. Certainly, life has a temporal quality, which can be serious but not necessarily grim. Despite public education the word *cancer* conjures up an immediate image of death and futility. Patients react to their diagnoses with an anxiety that is experienced as a stress, with little or no hope of resolution. For some patients, this word provokes prompt and necessary action; for others, delay and rumination. Clinically, many patients, upon being told they have cancer, experience overwhelming anxiety. They describe a feeling of being "stunned" or "fragmented." Some are emotionally paralyzed. Others call upon the defenses enumerated earlier in various combinations and utilize one, several, or all the defense mechanisms to cope with this stress.

Fear of a "lingering, painful death" arouses anxiety. Guilt also becomes prominent. Finesinger *et al.* (1951) found that 93 percent of the patients studied experienced guilt. In another study forty patients out of sixty felt "It's my fault" or "I've done something wrong." They attributed the cause of the cancer to sin (aggression or sex), lapses, or outside agents. They feared mutilation. Some of the sequelae of this guilt and fear were a delay in seeking treatment, feelings of inferiority, inadequacy, dependency, rejection, and inhibition of communication.

Patients meeting their illness with the defense of regression can pose a paradox for helpers. They become very dependent and seemingly grateful. Unfortunately, this gratitude is superficial. They feel a great need for doctors and see themselves as passive and vulnerable, which they deeply resent. This resentment is beyond their awareness. Guilt follows, because the doctor has been "so nice." Thus what the physicians see is an irritable, demanding, or withdrawn patient. It is incumbent upon doctors to be aware and not take patients' behavior personally.

Most dying patients (and "normal" people, too) entertain suicidal fantasies, but rarely act upon them. Although suicide would ostensibly avoid the pain of dying, the unconscious fantasy would be punitive. "Cheating" death, in a way, would be "cheating" and punishing those around them (family, friends, and doctor) who assume responsibility for the disease by not magically curing them. Then "they will be sorry." Patients thereby attempt retaliation. Prepared by their guilt in feeling "there but for the grace of God, go I," the family concur in this retaliation. There are patients, together with their families, who, upon being told the awesome diagnosis, flee their doctors. They seek repeated examinations from many doctors in many cities. Some finally find quack treatment centers.

Anxieties even emanate from fear of death, its searching questions, and fear of the unknown: "Will I rot after I am buried?" "Is there a Judgment Day?" Also, some fears are centered on losses: being separated from nurturing people who will be missed; the loss of body image, "Will I become emaciated?" "Will I smell bad?"; or the loss of control, "Will I reveal secrets as I weaken?" "Will I not have any say in what is done with my body while I'm still alive?"

Patients also fear regression because it implies role reversal and dependency. It can be a useful defense mechanism if it permits cooperation with therapy. There are those who resist regression completely, refusing to participate in their treatment and rejecting all help. There are those who capitulate to the defense by overdependency, becoming childlike in their clinging and, at the same time, resenting the dependency. There might even be a paradoxical response to "good news." Frequently, when patients are told that their biopsy was negative or that they are now in a "solid" remission, they will feel a great sense of elation followed by a period of depression. The suggested explanation is that these patients have their defenses (their "troops") always on the ready, only to find the effort no longer necessary. Also, they remain insecure, believing that "I'm OK now; but when will the axe fall? I have to sweat it out." One patient who had battled a breast cancer, recurrences, and metastases for six years, was told by an oncologist that with a "new" treatment, she "could be cured." After a day of high spirits, she became severely depressed. Her way of life had been geared to a total commitment of time and effort to fighting her cancer. Now she would no longer have anything to do and her life would be meaningless (Schnaper, 1979).

Care of the patient with cancer

Patients cope with stress: they have cancer, are anxious, and fear isolation. Despite the fact that they are patients with cancer, they are essentially patients and should be regarded as such. They can be irritated by hospitalization and treatments and displace this irritation onto the food and boredom. The dietician and the occupational therapist can address this outlashing through their skills. Family visits should be encouraged.

Oncologists should inform patients in a manner that is clear, unhurried, supportive, and accepting of patients' utilization of defense mechanisms. Oncologists should not take personally their patients' dependency, demandingness, or therapeutic recalcitrancy, but rather understand that these behaviors are the patients' response to regression. In the same vein helpers meet the families with calmness and a willingness to suppress personal annoyance or restlessness.

This is not to suggest that helpers be all-accepting and permissive, because such "passiveness" would not be in the patients' best interest. Also, because cancer patients have a life-threatening illness, it does not mean that they suddenly become holy or good. People die as they lived. If they were infantile or rigid, they will be the same during the progress of the disease. If they were flexible in coping, they will do likewise with illness (Schnaper, 1975a). In a sense, instead of "dying of cancer," they can "live with cancer" (or "alongside" of cancer). Whether they are "good" patients or not, they remain patients as well as humans. This recognition dictates that they be treated with concerned respect and appropriate therapy.

As time and treatments unfold, issues arise. Early on, physical and emotional complications such as infections, pain, body-image changes, depression, and more develop and continue. Helpers are not without resources. There are procedures and medications to combat infections and alleviate pain, tranquilizers for anxiety, and anti-depressants when appropriate. Yet, most beneficial to patients are their human contacts: family, friends, and helpers of all levels. Requests for visits from ministers or lawyers should be granted and, at times, even encouraged.

Simultaneously, there are patient-patient interactions. These go on in the inpatient areas as well as in the outpatient waiting rooms. Some feel threatened by the remission of another patient. Some are threatened by another's relapse. Some form close relationships, and still others keep their own company. All are very human reactions: resenting that other patients are "getting well, while I am not"; being frightened that others are relapsing and wondering "Am I next?"; feeling closeness with other patients; sharing a common experience; or getting too close to many who soon die so that "it hurts."

Even patients' denial of death can be useful. Denial in this instance can be equated with hope. Hope is crucial to acceptance of therapy and all of its potentially humiliating and painful side effects. To blatantly attack all use of denial could deprive patients of hope. Hope of cure can be realistic; insulin and the poliomyelitis vaccine give testimony to this fact. Skillful helpers walk the thin line between repeatedly and consistently directing patients toward reality and at the same time permitting patients the integrity of denial. If there is insistence on starkness, patients will lose all hope. An overemphasis on denial leaves patients feeling inadequate to deal with illness and the demands that must be met.

Guidance of patients should be through short, simple statements addressed to what they are saying or asking. Whatever is *really* being asked requires an answer, and it must be direct. If doctors are comfortable with themselves, the explicit and implicit demands of patients can be differentiated.

"Involved" helpers permit their patients to talk freely and openly about very private matters. In this way, despite the absence of a cure, patients' suffering is ameliorated. This is the "art" of medicine in its ultimate sense as well as an essential function of counseling.

During the course of the patients' illness, and even at the end, helpers *listen*. Listening is an art that is tedious and, at times, difficult. By listening, helpers permit patients to talk about anything and everything personal and/or seemingly inconsequential. Families should also be encouraged to listen to their ill relative. Some specialists who study "death and dying" advocate that families press patients to discuss their "feelings" about death. Most patients will discuss their thoughts and feelings about death (usually intellectualized denial) with their helpers, but many patients are not eager to discuss death with their families. Some patients fear guilt feelings for further "burdening" the family with their illness.

The minister's task is to help the patient live, and to live as well as possible until the moment of death. Orville Kelly's advice in *How to Live with Illness* to patients with a terminal illness is soundly in this tradition.

1. Talk about the illness. If it's cancer, call it cancer. You can't make life normal again by trying to hide what is wrong.
2. Accept death as a part of life.

3. Consider each day as another day of life, a gift from God to be enjoyed as fully as possible.
4. Realize that life is never going to be perfect. It was not before, and it will not be now.
5. Pray! It is not a sign of weakness; it's a sign of strength.
6. Learn to live with your illness instead of considering yourself dying from it. We are all dying in some manner.
7. Put your friends and relatives at ease. If you don't want pity, don't ask for it.
8. Make all practical arrangements for funerals, wills, etc., and make certain your family understands them.
9. Set new goals. Realize your limitations. Sometimes the simple things of life become the most enjoyable.
10. Discuss your problems with your family. Include the children if possible. After all, your problem is not an individual one.
11. Make each day count.

Clergy can be greatly helpful to patients and families both during the course of illness as well as at the end. The listening continues and at the very end the clergy offer sadness as well as hope, not tears (this belongs to the family) but the nonverbal sadness one friend feels for the other on parting. Ministers, when indicated, bring hope in a religious sense, and the response requires sensitivity on the ministers' part. They may even help patients accept a religious death without exerting their own convictions. The hope that should be conveyed is one of self-dignity, achieved by working through the difficult process of dying, just as one feels a sense of accomplishment by working through the equally difficult process of living.

Grief and mourning

From diagnosis to loss of consciousness or death, grieving in one form or another takes place. This ongoing process of grief is shared by the patient's family. All helpers can aid families and patients if they are attentive to their questions and the cues for help in grief resolution. At times, separately and privately, and at other times, together and publicly, but at all times, families and patients interact with grief (Parkes, 1972). Families play an integral part as patients move through different phases of the disease. Their reactions directly and indirectly affect the patients and helpers. They bring pressure on the providers to "spare" the patient and "not tell the truth." Implicit in this behavior is the guilt they themselves feel for having been spared the disease. A common reaction is resentment toward the diagnosing doctor. This is intensified if the patient is a child. Anger is felt toward the "messenger" rather than the message.

The grief process applies equally to patients and the survivors: the family's immediate response is shock and anguish, shared by the patient. "Why me?!" "Why him?!" "Why her?!" There are no answers to these questions, as no explanations or known etiological factors are forthcoming. Nonetheless, patients and their families look for explanatory fantasies: going out in the cold with wet hair, a neglected bee sting, a fall from a horse, an unforgiving attitude, frequent masturbation, etc. The initial shock response to the diagnosis introduces the grief reaction to patient, family, and friends. Death exacerbates the process for the survivors. Grief is the "normal" reaction to any loss or separation, e.g., divorce, a financial catastrophe, loss of a job, graduation, aging. Grief "work" is a psychological necessity—a "debt" that must be paid. The trauma must be assimilated and emotional ties severed. This separation must be resolved so that new relationships can be established. Mourning is manifest through the expression of the mental pain of grief.

There are overlapping phases to the grief reaction. Like all natural processes, the grief reaction can proceed in a variety of ways. Following shock, there is usually emotional release and tears. Emotion at first suspended, now reaches full impact with the realization of the loss. Fears are usual. Covert hostility is implicit in the protestations: "Why?" "Why?" "Why me?" "Why him?" "Why her?" At times one even hears the "Why me?" from a family member inferentially suggesting anger toward the patient for "putting me through this."

One observes the hopelessness, the loneliness, the helplessness, the sense of isolation, all combined under the rubric of utter depression. This period of depression can predominate and serve as painful expiation of guilt. Simultaneously, it can also provide a period of consolidation, an inventory of potential or actual loss shared by the patient and family.

Other phases can follow, though not necessarily in this order: panic with difficulty in concentrating; anorexia and insomnia as well as more serious physical symptoms; overt expressions of hostility toward the providers and/or family members; sadness at reminders of the potential loss or lost one; and difficulty with usual activities. After the patient's death, relatives experience a gradual waning of grief and mourning over a period of several weeks to two years. At the end of mourning, they feel a readjustment to reality: they are their "old selves" again. The stages may be summarized as *shock, turmoil,* and *resolution.* Most patients and/or their families begin the grieving process at the time of diagnosis. Some relatives postpone mourning until the death of the patient.

There are also pathologically morbid grief reactions: delayed or inhibited grief, chronic grief, overdependency, foolish behavior, and physical illness in response to grief. All require the intervention of the psychotherapist and need to be recognized by physicians.

In an effort to obviate later feelings of guilt and loss, some families move too close to the patient. They try to take over, telling patient and doctor what to do and not do. Other families anticipate the loss by withdrawing all interest in the patient. This is an attempt to protect themselves: "It won't hurt when he does die." These techniques are doomed, as mourning occurs regardless and is just as intense (Schnaper, 1969b).

It becomes the responsibility of helpers to be sensitive and alert to these grief reactions. They should encourage families toward a middle ground that avoids both extremes. This serves the patients' and the families' best interests. In this availability the care-givers stand by and resist the impulse to suppress mourning.

One defensive pattern for dealing with the spouse's cancer should be noted. The healthy spouse begins to complain of various aches and pains: headaches, backaches, leg or abdominal pain. Careful checkups are negative or the findings are minimal. In spite of medical reassurance the healthy spouse says, "I think *I* have cancer" or the equivalent. The concern for symptoms seems to be proportionate to the deterioration in the ill spouse's prognosis. The spouse's cancer is denied. The anxiety is displaced from the "horrible" (the ill spouse's imminent death) to the "terrible" ("my cancer"). The unafflicted spouse expresses verbally the guilt for "being selfishly preoccupied" and not thinking about the ill partner's serious illness. The healthy spouse hopes to die prior to the cancer patient. This would preclude witnessing the demise of the spouse with cancer. While these defenses find service in other serious illnesses, they appear to be peculiar to cancer in that they assume the diagnostic mantle of the patient's disease.

Reassurance of the spouse is helpful: but as the word implies, it must be repeated frequently. With some sophisticated persons, interpretation will work for a while. Like grief and mourning (which it is), it must run its course.

Helpers who include doctors, nurses, clergy (on the "frontline"), psychosocial professionals, etc., will have their own reactions of grief to deal with. Each will experience mourning in an individually determined way. As with the patient, so it is with the helpers. Helpers, being human, utilize personality and defenses, some to the patient's best interests and some otherwise. Some physicians and clergy find working with terminally ill patients difficult, if not impossible. They literally run away from the situation. If contact with terminally-ill patients or their families cannot be avoided, they limit their visit to thirty seconds and dash away. On the surface these helpers rationalize that they feel too deeply for patients' suffering. Also transference reactions can prevail: the patients remind them of ill relatives or friends from the past.

The helpers' defenses can manifest themselves in subtle ways. Emotional conflicts might be displaced, e.g., personal problems or problems in the family or marriage displaced into relationships with patients of the opposite sex. Projection is reflected when a patient's imminent demise is considered an attack on one's training or person. Helpers sometimes harbor omnipotent fantasies of being god-like (Schnaper, 1961). Patients, by their magical expectations, tend to reinforce helpers' fantasies and be very indulgent of helpers: they do not complain; after all, survival or salvation is in their helpers' power. If they perceive some coolness on the part of the helpers, they say "they're so busy" (rationalization); they understand that helpers must keep a "clinical distance" (another rationalization) (Schnaper, 1977, p. 883). There is danger that helpers become simply "providers."

The helpers' (as with all humans) feelings of omnipotence have roots in the past and ramifications in the present. Infants view the world as "my oyster." As they develop through a normal phase of ambivalence toward the objects in the environment, their feelings of power can also give feelings of pain. They are convinced that every wish is equated with the deed. Should they wish for someone to die (i.e., "go away"), they fully expect this to happen. At the same time, they are frightened that if the wish comes true, retaliation according to the *lex talionis* ("eye for an eye") is imminent (Schnaper, 1965).

The residue of this conflict between desire and fear persists in the helpers' unconscious. With awareness that their patient will die, they are compelled by unrealistic guilt and accountability to turn away before the patient dies, thus avoiding retribution. This is the same sense of omnipotence that is supposed to be able to kill or cure. Unfortunately, if this reaction is undisciplined, it can result in the rejection of persons in need and dying.

The role of the chaplain

From the beginning the duties of the chaplain (or minister) on the oncology unit (Andrews, 1981, pp. 11–12) have been primarily to visit with patients and families and to work with staff members. Support and encouragement are identified early by the unit's planners as ingredients needed for helping people cope with the stressful effects that cancer produces in their lives. The chaplain is looked upon as a source for spiritual guidance as well as for psychological and emotional understanding within specific situations. The chaplain's role is that of a minister dealing with crisis situations.

At first the role of the chaplain was basically to be a bedside visitor and to encourage people to ventilate anxieties, fears, and griefs. With the developing psychosocial expertise of the entire staff, the chaplain's role has expanded to include provision of more religious rituals, assessing psychological-spiritual needs of patients, teaching families and staff members, and training other ministers to work with people who are dealing with cancer. In addition to crisis intervention, the duties of the chaplain involve what Clinebell (1966, pp. 189–205) called "educative counseling."

The duties of the oncology unit chaplain include: day-to-day pastoral care of patients, families, and staff members; pastoral counseling with those who desire it; teaching staff, seminarians, and community ministers about the psychological-spiritual care of people living with cancer; and bereavement counseling as needed and desired by families and/or staff.

Burnout

Even those who work willingly and well with the critically ill and dying will have to deal with the cumulative effects of their service. The constant exposure to dying and death, with its painful twinges of failure, predisposes to depression. One's power, training, goodwill, resolve, and service are constantly being tested by repeated losses. All conscientious service implies a certain degree of stress. When stress becomes incorporated into the fiber of one's service over a long period of time, it diminishes the subjective work-gratification and sense of meaning, if not the performance. Other symptoms of burnout—besides loss of interest, blurring of creativity, and diminished productivity—are anorexia, insomnia, use of drugs, including alcohol, irritability, and withdrawal. Somatic symptoms such as increased heart rate and respiration, diarrhea, or constipation may also indicate anxiety.

There are various factors in intense patient-care units (particularly speciality units) that contribute to burnout. There is the constant crisis atmosphere, the intensity of the work itself compounded, at times, by lack of staff and double shifts. There are the sounds of people in pain, their moaning and crying, and the sight of blood, vomit, excrement, and torn or disfigured flesh. Death is present on too friendly terms. There is helplessness in spite of one's best efforts and anger almost without an object. There is a sense of loss. There is the weight of constant decision making and the fear of making a mistake. One's home life and social renewal take on great importance when faced with such intense work demands. Marital strife and family pressures, drinking habits (caffeine as well as alcohol), and ordinarily minor health problems can take on exaggerated significance.

Some helpers need a change of occupation. Others experience a transient "down" followed by renewed dedication. Friends and relatives of staff members find it difficult to understand how one can work on an intense speciality unit. There is no simple answer. Some conjectures about motivation are: an intellectual denial of one's own mortality; an effort to master death by increased knowledge; a need to rework a personal loss; and possibly, a response to the challenge and thereby a *proof* of one's omnipotence. Not to be overlooked is the conviction that one is doing interesting and important work.

The day-to-day coping with the stress is multifaceted, often subtle and always important. Management rather than treatment is the approach to the problem. Prevention is even better. Group meetings and one-to-one sessions within each discipline are useful. Research provides clinical distance, while nourishing a realistic sense of partipotence (partial omnipotence) at the same time. A sense of humor helps. Some well-placed vacations are necessary for the dedicated worker. A wide variety of interests and hobbies can help balance the narrow focus of critical care. Knowledge of relaxation techniques, a healthy sexual life, rotation through job responsibilities, support by colleagues and superiors can all rekindle work interest. Burnout attacks the sense of self; therefore anything that contributes positively to the sense of self, worthwhileness, and pride in one's endeavor fights burnout. There is no value judgment to burnout. It can happen in any profession and happens most frequently among the most conscientious workers.

Conclusion

The chronically ill, who are not technically critically ill, also beg our particular humane care. While aging does not cause chronic illness, the elderly are very susceptible to such illnesses. Aging in itself brings about a gradual loss of vision, hearing, appetite (taste and smell), and elasticity of tissues, and depression is frequent.

Some chronic illnesses can be controlled; others are fatal. Included in the former would be diabetes, rheumatic fever, tuberculosis, and mental illness. In the latter group would be the critical, life-threatening illness and traumata that have been the thrust of this presentation. Many physical handicaps (blindness, amputation, deafness, etc.) may or may not be a deterrent to a successful life. The fact of chronicity should not engender an attitude of hopelessness. The crucial consideration is how patients cope and how those in the environment deal with them (Schnaper, 1978).

Notwithstanding the expertise and clinical acumen of the helpers and technological ingenuity, many of our critically ill patients will unfortunately die. It is our humane concern that demands that we approach them with spiritual, psychological, as well as physical support.

Today, the highly honed skills in the discipline and practice of medicine are aided by ever-increasing technological advances. To limit medicine to technology is to exercise dehumanization. We should aim at comprehensive medicine. Comprehensive patient care encompasses the various clinical disciplines *plus* the humane involvement in all aspects of the *person* while he or she is a patient, critically ill or not.

The science and art of medicine are not antagonistic. They are complementary. The melding of medicine's art and science allows the care-givers to know patients as persons, to know their family, work, interests, and concerns. Their religious concerns are important and even crucial as the struggle with death intensifies. Humane treatment of the person-patient demands our interest and involvement beyond the technical expertise no matter how masterful.

While retaining our clinical objectivity, we need to react emotionally along with the critically ill person. All helpers need to develop empathy as well as technical skill. Every patient is a person. No person is a "case." The training of physicians emphasizes the medical-biological model of life and death; the training of clergy emphasizes the philosophical-social-psychological model of life and death. Both models are necessary to understand the critically ill. They are engaged in an all-encompassing battle against the forces of death. The terminally ill are losing the struggle. To understand the critically ill person is also to grieve and gain insight into our own feelings about death and life. Those who are experiencing separation and loss need ordinary, calm, unangry, unfrightened human contact, and not pseudoscientific theories. We benefit, through humaneness, as much as we hope that our critically ill fellow human will benefit (Schnaper, 1975a).

REFERENCES

Andrews, William Paul. *Developmental Tasks of Terminally Ill People.* Unpublished doctoral dissertation. Louisville Presbyterian Theological Seminary, 1981.

Braceland, F. J. Emotional accompaniments of cardiac surgery. *Postgraduate Medicine* 55, 130–35, 1974.

Clinebell, Howard. *Basic Types of Pastoral Counseling.* Nashville: Abingdon, 1966.

Collins, J. A., & Ballinger, W. F. The surgical intensive care unit. *Surgery* 66, 614–19, 1969.

Finesinger, J. E., Cobb, S., & Abrams, R. D. Psychological mechanisms in patients with cancer. *Cancer* 4, 1159–70, November 1951.

Hay, D., & Oken, D. The psychological stresses of intensive-care unit nursing. *Psychosomatic Medicine* 34, 109–18, 1972.

Miller, H. Accident neurosis. *British Medical Journal* 1, 992–98, 1961.

Mueller, A. D. Psychologic factors in rehabilitation of paraplegic patients. *Archives of Physical Rehabilitation* 43, 151–59, 1962.

Parkes, C. M. *Bereavement: Studies of Grief in Adult Life.* New York: International Universities Press, 1972.

Rome, H. P. The irony of the ICU. *Psychiatry Digest* 10–14, May 1969.

Ruesch, J., & Bowman, K. M. Prolonged post-traumatic syndromes following head injury. *American Journal of Psychiatry* 102, 145–63, 1945.

Schnaper, N. *What* preanesthetic visit? (editorial). *Anesthesiology* 22, 486, 1961.

Schnaper, N. Should an adopted child be told that he is adopted? *Maryland State Medical Journal* 13, 34, 1964.

Schnaper, N. Care of the dying patient. *Medical Times* 93, 537–43, May 1965.

Schnaper, N. Emotional reponses of the surgical patient. In *Tice's Practise of Medicine,* vol. 10. Hagerstown, Md.: Harper & Row, 1969. (a)

Schnaper, N. Management of the dying patient. In E. T. Lisansky & B. Shochet, eds., *Modern Treatment.* Hagerstown, Md.: Harper & Row, 1969. (b)

Schnaper, N. Death and dying: Has the topic been beaten to death? (editorial). *Journal of Nervous and Mental Disorders* 160, 157–58, 1975.

Schnaper, N. The psychological implications of severe trauma: Emotional sequelae to unconsciousness. *Journal of Trauma* 15, 94–98, 1975.

Schnaper, N. "Down the tube?" No: "rescue"—the language of oncology (correspondence). *New England Journal of Medicine* 296, 883, 1977.

Schnaper, N. Management of the chronically ill patient. In G. V. Basil, L. Wurmser, E. McDaniel, & R. G. Grenell, eds. *Psychiatric Problems in Medical Practice* (vol. 6 of *The Psychiatric Foundations of Medicine*). Boston: Butterworth, 1978.

Schnaper, N. Good news in cancer sometimes bad (correspondence). *New England Journal of Medicine* 300, 144, January 1970.

Weinstein, E. A., & Lyerly, O. G. Confabulation following brain injury: its analogues and sequelae. *Archives of General Psychiatry* 18, 348–54, 1968.

3

The Affective Disorders: Depression and Beyond

In the first edition of this book, Francis J. Braceland wrote eloquently about depression as an enigma; although recognized for centuries, and eminently treatable, it demonstrates many variations, and protects obscure origins. The focus of this chapter is quite different from that of the previous edition. This is not due to a disagreement with what was presented by my predecessor, nor is it an elucidation of the enigma. It is merely a reflection of the current emphasis on the biochemical dimension of moods and a shift in psychiatry toward a more well-defined role within medicine than a decade ago.

Mental disorders count as one of the four major public health problems in this country. Affective disorders, especially depressions, are the most common type of mental disorders among adults. The term *affective disorder* is a general one and refers to a mental disorder that fundamentally affects a person's mood. These mood changes — depression or elation — differ from swings in mood chiefly in degree and duration. They may occur without apparent cause, seem disproportionate, or even persist for a long time. Usually with these mood changes there are also disturbances in thought or behavior. The degree of abnormality of activity, affect, and thought in the person bears some relationship to the immediate social environment. Some estimates indicate that as many as 30 percent of the population develop a depressive episode during their life. Further studies reveal that about 15 percent of these persons are depressed at any one time, and that depressions occur two to four times more frequently in women than in men. Many, however, never see a physician, and perhaps only 20 to 25 percent of all depressed people receive treatment.

This chapter discusses the degrees and types of mood disturbances, especially depression. It will outline the symptomatology of the affective disorders and trace their clinical course. It will also consider the multiple causes — genetic, biological, stress, and psychodynamic — as they are currently understood, and will review the treatment modalities. Illustrative clinical examples are included.

Degrees and types of mood disturbances

We all experience a variety of moods. These include feelings of contentment, happiness, glee, excitement, elation, or, on the other hand, feelings of frustration, disappointment, unhappiness, loneliness, or despair. Moods and these feelings are considered "normal" if they are appropriate, porportionate, and manageable affective responses. For instance, grief, or uncomplicated bereavement, is a normal, appropriate, and affective response to the sadness of a recognizable external loss, and self-limiting, it gradually subsides. Aristotle considered melancholic mood to be the ordinary concomitant to superior intelligence and achievement. Ministers and psychotherapists know that growth and interior transformation are not accomplished without a degree of depression.

Depression, the most common mood disorder, was described clinically first by Hippocrates in the fourth century B.C. Braceland pointed out that Aretaeus, in the second century A.D., "described the illness and noted its association with mania, thereby delineating the manic-depressive cycle. In the same century, Plutarch gave a vivid account of it, in many ways comparable to present day descriptions of the disorder. In fact, the cardinal signs of the illness as delineated today have their counterparts in these three ancient descriptions of the same illness." Cases of affective disorder fall along a continuum from mild, short-lived, subclinical depressions and elations on the one end to severe delusional depressions and delirious manias on the other. Many clinicians who deal with affective disorder patients find it convenient to classify the disorder in line with the third edition of the *Diagnostic and Statistical Manual of Mental Disorders* (DSM III).

The most severe mood disturbances are listed (DSM III) as *major affective disorders* and involve either a depressive episode or a manic episode. A distinction is made between persons who suffer only a single mood (unipolar) and those who experience both manic and depressed episodes. The latter suffer a bipolar disorder. Those who have only a severe depression are said to have a *major depressive disorder*. A chronic mood disturbance involving numerous periods of depression and hypomania which are not of sufficient severity and duration to be considered a bipolar disorder are called *cyclothymic disorders*. When one suffers a loss of interest or pleasure in almost all usual activities and pastimes or is chronically depressed to a marked degree, that patient is said to have a *dysthymic disorder*. Any patient who has an affective disorder that cannot be classified in any other way is categorized as having an *atypical affective disorder*.

These diagnostic categorizations are attempts to bring about a certain amount of precision and standardization to a vague area. Each diagnosis holds implications for treatment. Although depression is common, casual diagnosis should not be tolerated. Precision is important not only to facilitate the comfort of the patient but also, because of the significant medical implications, it is sometimes involved. For instance, depression is frequently the first manifestation of serious physical illness. Second, depression is a common way for a patient to react to the development of a physical illness. In 1982 Sara C. Charles, M.D., suggested that "depression is one of the most commonly overlooked diagnoses in clinical medicine." Depression can also be a side effect of medical (especially drug) therapy. Ministers and pastoral counselors are sensitized to "moral problems" (acting out) that mask depression (as well as mania). Depression is really a syndrome that modern researchers suggest has multiple causes. In addition the boundary between normal mood and abnormal depression remains ill defined.

In an attempt to bring greater accuracy to diagnosis, a distinction is made between *primary affective disorders* and *secondary affective disorders*. The first refers to either the first psychiatric episode, or if there were previous episodes of psychiatric illness, they also were only episodes of depression or mania. The term *secondary* indicates that another psychiatric illness has been diagnosed (i.e., schizophrenia or alcoholism) or that the condition has developed from other medical or pharmacological conditions.

Formerly, a distinction was made between psychotic and neurotic depressions. Perhaps early treatment has had some effect, since the frequency of depressions of psychotic proportions has decreased in recent years. Even the term *psychotic* has lost its popularity; it has become synonymous with severe impairment of social and personal functioning. Description of the level and kind of impairment has more precision and usefulness to the clinician.

Another dichotomy used to delineate depressions was the determination of its source: from within (endogenous) or from some external stress (reactive). Although there are personality implications involved, distinctions based on biochemical reactions now seem to hold the ascendancy for exploration.

GRIEF

Depressive feelings that are part of grief reactions are personal, objective in the sense that they are caused by external events, and seemingly understandable. Ministers are confronted frequently with grief reactions of parishioners. Ministers are primary resources upon a death in a family. Just because the cause of the depression and mourning is understandable and, like most depressive reactions, self-limiting, its significance should not be minimized or overlooked. There is a healing process of value in working through and assimilating the grief experience. A minister can be a key resource in aiding a person in this salutary process. Grieving can develop into a clinical depression, even of major proportions, if it sets off a chain of guilt and recrimination, based on unresolved ambivalent feelings or sins, real or imagined. A minister can be a potent resource in short-circuiting such complications.

SUICIDE

Although the possibility of suicide is frequently raised by depressive disorders of all types, suicide is not exclusively limited to people with such diagnoses. Nearly everyone over the period of a lifetime has had death wishes and suicidal thoughts at one time or another. The number of suicidal attempts is much smaller than the number of people who have contemplated suicide, and the percentage of successful suicides is even smaller. It is variously estimated that attempts are five to fifty times more common than successes (the most common estimate seems to be ten attempts for every successful suicide).

M. R. Wilson and N. Soth discuss suicide in depth in the following chapter. It is sufficient here to note the following factors when evaluating the person for suicidal risk: most suicidal patients will admit their intentions. Ask! When estimating the possibility that a person will attempt suicide, the following questions are helpful: Have you thought of suicide? Have you thought of what way you would take your life? Have you already made preparations? Do you trust yourself?

Symptomatology of affective disorders

The symptoms of the affective disorders can be conveniently discussed under the two headings of depression and mania (elation).

DEPRESSION

The signs of depression comprise psychological and physical (somatic) symptoms. The chief clinical complaints of patients with depression include:

1. *Depressed mood.* The vast majority of depressed patients complain of this, and the symptoms include feelings of sadness, gloominess, dejection, and, in more serious cases, hopelessness and despondency. Their behavior is consistent with the verbally expressed depression. A small number of patients do not spontaneously complain of depression, but the disorder is manifested as two other symptom complexes. Such covert depression may appear as (a) chiefly hypochondriacal symptoms or (b) neurasthenic symptoms of exhaustion, fatigue, or weakness. A few people who are depressed do not complain of depression, and such cases are called smiling depression. Another small fraction of patients may complain of pleasurelessness (anhedonia) and say that previous interests no longer produce gratification.

2. *Anorexia.* Most depressed patients suffer loss of appetite and often lose weight, although a small number will overeat and gain weight.

3. *Insomnia.* Most patients experience some type of sleep disturbance. This may involve difficulty falling asleep (initial insomnia), difficulty staying asleep (interval insomnia), or early morning awakening (terminal insomnia). A few sleep excessively (hypersomnia).

4. *Psychomotor retardation* or *psychomotor agitation.* Depressed patients may appear retarded or depressed. Retarded depressions are manifested by decreased activity, including slowed speech and verbal frugality; inactivity. In stuporous depression the patient may be mute, immobile, and severely regressed. Agitated depressions are manifested by increased psychomotor activity, and this is evidenced in restlessness, jitteriness, pacing, wringing of the hands, and in difficulty in concentration (the patient reports that thinking is slowed down or that his or her mind is a blank, and often complains of loss of memory).

5. *Anxiety.* Many depressed patients complain of tension, apprehension, or uneasiness. This symptom must be distinguished from agitation, since the latter responds to certain kinds of neuroleptic agents, whereas anxiety responds to benzodiazepines (antianxiety agents).

6. *Lowered self-esteem.* This is usually accompanied by feelings of inadequacy, incompetence, and poor self-concept.

7. *Diminished sexual interests.* This is common during depressions, but not offered as a presenting symptom. Depressed men are sometimes impotent.

8. *Diurnal variations.* Many feel better in the evening than in the morning. There is no good explanation for this; superficially it would appear that the patient feels bad on arising in the morning because he or she has to "face the day" in a depressed state.

9. *Suicidal thoughts.* Many patients have suicidal thoughts, but only a few have suicidal urges (see the chapter on suicide in this volume).

Adolescent response to depression can vary. Acting out behavior, overeating, and oversleeping are not uncommon (see the chapter on adolescence in this volume).

Depressed patients may also complain of physical (somatic) symptoms. These may be manifested as mild physiological responses of any body system, hypochondriacal preoccupation, definite physical symptoms, or somatic delusion. Often it is the somatic symptom that first concerns the patients and leads them to seek medical examination. Depressed patients may complain of any one of a variety of physical complaints, such as headache, cramps, nausea, constipation, or indigestion.

A particularly depressed person usually has a constellation of the above-mentioned symptoms, but does not manifest all of them. We might speak of three depressive syndromes: ideational depressions (depressed mental content and few, if any, physical or motor symptoms); retarded depressions, which are manifested by decreased physical and mental activity; and agitated depressions, which are disclosed by increased psychomotor activity.

MANIA

In general mania (or, elation) is characterized by flight of ideas, elated or grandiose mood, and psychomotor excitement (generalized physical and emotional overactivity). An individual with mania excitement seems to be running away from recurrent depression. Elations are manifested on a continuum from hypomania to delirious mania. These are far less frequent than depressions. For convenience, they may be divided into the following:

1. *Cyclothymic disorder (also called cyclothymic personality or cyclothymia).* This disorder is characterized by recurring and alternating periods of depression and elation not readily attributable to external circumstances. This is more a personal "type" rather than a clinical illness.

2. *Hypomania (mild mania).* This is characterized by increased happiness or optimism. The thought process, rather than its content, is disturbed. Each individual act seems normal, but when it is considered together with other acts, the patient's deviation becomes evident. Char-

acteristically, such people are active, ebullient, socially aggressive, talkative, boisterous, and flippant. They behave with heightened emotional tone and are effusive and euphoric. They are impatient and become irritable when frustrated. They are superficial and insensitive in relationships with others. They are also intolerant of criticism, distractible (respond quickly to stimuli, but their attention is not held), and their speech is loosely associated (they pass rapidly from topic to topic). They may be openly erotic in speech or behavior. They usually remain oriented, lucid, and do not have delusions. Persons with chronic hypomania may accomplish much, although at times they may embark on schemes that either fail or that they abandon. They usually refuse to accept that they are emotionally ill.

3. *Acute mania.* Such patients are obviously psychotic. They are loquacious, often incoherent, and there is a marked flight of ideas. Characteristically, they are extremely distractible and often disoriented. They tend to rhyme, pun, and make "clang associations" (plays on words related by sound), and show marked psychomotor excitement. They shout, throw things, and continually move about. In addition, they are noisy, haughty, arrogant, and demanding, verbally abusive, expansive, and overactive. At times they may be combative and sometimes sexually indecent. Emotionally they are aggressive, irritable, and self-exalting. Sometimes they have delusions of grandeur, often in relationship to wealth, sexual prowess, or power. Paranoid traits are often evident, and sometimes they express hallucinations.

4. *Delirious mania.* This is characterized by marked aggravation of the conditions described above. Since the advent of modern psychiatric treatment, delirious manias are rarely seen.

Clinical course

Generally, depression can be said to have an onset that is variable, with symptoms developing over a period of a few days to weeks. Many depressive episodes are self-limiting and remit without specific treatment. With treatment, the duration of episodes has been reduced from several months to a few weeks. It should be kept in mind in dealing with depressive people that one can usually be optimistic that the depression will remit. It is estimated that at least half the individuals with a major depressive episode will have another one. About 15 percent of depressive disorders run a chronic course, and such people continue to experience depressed mood, sleep disturbances, and various bodily symptoms.

Generally, people who have manic episodes also have episodes of depression. Before the advent of the psychotropic drugs (neuroleptic agents, antianxiety agents, lithium) and electroconvulsive therapy, the episodes were usually longer. Manic episodes are often recurrent. Before the introduction of lithium therapy, only about 25 percent of the manic patients had a single episode. The prophylactic administration of lithium therapy often will prevent further attacks.

These disorders are characterized by one or more episodes of depression or elation. The major affective disorders are divided into two classes: bipolar and unipolar.

The bipolar disorder, formerly called manic depressive disease, is characterized by episodes of both elation and depression:

Example: Bipolar affective disorder. A well-respected thirty-four-year-old secondary school teacher was brought to a psychiatrist's office by her husband who was concerned about her increasing depression. Her marital situation had deteriorated markedly, and she had reached a point where she was no longer able to work. The patient was retarded and profoundly depressed. She could answer questions only with yes or no, but admitted she had suicidal thoughts of running her car over a nearby bridge. She was hospitalized for a month and did well on antidepressant medication. Following discharge from the hospital, she returned to the classroom, but soon this reserved lady began to exhibit troublesome symptoms: she became increasingly talkative, even telling dirty jokes in the classroom; she began staying out late at night, and picking up men in bars. Within a week she had her yard relandscaped, initiated an expensive and elaborate remodeling project for her house, and started a business of her own at a local resort. She resisted lithium therapy initially, feeling she'd "never been better, and no one else knew anything."

She finally consented to lithium therapy. In a brief time her symptoms subsided and she returned to the reserved, regulated functioning of a devoted high school teacher. This woman's husband had been an active alcoholic for several years. He gave up drinking and joined Alcoholics Anonymous three months prior to his wife's first depressive episode. This family, in its struggle to adapt, used not only the hospital, but AA and their church affiliation as well.

Major depressions, or unipolar affective disorder, includes former cases of psychotic depressive order and involutional melancholia, and some cases of depressive neurosis (also called reactive depression). The number of episodes is variable. There are people who have had only a single episode of depression or elation, but more commonly a person has a number of episodes over a lifetime. Generally, the course and prognosis for major affective disorders with treatment is favorable, particularly since the introduction of antidepressant medications, electroconvulsive therapy, and lithium carbonate therapy. Many psychiatrists consider it desirable to offer prophylactic drug therapy to patients suffering from major affective disorders. Without the prophylactic treatment, the usual course with recurring episodes is a gradual loss of economic, psychological, and social positions in society.

Example: Unipolar affective disorder. A fifty-two-year-old woman was admitted to a hospital after she took a large overdose of her elderly mother's medications. The patient's mother had lived with her since her marriage, but during the previous year there had been a significant change in the mother. She no longer cooked the meals or took an active part in the running of the house, which she had previously done as long as she had lived with her daughter. There had never been a separation between mother and daughter. Meanwhile, the family reported that the patient (the younger woman) had lost twenty pounds over three months, had difficulty sleeping, and had seemed sad and preoccupied. She no longer enjoyed any activity and had been increasingly withdrawn.

The patient presented herself as a severely depressed woman, with no spontaneity. Motor activity was markedly retarded. She was delusional and refused to eat for fear someone was poisoning her food. She expressed suicidal wishes and her insight and judgment were markedly impaired.

She improved markedly with large doses of antidepressant medication and was discharged from the hospital. She did well for two and a half years when she went off her medication. When her mother died the following year, the patient was again in the hospital after slashing both wrists in a serious suicidal attempt. She responded well to medication and returned home. There was no evidence in the history of any manic symptoms.

Causes

Any consideration of the etiology of major affective disorders must take into account genetic, biological, psychodynamic, and social factors.

GENETIC FACTORS:

As with so many other diseases, medicine now seriously considers the familial component of the affective disorders. There is an increased frequency of affective illness, particularly bipolar affective disorder, in the relatives of affectively disordered patients. Generally, these studies indicate that families with histories of unipolar illness are at risk for unipolar disease, and families with history of bipolar disorder are more at risk for bipolar disorders. Studies of twins show a concordance of 68 percent for identical twins (monozygotic) in the incidence of bipolar disorder. Thus, from these studies, it is evident that there is a genetic factor in affective disorder and that studies support the use of a bipolar-unipolar classification.

BIOLOGICAL FACTORS

Certain biological factors seem to be important. Several studies consistently suggest that a norepinephrine deficiency is the major factor in depression. Conversely, mania, which one would assume would be due to a simple excess of norepinephrine, seems more complicated. Current opinion is that mania results from the relative preponderance of dopamine (both norepinephrine or both catecholamines).

ENVIRONMENTAL STRESS AND LIFE EVENTS

Most clinical psychiatrists believe there is a relationship between the onset of depression and environmental stress. Some believe that such events play the major role. Some recent research confirms a relationship between stressful environmental factors (e.g., death or losses) and the onset of depression.

PSYCHODYNAMIC FACTORS

In the past it was believed that the dependent person with a low self-esteem and a strong superego was more prone to depression. Subsequent clinical findings have not supported the existence of such a single personality type or constellation of personality traits. Also in the past it was assumed that hostility that was turned inward was important in the development of the depression. While this dynamic formulation enjoys wide clinical acceptance, research does not support it. Mania is often thought of as a "running away" from depression. One formulation suggests that mood disturbances may be considered a result of the manner in which the individual handles impulses, especially hostile and aggressive feelings. When the restraint of one's censoring forces (conscience or superego) is removed, these impulses are freely expressed leading to a manic episode. If the censoring forces become strengthened, the impulses are directed against the individual and depression results. In this case, the effects are due to a rigid superego. Thus, some have regarded manic depressive illness as a "disease of the conscience," and hostility can be said to be the common denominator in both depression and mania. At present, however, the psychodynamic hypotheses are chiefly of empirical value, assisting the therapist to formulate a therapeutic program.

From a pragmatic viewpoint it is perhaps useful to regard the major affective disorders as genetically determined disorders, but that specific psychodynamic factors interpreted as "loss" can precipitate episodes of mania or depression. However, once started, the episode does not respond to interpretation, and thus the person usually requires treatment with medication or electroconvulsive therapy. However, once the episode is controlled with appropriate medication or ECT, psychotherapy may be helpful in dealing with the secondary consequences of the illness and will foster avoidance of precipitance or help the individual deal with contributing underlying psychological problems.

Example: Chronic depression. A thirty-five-year-old clergyman was hospitalized because of a major depressive episode and suicidal thoughts. He responded well to antidepressant medication and psychotherapy within the hospital setting. Following discharge from the hospital he continued both medication and psychotherapy for one year. Two years later he presented himself to his spiritual director with renewed feelings of depression. Knowing the history of serious depression (his former psychiatrist had died in the meantime), the minister referred his client to a psychiatrist for further evaluation. The patient was placed again on Elavil, with improvement in his symptoms. The clergyman continued to see his minister regularly for spiritual direction, but every one of several attempts to discontinue medication resulted in a relapse into depressive symptoms after a short time. Since his symptoms interfered with his personal and professional functioning, a joint decision was made to support this patient indefinitely with an antidepressant. He has functioned well, with his chronic depression well controlled with the help of medication and a supportive director.

Treatment

DEPRESSION

There are many effective treatments for the depressive disorders, including drugs, various psychotherapy modalities, and electroconvulsive therapy. Most psychiatrists adopt a pluralistic approach to treatment.

1. *Pharmacological therapy.* Although direct stimulants, primarily the amphetamines, were used by physicians for the treatment of depression for many years, the modern pharmacological treatment of depressions

dates back to the early 1950s, when the tricyclic antidepressants and the monoamine oxidase inhibitors were introduced.

Of the types of antidepressant agents available, the monoamine oxidase inhibitors (MAOI), and especially the tricyclic antidepressants, are the most commonly employed. Generally, they are effective antidepressant agents and act by blocking the neuronal uptake of amines into the presynaptic nerve endings. Generally, they have an overall improvement rate of about 70 percent. There are many tricyclic antidepressant agents, and in general there are more similarities among them than differences. Among these are: Amtriptyline (Elavil, Endep); Desipramine (Norpramin, Pertofrane); Doxepin (Sinequan, Adapin); Imipramine (Tofranil, also available in generic form); Nortriptyline (Aventyl, Pamelor); and Protiptyline (Vivactil).

Perhaps the two most popular monoamine oxidase inhibitors are Tranylcypromine (Parnate) and Phenelzine (Nardil). These are used when tricyclic antidepressants have not produced remission.

Recently, some different classes of antidepressants have been introduced and are gaining popularity. Among these are Amoxapine (Asendin), Maprotiline HCI (Ludiomil), Trimipramine maleate (Surmontil), and, most recently, Trazodone HCI (Deseryl).

There are certain toxic and side reactions that might result from antidepressant agents. The tricylic and MAOI drugs often produce anticholinergic effects (dry mouth, sweating, blurred vision, feelings of sluggishness). These are usually not serious, and most people can tolerate the drugs in therapeutic doses. The changeover from the use of tricyclics to MAO inhibitors requires a waiting period of one to two weeks in order to avoid the rare but serious reactions that may ensue (for example, hyperpyrexia or convulsions). It is also important for people who use MAO inhibitors (Parnate and Nardil) to realize they must avoid certain foods and drink that have a high tyramine content, and certain other drugs, because of the dangerous reactions that will occur.

2. *Electroconvulsive therapy.* This treatment, which was used extensively before the advent of the antidepressant drugs, is still effective and will relieve a high percentage of depressions. However, it is much less used now. It is an empirical treatment that relieves symptoms, and there is no theory that satisfactorily explains how it acts. Recent neurobiological research suggests that it may alter amine metabolism in the central nervous system. Such a theory seems plausible in light of studies that indicate the catecolamines play a role in affective illness.

The technique is as follows: Sufficient electrical current is passed through electrodes applied to both temporal areas of the head to produce a grand mal seizure. A series of such treatments is given, the average being six to twelve. In recent years electrodes have been applied over the nondominant temporal hemisphere. This unipolar technique is said to produce less seizure confusion and memory loss. Certain medications are administered in conjunction with the treatment to allay apprehension and reduce physical risk. These are usually administered under the direct supervision of an anesthetist or an anesthesiologist.

The following drugs are given intraveneously: Atropine, to reduce salivation and inhibit vagal action; Succinylcholine chloride ("Anectine"), to modify the muscular contractions of the convulsive seizures; and intravenous Brevital or pentothal sodium, to put the patient to sleep just prior to the treatment. Thus, the patient is put under light general anesthesia for a brief period of time. During the procedure the patient receives oxygen under pressure. He or she usually awakens from this a short time after treatment without any memory of having received it.

ECT should be considered in treating severe depression with a high suicide risk, or when the patient is not taking adequate food or fluids, and when the use of other drugs or other therapy is either risky or will take an unacceptably long time. It is usually effective in depressions that have not responded satisfactorily to adequate courses of therapy with antidepressant drugs.

3. *Psychotherapy*. There are a number of psychotherapeutic modalities that have been employed in the treatment of depression. However, generally most psychiatrists employ an eclectic approach, often using eclectic-oriented psychotherapy with a judicious use of antidepressants. Generally some form of supportive psychotherapy is the most effective. This type of therapy deals predominantly with conscious material and is centered chiefly on bolstering the individual's strengths and assets. Supportive psychotherapy includes reassurance, unburdening, and clarification. Reassurance is the imparting or restoration of confidence and freeing the patient from fear or anxiety. It does not mean false reassurance. Reassurance cannot be imparted unless one is really self-assured. Unburdening, another element of supportive psychotherapy, is the therapeutic release of feelings through conscious free expression. This is "getting it off the chest" and sometimes referred to as ventilation and catharsis. Lastly, clarification, still another element of supportive psychotherapy, is the process by which the therapist helps the patient to understand his or her feelings and behavior and gain a clearer picture of reality.

A word of caution: Advice should be given very sparingly. One usually does not know all the nuances of the situation under consideration. Furthermore, the depressed individual does not want advice, but rather someone to listen with respect and understanding, and without criticism. Also, we should remember that most depressions remit (the advantage of treatment is that it shortens the periods of depression).

4. *Hospitalization.* Although most depressed patients can be treated outside of the hospital, some with severe depressions, suicidal urges, or medical conditions that require extensive evaluations should probably be hospitalized. With modern treatment, the average stay is three to four weeks.

5. *Maintenance therapy.* For those persons with recurrent episodes or chronic symptoms, maintenance therapy consisting of antidepressants, or combinations of antidepressants and other psychotropic drugs, plus supportive psychotherapy, seems to be effective.

MANIA

Persons with mild elations (hypomania) can often be treated as outpatients. However, the minister who is seeing a hypomanic should be aware that such a person may be a victim of his or her own expansive behavior and poor judgment. Hospitalization is indicated for acutely manic patients. Aside from specific treatment for the episodes, patients often need protection from the social consequences of their expansive behavior and poor judgment.

Lithium carbonate shortens periods of elation and helps prevent attacks of either depression or elation when administered as part of a maintenance program. Other psychotropic drugs, especially the phenothiazines (such as Thorazine and Mellaril) and butyrohpenone (Haldol), are effective in controlling the maniacal symptoms. In clinical practice, since it usually takes several days for lithium to become effective, lithium and phenothiazine or Haldol are often prescribed simultaneously. When the elation comes under control, the phenothiazine or Haldol is gradually withdrawn.

In bipolar disorders, the goal is to prevent recurrences of acute episodes, relieve chronic low-grade disturbing symptoms, and improve the patient's adjustment. The most effective clinical approach to this seems to be combined drug therapy and psychotherapy. The medications used are lithium carbonate, or other antipsychotic medications, and supportive dynamic psychotherapy. Antidepressants must be administered judiciously to people who have manic episodes, since it is possible to "push" the patient into an elation in the course of long-term maintenance therapy. Occasionally electroconvulsive therapy is used on a maintenance basis to prevent relapses. Such treatment is given at intervals of four, six, or eight weeks for several months or years. This treatment has proven effective in certain cases.

Thoughts for the minister

1. Affective disorders, especially depression, are a major health problem. Anyone involved in the helping professions can expect to see many persons so afflicted. Ministers are not only no exception, but are the first line of defense for many sad, aggrieved, and frankly depressed people. Although ministers alone should not have to bear the full weight of diagnosis, they should be sensitive to the boundaries of what is bearable to the patient and supportable by counseling alone. A minister sensitive to the varieties, pressures, and effects of mood disturbance can be of tremendous help to young and old alike. For instance, depression in the elderly can mimic the symptoms of senile dementia, i.e., forgetfulness, lack of personal hygiene, retarded affect, etc. The treatment for each of these disorders is quite different and depression in the elderly responds well to treatment. An aware, informed pastor can be instrumental in providing help or initiating intervention for a situation otherwise overlooked or unattended.

2. Deeper and longer-lasting forms of depression require expert attention. The development of drugs which can alter mood and the refinement of understanding of the biochemical components of mood disturbance make medical intervention desirable in many cases and lifesaving in some. In the area of affective disorders, a cooperative relationship between ministry and medicine is ideal, since often both supportive therapy as well as medication is indicated. The consistent, hopeful involvement of the pastoral minister should be something the patient plagued with overwhelming inner feelings of helplessness and hopelessness ought to be able to count on, whether a period of hospitalization or medication is prescribed by a physician or not. But a patient has a right to the most effective and efficient treatment available. Treatment is usually maximized when several resources are mobilized: medical, familial, as well as spiritual.

3. Generally affective disorders respond favorably to treatment. This is important to keep in mind, since those who are afflicted with an affective disorder feel caught and doubt that things will ever be different. The depressed feel hopeless, the elated feel too good; neither experience the inner push to change. The confident knowledge of the pastoral minister that "this too shall pass" can act as a lighthouse to a ship in a storm. It does not diminish the turmoil, but it provides the promise of a safe harbor.

4. Many cases of mild depression never reach mental health professionals. These people, however, are in pews on Sundays, in parish organizations, and in the pastor's study or counseling office with a variety of stories and requests. They can be helped where they are. Sensitive ministers, whether counseling specialists or not, can be attuned to the dynamics of the struggle and offer support to endure, overcome, and learn from the stresses of mood.

5. The minister can be of help to the depressed person by showing concern and offering support and reassurance. Pastoral counseling can be of specific and crucial aid through these crises. Depressions often mark the turning point in people's lives and result in an alteration in life-style. Pastoral counseling can be the ministry of choice for that moment in a person's development.

6. Although the minister must be aware of the possibility of suicide in the depressed person, the prognosis for most depressive episodes is good. The weight of sad and oppressed feelings of a depressed and suicidal patient is difficult to bear for the family or a counselor. But hope, the one commodity which the patient lacks so completely, should not get buried in the supporting system. There is hope. Although the depressed person can only see it fleetingly and, in anguished moments, is tormented at the prospect of never experiencing it, all memory of it being obliterated, hope should stand in the minister. Those who work with the troubled and afflicted should take care to refresh themselves, keep their perspective, and order their personal priorities in order to serve refreshed and genuinely hopeful for the eventual outcome of a very stressful experience.

REFERENCES

American Psychiatric Association. *Diagnostic and Statistical Manual.* 3rd ed. 1980.

Eaton, M. T. Jr.; Peterson, M. H.; & Davis, J. A. *Psychiatry.* 4th ed. Garden City, New York: Medical Examination Publishing, 1981, (especially chapter 9).

Kaplan, H. I., & Sadock, B. J. *Modern Synopsis of Comprehensive Textbook of Psychiatry* III, 3rd ed. Baltimore: Williams and Wilkins, 1981 (especially chapters 16 and 17).

Kolb, L. C., & Brodie, H. K. H. *Modern Clinical Psychiatry.* 10th ed. Philadelphia: W. D. Saunders, 1982.

Rowe, C. J. *An Outline of Psychiatry.* Dubuque: William C. Brown, 1980.

4

Suicide

M. ROBERT WILSON AND NANCY BRITTON SOTH

Twenty-five thousand people in the United States kill themselves every year. Throughout the world the annual number of suicides is equivalent to the population of Edinburgh, Scotland, and the annual number of attempted suicides is equal to the population of London or Los Angeles (Battin, 1982, p. 1). The suicide rate goes up according to age groups: the older the person, the more likely he or she will die from suicide (Murphy, 1980, p. 519). Completed suicides are twice as high for men, although attempted suicides are twice as high for women. Although the rate of attempted suicide is higher among persons in certain psychiatric or social diagnostic categories, such as depressive reactions, schizophrenic disorders, and alcoholism, few diagnoses can predict a fatal outcome (Mintz, 1968, p. 271).

There are many reasons why people commit suicide. Loss can play an important part: loss of a loved one; a functional loss that might be physical or psychological (loss of a limb, for example); loss of position, status, or finances; or loss of normal social relationships (Pretzel, 1972, p. 70). Suicide may be the final result of aggressive impulses turned back on the self or efforts to destroy intolerable feelings or impulses within the self, such as those related to incest, homosexuality, or extreme hostility. It may be a desire to escape from real or anticipated physical pain, emotional distress, or from an emotional vacuum. The term *dyadic suicide* refers to a suicidal act taken in response to a human relationship. Such acts may be a cry for love and attention or may involve retaliation or a wish to punish another by engendering guilt. Other suicides may be more positive acts expressing a desire for rebirth, a desire to rejoin or merge with a dead or lost loved one. They can be attempts at atonement or expiation to make restitution or reduce feelings of guilt (Mintz, 1968, p. 274).

Very religious persons who wrestle with thoughts of suicide may take many preliminary actions to insure that life after death will be free of problems. They may stop going to church and become atheists, thereby disposing of heaven and hell, or they may finally presume that hell is better than life on earth. They can also look for evidence that God forgives everything (even suicide) and thus become more religious, ask God for forgiveness, and ask others to pray for them. Beliefs in reincarnation and life after death may also give encouragement.

Role of the minister in suicide prevention

As professionals devoted to the alleviation of human misery, ministers have an important role to play both in preventing suicide and in counseling the suicidal person. Yet, too many pastors neglect educating their congregations about suicide. Sermons on guilt or workshops to help people know the signs of suicide, or to make it more understandable, are absolutely vital in raising their level of consciousness. Any effort that can remove the stigma and mystery of suicide and cause it to be stricken from the list of taboo subjects will be of great value to those who have harbored thoughts of suicide, to those who have survived it (both attempters and surviving families), and to those who must comfort them. Pastors who can create an open and caring atmosphere (among the congregation) that can lower the threshold at which people will be free to call for help, have made a deep commitment to provide the emotional support necessary to prevent suicide.

Ministers will be helped in their own efforts if they can become familiar with the characteristics of suicidal persons and with what has been learned from counseling and rescuing them. There is a large body of knowledge regarding suicide and special considerations and procedures about which ministers should be aware. The information in this chapter is based upon professional experience and the research and writings in the field. Although some authors feel there is a real distinction between those who attempt suicide and those who complete it, that distinction has not been made here, since ministers must approach both cases with identical seriousness in initial treatment. Likewise, this chapter does not differentiate between counseling or intervention techniques for those who have actually attempted suicide and those who only contemplate it. The function of the minister in both situations is very similar.

Characteristics of the suicidal person

However misguided they may be, suicide attempts are efforts on the part of desperately unhappy human beings to solve a currently intolerable problem of living. These efforts may be directed toward bringing about a drastic change in their external world or in the internal world of their psyche. Suicides are not usually the result of a few isolated events in people's lives, but the end of a process of extremely painful events which lead victims into an irreversible desire to end their life.

There are three related factors that influence suicidal behavior: extreme stress, the individual's ego strength or ability to cope, and external resources. Stress refers to the external and internal events that press upon the individual; it must be seen not only in terms of severity but also in its meaning to the individual. Difficulties, stresses, or disappointments that might be easy for one person to handle may be intolerable for someone else; so we need to understand what "intolerable" means to each individual.

Ego strength is reflected in the person's ability to keep meaningful and realistic perspectives on emotions such as guilt, shame, or fear. When a person has not had the benefit of good childhood experiences or has not been able to build upon them or had enough satisfying experiences with people to make him or her feel worthwhile as a person, that individual may simply not have the inner personality reserves to bear with the struggle. So, he or she may need to turn to external resources of support that claim and maintain the person as part of the human community; often these resources are the important persons or groups in his or her life. The minister cannot always relieve the individual's stress, nor strengthen the individual's ego in a short period of time. The most important ministerial role is to provide external support and resources.

Counseling the suicidal parishioner

ASSESSMENT OF RISK

A crucial step in the management of suicidal persons is the assessment of risk. All authorities agree that it is a grave error *not* to ask depressed or troubled persons about their suicidal thoughts or feelings (Mintz, 1968, p. 277). Such inquiries should take place in private, since the presence of family members might inhibit truthfulness. The pastor (or minister) may be more reassured when such individuals admit they have thought about

suicide but would be "too frightened to do it" than if they become indig-
nant or flatly deny having thought about it at all. Seriously depressed
persons who deny any thoughts of suicide surely invite suspicion.

If individuals are truthful about their desire to commit suicide, they
should be asked how they plan to do it. If the answer is they don't know
yet, there may not be an *immediately* high suicide risk. The lethality of
means (a gun versus an aspirin overdose, for example) and the availability of means are crucial items to listen for. If there is talk of taking
sleeping pills, these persons should be asked if they have begun to save
the medication.

Another part of this assessment should include asking about others
who live with the suidical person, and, if possible, to learn if there is
something about them which may be unconsciously permitting (or in-
stigating) this act. Are they perhaps "calling the bluff?" Are they
themselves in need of guidance in managing this difficult task? Or, can
they, too, enhance the persons' external resources?

If these individuals are specific as to how they plan to kill themselves
and if the means are highly lethal and available, hospitalization should
be considered for the duration of the crisis. Hospitalization is but a temporary solution, and the work of prevention must still proceed.

SUICIDE PRECAUTIONS

If it is determined that such persons need not be hospitalized, every effort should be made to have firearms and potentially lethal medications
removed from the home. Although this seems obvious, reviews of cases
of suicidal outcomes reveal instances in which elementary precautions
were ignored and such inquiries were not made (Mintz, 1968, p. 289).
Having someone stay with the suicidal person is also helpful. If several
agree to be with him or her at all times, coordination among them is
vital. Such procedures have sometimes been described as useless, since it
is said that if someone intends to commit suicide, he or she can surely
find the means. This ignores several important considerations: the
message communicated by this type of care; the fact that intense suicidal
impulses are almost always episodic; and the fact that a suicidal person
might take barbiturates if available, but would not try hanging or jump-
ing out a window. Making unavailable the specific or previously selected
means for suicide can often prevent its occurrence.

COMMUNICATION OF SUICIDAL INTENTIONS

The myth that those who talk about suicide seldom die is erroneous and
dangerous. Most suicidal persons communicate their intent to others.

This communication is often a cry for help; whether someone recognizes it and adequately responds to this plea may mean the difference between life and death. Suicidal individuals communicate this intent because they may be ambivalent about dying and their communication is a plea for help. Or they may be so preoccupied with death and suicide that, even without their knowledge, most of their conversation indirectly reflects this concern. They may do this because they want to prepare relatives and friends in order to reduce the shock, or they may only want to threaten and taunt the significant people around them (Lester, 1970, p. 241). Even this behavior should be given a degree of seriousness so that these individuals do not feel compelled finally to prove that their threats are real.

Recognition of this communication is the first step, and the minister must be aware—and help others come to an awareness—of all that stands in the way of such recognition. Talk of suicide will make us anxious and uncomfortable, especially if it involves someone for whom we feel responsible. (For the minister or pastor, this may include a vast number of people.) We feel rejected and powerless, and we may tend to deny or repress the fact that it was said. We may rationalize it by saying that the person didn't mean it. Our respect (and concern) for personal privacy may often preclude a timely rescue on our part.

INTERVENTION

How do we justify our "interference" into a person's private decision to end his or her life? Suicide prevention consists essentially in recognizing that potential victims are in the balance between a wish to live and a wish to die, and the minister, just as the physician, must throw his or her efforts on the side of life. Most researchers have found that the persons who had attempted suicide, whatever the degree of potential lethality of the method employed or the seriousness of their desire to die, later said that they were glad that their attempts at self-destruction failed. Although the suicidal individual is ambivalent, the minister cannot be; suicide prevention depends on the active and forthright behavior of the potential rescuer.

Since suicide often stems from a dreadful sense of isolation, psychological support is greatly desired. One of the most potent forces in time of crisis is the empathic presence of an understanding human being. An integral part of a person's climb out of suicidal depression is the firm and hopeful attitude of friends, family, and counselor that he or she will make it.

Intervention is also justified because suicidal impulses may be temporary. People are acutely bent on self-destruction for a relatively brief period in their lives. Although for a short time persons may want to kill themselves, the rest of their existence cannot be disregarded. They must be given a sanctuary or the means of preventing suicidal tendencies after this period. Postponing the determination to die may infuse these individuals with the possibility of a different kind of resolution to their predicament. This is not to say that for many the impulses will not arise again; sometimes they occur quite predictably in a given patient at particular times or in particularly definable situations. Frequency and intensity may vary.

We can also justify intervention because there may be a temporary distortion of perceptions. Suicidal persons may be depressed, disoriented, or even defiant. Since most suicide attempts are made by persons suffering from depression, the diagnosis of this condition may be an important first step in the prevention of suicide. The syndrome of depression is made up of symptoms that reflect the shifting of the individual's psychological interests from aspects of the exterior life with others to aspects of private psychological life and to some intrapsychic crisis within the self.

The extreme loss of interest in the world around them may cause their perceptions of reality to be temporarily distorted. No longer can they be alert to other possibilities for solving problems, and they may grossly distort communications that are coming to them. The depression causes an inability to perceive or create alternatives. A decision to kill one's self at this particular time is a consequence of misperception, which is usually transient, and therefore justifies intervention. Suicidal persons may also be so desperate that they are distorted, confused, and unable to make a rational decision. Such persons (particularly younger persons or schizophrenics) may often make errors in logic, particularly when it involves the self. They confuse the self as experienced by them and the self as experienced by others, and they mistakenly believe that even after suicide the self will be there to experience the anticipated results of this drastic action (Lester, 1970, p. 205). Errors in reckoning can be corrected—and further justify intervention.

Suicidal behavior might be regarded as a continuum, with one extreme being irrational suicides who kill themselves entirely because of inner emotional stresses (for example, psychotics whose voices command them to destroy themselves), while at the other extreme would be suicides who destroy themselves because of external stresses (the businessman experiencing severe financial reversal or the terminal cancer patient in extreme pain). Psychotics will always need more intensive treatment than the pastor can provide. Indeed, it should not be the task of any minister to assume responsibility for the care and handling of *any* seriously suicidal person.

CRISIS INTERVENTION

Although the minister (or pastor) should not carry the primary responsibility for the management of the suicidal person, he or she may be the first person who is consulted—the first line of defense, despite the intense professionalization in our society. The minister's role in counseling the suicidal person is distinguished by three periods. The first step is to establish a relationship with the suicidal person, one of mutual trust and respect with a free flow of information. If the suicidal person can make no emotional response to the minister after the first meeting, the hazards of remaining outside the hospital are greatly increased and an immediate referral to a psychiatrist should be considered. If the beginning of a relationship can be established, both minister and parishioner should begin to identify the focal point—the reasons for considering suicide. The counselor must listen carefully to what the suicidal person hopes to gain by the act. It may not be death, but something else that is intended: attention, love, revenge. The minister should listen carefully to ascertain what the suicidal individual *really* wants. The latter may have been so confused and disoriented that it may be a relief to articulate this. The minister also must evaluate the suicidal danger and respond. He or she can assess the person's strengths and resources and attempt to mobilize all of them—the individual's own resources and those of others.

A therapeutic plan must be developed by the minister and implemented: hospitalization, psychotherapy, and/or family counseling. The minister should be ready to call upon professional psychiatric, psychological, and social-work specialists; their treatment of a potentially suicidal person may mean the difference between life and death.

The minister who is experienced in counseling should be aware that such crisis therapy differs from traditional counseling in that the counselor must be much more active and make decisions on the basis of limited information under the pressure of time. Another difference from the usual counseling process lies in the question of confidentiality. Although confidentiality in every other aspect is tenaciously kept, when clients want to kill themselves, the secret must be shared. Since most suicidal persons feel completely alone, those who are close to the person must become involved. Providing suicidal persons with the confidence that something positive is being done alleviates their feelings of hopelessness and provides order and organization in their life. Authoritative intervention will provide the emotional support that they need to overcome the crisis, particularly if it is temporary.

In considering the three interrelated factors that produce suicide—extreme stress, lack of ego strength or coping ability, and lack of external support — the minister is best equipped to provide external support. Even persons with a weak ego structure may survive a suicidal crisis if they are able to accept their limitations and devise ways to obtain support from others. Many suicides have been averted by the assistance of those who made available to a suffering victim personal warmth in a supportive and helpful way.

In most relations with adults, it is important not to foster dependency; thus, the minister must allow suicidal persons to depend on him or her in the beginning but gradually help those persons to widen the circle of dependency. Some high-risk individuals have an inability to express dependency and thus could never obtain the support and gratification they need. At the same time, if suicidal persons are to make progress later, one cannot permanently give them the message that another person is responsible for their staying alive. Those who make a suicide attempt are socially isolated and in need of affirmation. So strong is their detachment that they often feel like trespassers in the land of the living. It is therefore important to restore in them a sense of their own identity and a sense that they belong. The minister and the Church community can be an important part of this process.

Persons who contemplate suicide may be afflicted with a lack of basic trust, the development of which begins in early childhood. Later experiences either strengthen or diminish this trust. Religion, of course, is an important way in which trust can be strengthened. A person who does not have strong religious faith may possibly derive trust from other beliefs; but suicidal persons have usually failed in this attempt. They have not found adequate support either from religion or other sources to develop this sense of trust. The minister and the Church can address themselves to the task of nurturing the sense of trustfulness within suicidal persons with the hope that they can discover some things in life which can be trusted.

FOLLOWING THROUGH

Improvement in suicidal persons does not mean that the danger is over. Many writers have warned that suicide in depressed patients is even more likely when recovery is beginning and not during the severely depressed phase. This is because in the depth of depression they simply do not possess the psychic or motor energy essential to carrying out a suicide plan. It often takes place when these persons are in a state of relative calmness in contrast to their earlier agitation. Hospitalization of suicidal persons is only a temporary solution to provide initial protection, although therapeutic ties can be initiated in this milieu. A most dangerous time may be the period of initial home visits from the hospital and the first few months (at least for ninety days) following discharge. Release from the hospital, of course, always means an increase in the opportunity for suicide as well as return to the environment where the illness began.

The minister may play a significant role in helping suicidal individuals after an attempt. These socially isolated victims must be resocialized and reclaimed into the human community, and the Church has a unique role to play. In a society where the prevailing ethic is individual responsibility *only* for one's own happiness, the Church is the only place where it is still permissible to be one's brother's and sister's keeper. It is advisable to arrange a visit on the day of the patient's discharge from the hospital, and to make regular appointments for counseling in cooperation with the person's therapist, and if possible, to encourage the person to share insights gained through therapy.

Family and minister should watch carefully for any signs of regression and should request consultation with the therapist when questions arise. While the therapist and the patient are responsible for developing inner resources, the minister and the congregation are uniquely qualified to provide external support. It may be possible to call upon these persons for some task that will provide a feeling of importance or belonging, while working gradually toward the goal of relative dependency. For the first three months, frequent contact with these persons should be initiated, if only by telephone.

FEELINGS TOWARD SUICIDAL PERSONS

Suicidal persons may have a strong conflict between the seeking of love and the seeking of rejection and may act so as to force rejection so that they can confirm their resentment of the world. The minister must realize that such hostility may be projected upon anyone who attempts to treat them.

There must be a way for the minister to work through his or her own feelings about suicide, a problem that involves struggling with the very fabric of human existence. Someone who questions the basic assumption that life is worth living can stir up intense anxiety and frustration. There seems nowhere to start, and arguments beginning with this assumption seem empty. In fact, empathy and being present for suicidal persons are much more effective than reason. Hendin has recently suggested that even urging suicidal patients to live for their families is misguided, since many such patients feel they are living only for the sake of others (1981, p. 470), i.e., an empty existence.

There will be feelings of great frustration, fear, and ambivalence (love and hate), even complete immobilization at times toward persons who want to kill themselves. Such persons make taxing demands on the minister's time, telephone at inconvenient hours, and unconsciously attempt to provoke angry rejection.

Objectivity must be developed to avert panic. If the minister's feelings are too intense or if he or she becomes afraid of them, the minister may either deaden them or let them take over and lose all assets in counseling. Consultation with a psychiatrist or other mental health professional will enable the minister not to be engulfed by his or her own feelings or by the suicidal person. No one should be expected to be isolated when dealing with suicidal persons. Identification and separation of his or her own feelings from those engendered by suicidal persons will enable the minister to achieve the balance necessary to stimulate development of alternatives.

There are some who will need more than their minister or the Church to help them rejoin the human community. Suicidal persons are often in a state of emotional bankruptcy. In contrast to high-risk suicidal persons who cannot express their dependency, there are dependent persons who have alienated their relatives and exhausted their friends. Conventional psychotherapy and pastoral counseling have been tried and have failed. Although they are not psychotic, they often need long-term inpatient care for the full development of ego strength. Group therapy will help them to develop more socially independent ways of relating to themselves and others, and they often establish dependent transference relationships to institutions. One might say that only institutions are large enough and inexhaustible enough to endure this form of dependency. Such persons are too much of a challenge for office treatment. A normal human reaction to their extreme dependence is rejection, and in response to this they hold the ultimate weapon, another suicide attempt.

Periodic consultation with a psychiatrist will enable the minister to obtain the help needed to continue rehabilitation with suicidal patients, as well as to know when his or her own capacities have been exhausted.

COUNSELING THE SURVIVING FAMILY

Counseling the family survivors of suicide is a sobering task. The minister has had full experience with normal grief reactions, but for the survivors of suicide the grief process is intensified and more difficult at every stage.

The greatest problems may be the survivors' feelings of guilt. There is no question that many suicides are an attack on someone else; some suicides have been interpreted as "retroflexed" murder or inverted homicide. Persons who commit suicide have finally had the "last word," and survivors are left with strong feelings of frustration, resentment, and anger that are almost impossible to discharge without professional help.

The surviving family may also be estranged from others because of guilt and shame, so that there may be a loss of the usual social support that most grieving families may rely upon. The stigma and superstition about suicide remain strong even today. The minister can perform a true service by educating his or her congregation about suicide and by attempting to relieve the shock and stigma of such an act, so that all may respond to the survivors' personal catastrophe rather than ignore it. Since suicide produces so much anxiety, it is tempting for many simply to stay away from suicidal persons. A free discussion with friends and members of the congregation in order to mobilize social resources for the survivors is essential, and the minister can provide them with the initial courage to reach out in a caring way.

Providing aid for the family is a long and painful process. It may be described as having three phases: psychological recuscitation, rehabilitation, and renewal (Pretzel, 1972, p. 174). Resuscitation—i.e., attention to and care of the family—should take place within the first twenty-four hours. The minister should assist in the initial shock of their grief and establish rapport so that a return to normalcy can take place. Basic emotional issues will include blame, feelings of guilt, and even hostility. If survivors need to distort the facts or even deny a suicide, the minister may permit this distortion for a time. To the extent that family members need some defensive explanations of what happened, the minister may permit this, seeking neither to confirm nor deny the family's version, but accepting it as necessary for the time being.

The rehabilitation phase takes place within the next few months. The experienced minister can facilitate the mourning process at this time. Concern for the integrity of the family is important, as well as awareness of any social and emotional problems that may be developing. In the stage of renewal, the family works to gain control of its unity and integrity, and the minister will need to provide help only on request.

A surviving child is especially vulnerable to the shock of suicide. There are the same intense feelings of shock, guilt, and anger, and also a rage over the rejection and abandonment of the parent (Pretzel, 1972, p. 146). Family life prior to the parental suicide was probably in upheaval, and surviving relatives may be too preoccupied to provide the child with the support and guidance he or she so desperately needs. Another life is seriously at stake and professional psychiatric help may be needed.

Suicidal death inevitably brings up serious emotional conflicts, and yet the family may feel too frightened and vulnerable to seek help. The minister can assist by encouraging the survivors to seek psychiatric help, being careful to assure them that he or she is not in any sense abandoning them, and that this suggestion is by no means an abdication of pastoral care. The minister may also take the initiative to find a qualified therapist.

Special populations

ADOLESCENT SUICIDE

Suicide is a leading cause of death for adolescents in the United States; the rate for fifteen to nineteen year olds doubled between 1968 and 1976. Approximately five thousand deaths per year are attributed to suicide among teenagers (Crumley, 1982, p. 158). Suicidal adolescents may often be seeking a magical restoration of childhood, so that they might fulfill overlooked and/or unmet childhood needs and wishes.

Artistic creations, written compositions, essays, poetry, and lyrics by potentially suicidal adolescents will often depict themes of despair, isolation, and self-destruction. However, we must remember that the *normal* early adolescent is undergoing a grief reaction, mourning the loss of childhood and, to them, the omnipotent and omniscient parents of childhood. But at the same time, adolescents' pride prevents them from revealing this grief to others. Simultaneously, they "decathect" their world, withdraw their feelings. The transition from this period of normal mourning to pathological melancholia, depression, and suicidal potential is a common route traveled by many teenagers.

The basic dynamic in most adolescent suicides is one in which the adolescent regards him- or herself as being fundamentally bad. The symptoms of depression are harmonics of this dynamic; e.g., my behavior is bad (delinquent); my body is bad (hypochondria); I am a bad person (suicidal). Adolescents' degree of social isolation is often what determines whether they may make a suicidal gesture or a real attempt. As long as there is someone to whom they can turn for help or even against whom they can vent rage, suicide may be averted. If they believe that no one cares if they live or die, then suicide becomes a real possibility.

The adolescent suicide attempt should be viewed as a cardinal symptom of a serious psychiatric disorder (Crumley, 1982, p. 158). The seriousness is related neither to the physical lethality of the means for suicide nor even to the surface triviality of circumstances that preceded the event. Suicide attempts or gestures are their desperate communications to others, while true suicides are well planned with no chance of survival. Gestures and attempts, however, have associated dangers. They can misfire and the adolescent can die, and if *not* taken seriously by loved ones, this further proof of not caring will cause a final suicide attempt.

Adolescent suicide attempts must never be minimized, nor should any adolescent symptoms. A suicide attempt represents true internal pain, decreased reality testing, long-standing pathology, and increased lethality over time. Behind such attempts may be a depressive syndrome, poor adaptation, or personality disorders. Such attempts usually result from adolescents' feeling that they have been subjected to progressive isolation from meaningful social relationships. When strong feelings of hopelessness are present, adolescents may feel that they have been let down by someone on whom they have been depending. The hopelessness might follow a loss, such as the breaking up of a teenage romance. However, suicidal adolescents have usually had a long history of problems from early childhood. Adolescence itself brings a great escalation of problems, but these are also quite beyond those normally associated with the age period.

In order to discharge their misery and also to cry for help, adolescents use a number of "adaptive" techniques, usually taking the form of behavior problems. Jacobs, who studied adolescent suicide attempters, found that thirty of fifty had attempted all of the following categories of behavior: rebelling, withdrawing, running away from home, and suicide (Jacobs, 1971, p. 81). Usually adolescents who attempted suicide had tried these other forms of behavior first. When interviewed, they revealed that they had hoped such behavior would bring them the parental assistance they wanted.

There is not only a progressive failure of these attempts at adaptation, but Jacobs (1971, p. 27) found that there was a chain reaction dissolving any remaining meaningful social relationships in the days and weeks preceding the event. Such hopelessness and isolation deepens an internal process whereby adolescents justify suicide to themselves and gradually bridge the gap between thought and action. Adolescent suicide attempts may also be anger which is internalized in the form of guilt and depression, or for the more disturbed adolescent, reactions to a feeling of inner disintegration.

Treatment approaches will differ with the age of the adolescent. For early adolescence (ages 12–15), the more effective intervention will be through the peer group or through older teens, due to this stage of secondary narcissism (self-involvement) and their related acceptance of those who are most like themselves. In mid-adolescence (15–17) and late adolescence (17–19), individual therapy is more effective than the peer group. Adolescents are ready to seek more intimate one-to-one relationships and be more selective. They are then much less suspicious of adults.

A teenager has normal dependency needs, so that the minister must allow the development of appropriate dependency upon him or her, the Church, and the group. But what can the minister do if the adolescent is so socially isolated that he or she is not in contact with others or with the Church? One role is to educate the parents as to the seriousness of escalating behavior problems and the recent research that indicates that phenonema such as mood swings and poor family relationships are not necessarily normal ingredients of adolescent development (Offer, 1981, p. 152). Emotional turmoil is not just a part of normal growing up. Nor do we help adolescents who seek our counsel when we tell them not to worry about their problems because they are a normal part of adolescence and will be outgrown.

SUICIDAL CRISIS AND THE COLLEGE STUDENT

College students are more vulnerable to suicide than nonstudents of their age group. Most of what is known about adolescent suicides pertains to them as well. There are, however, new forms of external stress. Higher education provides a metamorphosis for most students, and the change can be frightening and painful. There are the problems that students bring with them and many that they may find there: separating from family, loss or modification of values and ambiguity about religion, excessive competitiveness and fear of failure, identity diffusions, and fear of homosexuality. The pastor and the Church may provide a haven for the young person who is suffering in the college environment.

SUICIDE AND THE ELDERLY

In America suicide is most prevalent among the elderly, especially among white males. Whereas at younger ages the suicide rate for males is twice that for females, among the aged the ratio is ten to one (Knight, 1968, p. 255). The potential for completed suicide increases with age, loss of a loved one, lowered interpersonal, social, and financial resources. In an older person, a depressive reaction carries with it some danger of suicide.

Elderly people contemplating suicide may give warning signals: withdrawal or rejection of loved ones, putting effects in order, and leaving letters with specific instructions. Suicidal behavior among the elderly is not usually a free moral choice, but is most often a symptom of culturally, psychologically, and biologically determined psychiatric disorder. Many of us make the mistake of thinking that little can be done in psychotherapy and other forms of treatment for older suicidal people. Increasing the knowledge and sensitivity of all persons likely to come in contact with older suicidal persons can prove to be effective both in therapy and prevention. All of the methods for suicide prevention and counseling pertain to the elderly as well. With an ever-increasing older population having access to affordable medical care, prevention and treatment of suicidal behavior is not only possible but a grave responsibility.

RATIONAL SUICIDE

A society that has legalized abortion, has developed *in vitro* fertilization, and seriously debates the question of euthanasia must also examine the individual's right to die. In a collection of essays entitled *Suicide: The Philosophical Issues,* Mary Rose Barrington argues that birth planning logically involves death planning: "It no longer makes sense to speak of a 'natural' end when very little is natural about our present existence. It is only the human animal that allows its fatal illness to spread over such extended periods."

The concept of rational suicide has gained more public attention and possibly more respect in the last two decades. Rational suicide is suicide in which the individual is not insane and in which a decision is reached in an unimpaired and undeceived fashion with full knowledge of the consequences. The person's motives might be justifiable or at least understandable by the majority of his or her contemporaries in the same cultural or social group.

Dyadic suicide, or suicide that involves a human relationship, is never completely rational: but there are some forms of suicide which, although we may not condone them, are not irrational. Many of us may acknowledge the rationality of surcease and suicide in cases where pain and suffering, either mental or physical, serve no further purpose. At the same time, it is still not clear what degree of pain and suffering must be reached before it becomes rational to avoid them by death. Some psychotherapists have had to face the truth that insistence on a continued life for deeply troubled and psychologically impaired patients may mean insistence on a continued unremedied and unremitting suffering with no opportunity for normal life satisfaction. Although these persons are few, if such patients committed suicide, their acts would not be called "rational," but many would feel that there seemed to be no answer but death.

The minister and the Church will continue to wrestle with the issue of whether it is morally permissible for individuals to choose to die, to acquiesce in another's death, or to bring about their own death. For those others who may not be completely rational nor masters of their own fate and who desire to succumb in the midst of their struggle, we must always be there to fill their emptiness with abundance and replenish their desire to live.

REFERENCES

Battin, M. Pabst. *Ethical Issues in Suicide.* Englewood Cliffs, N.J.: Prentice-Hall, 1982.

Crumley, Frank. The adolescent suicide attempt: a cardinal symptom of a serious psychiatric disorder. *American Journal of Psychotherapy* 36 (2): 158–65, 1982.

Hendin, Herbert. Psychotherapy and suicide. *American Journal of Psychotherapy* 35 (4): 469–80, 1981.

Jacobs, Jerry. *Adolescent Suicide.* New York: Wiley, 1971.

Kiev, Ari. Psychotherapeutic strategies in the management of depressed suicidal patients. *American Journal of Psychotherapy* 29 (3): 345–54, 1957.

Knight, James A. Suicide among students. In H. L. Resnick, ed. *Suicidal Behaviors: Diagnosis and Management.* Boston: Little Brown, 1968.

Lesse, Stanley. The range of therapies in the treatment of severely depressed suicidal patients. *American Journal of Psychotherapy* 29 (3): 308–26, 1975.

Lester, David. *Why People Kill Themselves: A Summary of Research Findings on Suicidal Behavior.* Springfield: C. C. Thomas, 1970.

Mintz, Ronald S. Psychotherapy of the suicidal patient. In H. L. Resnick, ed. *Suicidal Behaviors: Diagnosis and Management.* Boston: Little Brown, 1968.

Murphy, G. E., & Wetzel, R. D. Suicide risk by birth cohort in the United States, 1949 to 1974. *Archives of General Psychiatry 37* (5): 519–28, 1980.

Offer, Daniel; Ostroy, Eric; & Howard, Kenneth I. Mental health professional's concept of the normal adolescent. *Archives of General Psychiatry 38* (2): 149–52, 1981.

Pokorny, Alex D. Myths about suicide. In H. L. Resnick, ed. *Suicidal Behaviors: Diagnosis and Management.* Boston: Little Brown, 1968.

Pretzel, Paul W. *Understanding and Counseling the Suicidal Person.* New York: Abingdon, 1972.

Resnick, H. L., ed. *Suicidal Behaviors: Diagnosis and Management.* Boston: Little Brown, 1968.

Shneidman, E. S., & Farberow, N. L., eds. The logic of suicide. In *Clues to Suicide.* New York: McGraw-Hill, 1957.

Toolan, James. Suicide in children and adolescents. *American Journal of Psychotherapy* 29 (3): 339–44, 1975.

Weiss, James. Suicide in the aged. In H. L. Resnick, ed. *Suicidal Behaviors: Diagnosis and Management.* Boston: Little Brown, 1968.

5

The Paranoid Parishioner

WILLIAM W. MEISSNER

Confrontation with paranoid individuals can be most disconcerting and frustrating, whether we are pastors, lawyers, police, religious superiors, or even psychiatrists. Whatever our position and role in life, the confrontation with paranoia brings us face-to-face with the uncomfortable and disturbing irrationality that lies embedded in human nature. Anyone who deals with human beings, particularly when these dealings are personal, intense, and meaningful, encounters the risk of running afoul of the elements of paranoia.

For psychiatrists, who are schooled and experienced in dealing with the problems of mental illness, paranoia remains one of the most confounding, difficult to understand, and resistant to treatment of all the forms of mental disturbance. When psychiatrists begin their psychiatric experience as first-year residents and first come into close, personal, hand-to-hand contact with paranoid patients, the experience can be unsettling and confusing. One of the basic lessons that every psychiatrist must learn in dealing with such patients is that humility is the order of the day. Any hope of helping these patients find their way out of their difficulties travels a long, difficult, tortuous, and problematic road that must face and alter some of the most basic parameters of the patient's psychological structure and self-organization. The history of psychiatric attempts to treat paranoid disorders is not a happy one. The task is exceedingly difficult and the results far from uniformly gratifying.

If such be the state of affairs among trained medical professionals, whose life work centers on the understanding and treatment of emotional disorders and mental illness, what must we say of good-hearted pastors, the ministers of souls, who inevitably stumble upon frank and sometimes not so frank manifestations of paranoid thinking and disturbance among those members of the flock to whom they try to bring counsel, guidance, and spiritual assistance? It is essential for pastors, and particularly pastoral counselors, to learn the lesson of humility that psychiatric residents must master. For pastors, their best resource in this arena is a healthy sense of their own limitations and the inherent difficulty of dealing with and trying to be helpful in the face of paranoid psychopathology.

Depending on the context in which the paranoid manifestations arise, pastors are best off if they set themselves minimal goals and learn to settle for a modest, even minimal, contribution that may have some hope of setting in motion the process which may lead patients ultimately in the direction of resolving some of their difficulties. By and large, with very few exceptions, the treatment of paranoid disorders and paranoid personalities is a difficult and challenging task that belongs to psychiatrists who have the training and experience to undertake it. The role of the pastors and even the pastoral counselors in this connection is to facilitate the engagement of patients in a meaningful and productive course of psychiatric treatment.

The paranoid characteristics

The first question we must ask is "What do paranoid individuals look like?" What are the characteristics that allow us to identify these individuals as suffering from paranoid pathology? From one point of view, the question is easy to answer insofar as the paranoid manifestations are often dramatic and striking; but in another sense the answer is difficult, since these same characteristics tend to shade off into various grades of expression that might easily be found in a relatively normal population. We can speak here of a paranoid style that represents a manner of construction of life experience and an organization of the perception of reality which both permits a partial testing and validation of the subject's experience, but which at the same time involves distortions in the individual's reality experience. The paranoid state of mind can be seen as an organization or system of coherent beliefs which allow individuals to interpret and organize their reality in such a way that it serves certain adaptive needs. The manner in which individuals organize their experience serves specific defensive needs, particularly in defending against underlying anxiety or depression.

PROJECTION

What, then, are the characteristics of paranoia? One dominant characteristic of the paranoid style is the tendency to displace responsibility from the self and to place it on others. In this sense, paranoid individuals see their difficulties not in terms of their own internal conflict or inadequacies, but rather in terms of forces and external influences that surround them and cause difficulties. Instead of blaming themselves as depressive individuals might, paranoid persons blame others for their unhappiness. By this means they avoid the self-blame that is so painful and threatening, while at the same time it allows them to maintain a certain measure of self-esteem and self-justification. The blaming maneuver allows paranoid individuals to feel that their own behavior, feelings, or beliefs are indeed right, true, and good, so that others who do not see things their way or do not agree with their view of reality may be regarded as wrong, stupid, devious, or even malicious.

SUSPICIOUSNESS

The trait of suspiciousness is pervasive in paranoid personalities. Paranoid suspiciousness and guardedness serve an important self-protective function and allow individuals to preserve the rightness of their interpretation of reality. Paranoid suspiciousness is usually quite insistent in its effort to assimilate the available data in reality to the paranoid beliefs. This is not mere intellectual curiosity, but a constant pressure that requires the data of reality to be modified, distorted, or reinterpreted in a manner that will make them consistent with the paranoid beliefs. Clinically, paranoid patients are quite resistant to any attempts at clarification, testing of reality, or interpretation that are not consistent with their paranoid convictions. Any such efforts on the part of counselors or therapists only serves to cast them in the light of persons who seek to attack the paranoid patient at the point of greatest vulnerability.

GRANDIOSITY

Paranoid grandiosity is a general feature of paranoid states, but the intensity and degree of pathological distortion involved in the grandiosity is subject to considerable variability. Freud noted the role of grandiosity in paranoid states in helping to preserve the individual's self-esteem. The paranoid retreat to grandiosity not only involves a denial and a distortion of the perception of reality and particularly of these individuals' own inadequacies or limitations but also serves as a basis for the assertion of their own specialness and rightness.

DELUSIONS

In its most pathological form, paranoid grandiosity expresses itself in terms of delusions of an identity that has characteristics of being special, extraordinary, unique. Psychotically paranoid individuals may identify themselves with important historical or religious figures — Jesus, the Blessed Virgin, one of the saints — or with important political and public figures. The grandiosity, however, can be seen in more subtle forms as, for example, in ideas of reference in which patients are convinced that others are watching them, thinking things about them (usually uncomplimentary things, accusing them of certain sins, and particularly homosexuality). Such ideas may take an even more elaborate form, as when patients are convinced that they are the object of a far-flung and complicated plot involving communists or Nazis, the CIA, or the FBI, or even involving a far-flung international conspiracy. Hitler's delusions about a worldwide Jewish conspiracy would be a well-known example. In such delusions, patients become the focus for intense interest and conspiratorial effort on the part of many individuals, a position which makes these paranoid individuals of considerable importance and interest on the part of others — even though that interest may be malicious and destructive.

The paranoid delusions and the individuals' conviction of their reality is particularly strong and unyielding, particularly when the illness has progressed to a psychotic level. Paranoid patients are highly sensitive to any hostility, impatience, or irritation that may come their way, especially when the nature of their behavior or the stubbornness of their beliefs may accomplish little more than to elicit such reactions from people around them. Thus, paranoid individuals are unable to modify their beliefs in response to their ongoing experience of reality. But, as Freud pointed out, the delusional beliefs are usually not without a basis in reality, the so-called kernel of truth, which gives paranoid individuals sufficient ground to cling to their beliefs. At the same time, the paranoid conviction may also be based on a set of psychological pressures which make any admission of error or any yielding in their conviction somehow threatening or painful. The admission of error or inconsistency in their theoretical formulation means that these patients must also admit some sense of personal defect.

PARANOID PSEUDOCOMMUNITY

The last characteristic of paranoid individuals is what has come to be known as the paranoid pseudocommunity. As these patients' delusions evolve and become more consolidated, ideas of reference or persecution may be referred to nonspecific groups or to isolated individuals; but these delusions gradually become organized into a more unified and broadly extended conspiracy, which aims to work some harm against the patient as the intended victim. Thus, patients create an imaginary organization composed of real and imagined persons whom they represent as united in a conspiracy to carry out some malicious action against themselves. The formation of the pseudocommunity marks a phase of final crystallization of a paranoid psychosis.

Diagnosis

It may help at this point to review the recent diagnostic categories pertaining to paranoia as contained in the *Diagnostic and Statistical Manual* of the American Psychiatric Association (DSM III). The predominant feature of paranoid disorders in this classification is persistent persecutory delusions or delusions of jealousy. These delusions may be simple or elaborate but usually involve a single theme or a series of connected themes as, for example, being the object of a conspiracy, being cheated or spied upon, being followed by suspicious individuals, being threatened by persecutors, being poisoned or drugged, or feeling maliciously maligned, harassed, or obstructed in the attainment of longterm goals. In such individuals, even small slights may be exaggerated out of all proportion and become the nucleus of a delusional system. Delusions of jealousy may occur without any clear persecutory theme. In such cases, without any basis or relevant evidence, spouses will become convinced that their mates have become unfaithful. Offended spouses will then begin to collect small bits of "evidence" to bolster their delusional case.

The paranoid syndromes may be associated with anger and resentment that can escalate to frank physical violence. Ideas of reference are common and often accompanied by tendencies toward social isolation, seclusiveness, or behavioral eccentricity.

PSYCHOSIS

An important distinction between psychotic forms of *paranoia* and *paranoid schizophrenia* must be made. Paranoid signs and symptoms are often a prominent part of schizophrenic illness and take the form of persecutory or grandiose delusions or hallucinations with persecutory or grandiose content. Delusions of jealousy may also occur in schizophrenic patients. However, paranoid schizophrenic patients also show the stigmata of the schizophrenic process, which may manifest itself in a variety of disorganized symptoms, such as an unusual degree of agitation, anger, argumentativeness, or violence, or feelings of fearfulness and terror, along with concerns about autonomy, gender identity, and sexual preference.

The diagnostic discrimination between these psychotic forms is often difficult but has considerable implication for the prognosis. Theoretically, the relationship between paranoia and schizophrenia is a matter for considerable controversy. The classic diagnostic approach treats paranoid schizophrenia as one of the forms of schizophrenic illness; but more recent studies have demonstrated differences in level of functioning and psychological organization between paranoid and other forms of schizophrenia. These findings have led recent students of the subject to try to distinguish these illnesses more definitively.

Besides the paranoid psychosis, the DSM III describes two other forms of paranoid illness, namely, the *shared paranoid disorder* and the *paranoid state*. In the shared paranoid disorder, the delusional system develops as the result of a close relationship with another person who already has an established paranoid psychosis. Usually, when the second individual can be separated from the individual with the primary disease, the second individual's delusional beliefs diminish or disappear. Such shared delusional systems at times may involve more than one person. Such a phenomenon may be at work in some religious cults, for example. In contrast, the paranoid state is a more or less acute condition that arises as a result of some recent traumatic change in an individual's living or work situation. Such paranoid states usually occur with a relatively sudden onset, but are time-limited and rarely become chronic. Such states may occur in recent immigrants or refugees, prisoners of war, military inductees, or even in young people or college students who may leave home for the first time.

PARANOID PERSONALITY

The paranoid style may also be expressed in the form of a personality disorder, that is, a form of personality organization in which the paranoid features have become embedded as a longstanding and relatively consistent fashion of dealing with reality and personal relationships. In the paranoid personality the suspiciousness and lack of trust found in other forms of paranoia become pervasive and long-standing characteristics. These individuals are usually hypersensitive and easily feel slighted or offended. They are constantly scanning the environment for even minimal clues that may serve to validate their prejudicial ideas or biases. They have a limited range of affective experience and generally feel little in the way of anxiety or depression. Such persons become hypervigilant, constantly scanning and searching the field of reality to detect and defend themselves against any possible threat. They are incapable of accepting blame and avoid it under any circumstance in whatever way possible, even when such blame may be warranted.

Putting such individuals in a new or unfamiliar set of circumstances presents them with an intense challenge. They are forced to intensely survey the new context and search for the available clues that will confirm their attitudes and biases. The selection and emphasis on such confirming details invariably makes it impossible for them to appreciate the broader meaningfulness of a given context and the modifying or countervailing aspects of the broader picture. It is by no means surprising that their ultimate conclusion proves to be exactly what they expected in the first place and what they were looking for. Paranoid individuals are generally argumentative and easily aroused to agitated contentiousness. They are experts in making mountains out of molehills. To others, they may appear tense, anxious, guarded, even devious, sensitive to any least innuendo or any perceived hostility, and ready at a moment's notice to counterattack. They are ready at all points to criticize and devalue others, but any criticism of them is simply unacceptable. In their relationships with others, they may seem to be cold or unfeeling and lacking any sense of humor or spontaneity.

Paranoid individuals may often be seen as energetic, ambitious, hardworking, and competent. Generally, they tend to be intelligent and intellectual; but they are often also hostile, stubborn, rigid, and unyielding. They are often inflexible in their judgments and unwilling to compromise. Their capacity for intimacy is severely limited, since the capacity for trust is at best fragile. They have an excessive need to be self-sufficient with an exaggerated sense of their own self-importance, such that participation in group activities is either uncongenial or threatening.

It can be readily seen that the characteristics of paranoid personalities may be found in varying degrees in a great many people. The diagnosis, therefore, can be made only when there is a cluster of such characteristics and when the level of difficulty they create in the patient's life becomes sufficiently maladaptive or disruptive. The diagnostic problem, however, is that such paranoid traits may be manifested in minor degrees in a significant portion of the normal population. Consequently, drawing the line between pathology and normality is sometimes a considerable problem. Because of the nature of the disease, paranoid manifestations are frequently quite subtle and form a relatively hidden or latent portion of the patient's personality that may emerge only under special circumstances or stresses or after lengthy periods of treatment.

CENTRALITY

Consequently, we can think of a number of indices that might reflect the subtle and more or less minimal operation of paranoid factors and may serve as clues for an underlying as yet not readily identifiable paranoid illness or may reflect minimal levels of a paranoid personality style that has not yet reached pathological proportions. One such indicator of the paranoid process is the notion of "centrality." This expresses the quality of these patients' thinking that places them in the center of interest or attention from other people. The feelings of centrality may serve as a subtle expression of their feelings of being impinged on by outside forces, of a sense of being a passive recipient of external influences to which they are subjected and over which they feel they have little or no control.

HYPERSENSITIVITY

These individuals' hypersensitivity is another subtle indicator. They may seem more than unusually reactive to comments or opinions of other people; there often are feelings of being slighted or wronged or mistreated. Such sensitivity is not uncommon within the normal spectrum of behaviors and may often have reasonable justification in reality. When individuals present a facade of excessive self-sufficiency, one senses an underlying sense of vulnerability and susceptibility which is being defended against and countered by the hyperadequate facade. Both the hypersensitivity and the hyperadequacy reflect different aspects of an underlying vulnerability. By the same token the characteristic preoccupation with hidden meanings reflects the same underlying issues. In terms of the inherent dynamics of the paranoid position, things cannot be taken at face value; but the hidden, subtle, and fragmentary implications must be exposed in order that patients' experiences be consistent with their paranoid view of reality. The meanings that are thus divined behind the apparent data of reality are always overladened with threat, harm, or deleterious implication for paranoid individuals.

AUTONOMY

Another subtle and pervasive concern of paranoid individuals is the concern over autonomy. This may take various forms of expression and is often extremely subtle. Such concerns may emerge as a fear of loss of control, but often these may be expressed in avoidances or even unexpressed and silent inner reservations that resist the suspected others' attempts at influence of persuasion. Paranoid autonomy is a threatened and fragile autonomy.

EXTERNALIZATION

We have previously noted the tendency to blaming in paranoid individuals, but this characteristic may be extremely subtle. It is closely related to the tendency to externalize, that is, to formulate and understand problems and difficulties in terms of external circumstances, forces, events, persons, etc., rather than in terms of one's own internal difficulties or limitations.

INADEQUACY

Feelings of inadequacy or deficiency are pervasive in paranoid individuals. They may take the form of complaints about being too short or too tall; they may express concern about genital size or adequacy; or it may be more diffuse and nonspecific in form as in concerns about being somehow "different." Some paranoid individuals express feelings of being outsiders, of not being a part of the social, political, or cultural contexts in which they live.

AUTHORITY

The whole question of authority relations is particularly problematic. Individuals with a paranoid predisposition tend to be excessively concerned over problems of power and powerlessness. The concerns over authority may be expressed in a form of personality functioning that is described as authoritarian. Such individuals tend to be conventional, that is, rigidly adhering to conventional middle-class values; they tend to have a submissive and uncritical attitude toward the idealized moral authorities in any social group. They can be extremely sensitive and reactive against anyone who would violate conventional values, and tend to adopt excessively punitive responses to such violations. Their thinking falls into more or less rigid categories, tending toward superstition and stereotypical thinking. They are preoccupied with issues of control, power-submission, and strength-weakness, and have a strong tendency to identify with figures who seem powerful and influential. Such individuals tend to have a generalized hostile attitude, seeing the environment as though it were hostile and threatening, and expressing the belief that, unless control and rigid constraints are maintained, dreadful or destructive consequences would follow. Projection in such individuals is a major form of defense.

These attitudes can find ready application in religious contexts. They can be reflected in excessively rigid and dogmatic stances, in prejudicial attitudes toward other religious groups, in moral rigidities and stereotypical thinking, in rigid and unthinking adherence to authoritative moral directives, and in forms of superstition and fanatical investment. Moreover, since pastors or ministers are authority figures, they may become the object of such authoritarian attitudes and will experience passivity and willing compliance not only with their religious or moral teaching but also with any pronouncement they might make. Wise pastors know that such superficial compliance is accompanied by its underlying measure of rebellion.

To clinical psychiatrists, all of these indices may suggest the first stirrings or the minimal reflections of an underlying process. But in the broader nonclinical context, these same indices are the stuff of everyday human experience. Who is there among us, who, at one time or other, in one degree or other, might not manifest one or other of these indicators? The conclusion can be fairly drawn that manifestations of paranoid mechanisms and paranoid dynamics are not restricted to individuals who can be diagnostically labeled as paranoid, but rather may extend in varying degrees of subtle manifestation and intensity throughout most of humankind.

ENVY AND JEALOUSY

This overall impression receives considerable reinforcement from a consideration of certain pathological conditions that may not be explicitly paranoid of themselves, but are nonetheless closely related. The first of these are envy and jealousy. Such feelings are relatively common stuff in human relationships. Early views of envy and jealousy connected them with an inner sense of deficiency that involved feelings of self-dissatisfaction and self-criticism. Early psychoanalytic thinkers related such feelings to unconscious guilt feelings and usually related them to unconscious oedipal wishes. The unconscious guilt created a sense of lack in self-love and self-esteem, leaving the jealous person sensitive to any criticism and excessively yearning for approval or recognition. For such individuals, the loss of love is equivalent to a loss of their own self-esteem. More recent views have emphasized the vulnerability of such individuals to recurrent losses, which may contribute to inner conflicts that could only be defended against by primitive forms of projection and denial, thus enabling the individual to avoid the intense experience of grief and rage. Jealous and envious individuals suffer from significant narcissistic vulnerability.

The continuity between states of envy and jealousy and paranoid states is not difficult to discern. Not only are mechanisms of denial and projection at work, but there is a sense of wounded narcissistic expectation and injustice which serves to displace the blame for the individual's lack or loss to other persons or even to impersonal forces in the social environment. Envious persons begin to feel not only that they have a right to the possession or state of well-being that is desired, but that other persons' possessing it is equivalently an injustice that they have suffered at the hands of those other persons.

THE GRUDGE

Another state of mind which mimics aspects of paranoia is the attitude of vengeance or holding a grudge. The grudge has certain consistent characteristics: it occurs in the context of a close, positive relationship; the degree of resentment is usually out of proportion to the wrong committed; grudge holders often feel urged to defend or publicize the wrong committed against them; there is a tendency to phobically avoid the object of the grudge; and finally, the thought content is usually distinctively paranoid in quality. The injury, whether real or imagined, is narcissistic, that is, an injury to self-esteem is interpreted as a humiliation. At a greater degree of intensity, the seeking of revenge is associated with pain and rage, secondary to loss. Vengeful people are unforgiving, remorseless, ruthless, and inflexible. At the extreme, vengeful persons live with but a single object in mind, to get even. They seek revenge against all odds and no matter what the cost and experience no guilt, no concern for possible moral or other consequences of their revenge. Here again, the paranoid motifs of injured narcissism and victimization at the hands of persecuting objects are evident.

PREJUDICE

Another common and very widespread phenomenon that reflects the continuities with paranoid dynamics is that of prejudice. Prejudice is a very complex phenomenon, with many intrapsychic, social, economic, and even cultural determinants. Our emphasis here is on the psychic mechanisms in prejudicial attitudes, which mimic or approximate those of paranoia. A moment's reflection on social conditions of our time heightens the realization of the multiple forms of prejudice in our society — racial, sexual, religious, economic, and even cultural. It also brings home the realization that prejudicial attitudes are for all practical purposes endemic in the population and, given the right combination of circumstances and influences, any one of us may develop frankly prejudicial attitudes on one or other of these scores, depending on the extent to which they impinge on our own narcissistic vulnerability.

Prejudice carries with it an inherent antipathy, suggesting that it is related to underlying fear and anger and that hostility and rejection are expressing underlying unconscious needs. Study of prejudicial attitudes has revealed the underlying projective mechanisms that contribute to the distorted perceptions and interpretations in prejudicial attitudes. Prejudicial devaluations are based on underlying projections in which attributes of the subject's own personality are denied and projected onto the object of prejudice. For example, Caucasian individuals who regard intelligence as a part of their own ideal for themselves may tend to look disparagingly on blacks as stupid in an unconscious attempt to minimize their own feelings of intellectual inadequacy.

BELIEF SYSTEMS

There are also extremely important contexts of human endeavor which tend to mimic aspects of the paranoid dynamics but in themselves are decidedly nonpathological. Religious belief systems and value systems are such entities. The belief system organizes the understanding of some aspect of reality in terms of a coherent schema of explanation. The explanation is not supported scientifically by explicit evidence, but adherence to the explanation is urged on other grounds. The belief system requires assent, not on the basis of evidence but on the basis of inner needs that the belief system satisfies and responds to. Religious belief systems answer to some of the most basic and fundamental needs and insecurities in human beings. Religious beliefs respond to our insecurity about the meaning of life and the confrontation with death.

Such belief systems may enjoy varying degrees of closedness or openness. The more closed the belief system, the more one sees a rigidity in adherence to it, the greater becomes the insistence on maintaining the totality of the belief system with all of its parts, and the greater grows the degree of intolerance to other beliefs. The degree of dogmatism or closedness is associated with a need to adhere to the belief system as a whole. No single part can be challenged or questioned without posing a threat to the whole. Individuals need the support and security of a complete, totally integrated, unshakable and unquestionable view of their world and its meaning. If doubt is cast on any portion, this threatens the individuals' inner stability. This is the same quality of rigidity and peremptoriness that we have identified in the paranoids' need to maintain their delusional projective system.

Paranoid individuals find it essential to their sense of inner equilibrium to bring all data into congruence with their delusions and to maintain them even in the face of contradictory evidence. There is, thus, an analogy between the paranoid delusional system and belief systems, particularly religious belief systems, which involve such basic and fundamental needs. Consequently, there is little surprise that in the area of religious beliefs, greater degrees of rigidity and dogmatism are found. This by no means implies that religious belief systems can be reductively regarded as equivalent to paranoid delusional systems, but it does alert clinicians as well as pastors to the likelihood that religious beliefs held with excessive dogmatism, rigidity, and stereotypical thinking can become the vehicle for underlying paranoid dynamics.

Paranoia in the pastoral context

The guises in which paranoid manifestations can present themselves to pastors are protean and multiple. There is practically no phase of the pastoral ministry which does not, in one way or other, lend itself to paranoid distortions or serve as a channel through which pastors may begin to come in contact with paranoid difficulties. Priests or ministers may find paranoid attacks coming their way because of the hidden implications of something they might have said whether in a sermon or in casual conversation. They may be angrily and argumentatively accosted and challenged on the basis of some attitude or belief that was expressed. Paranoid individuals may become upset by something that happened in the liturgical setting, some text, some spoken word, some gesture to which they attribute a special meaning, often hostile, malicious, and threatening. Paranoid individuals often hold strong religious convictions, holding fanatically and stubbornly to dogmatic positions or moral beliefs and attitudes, and presenting these argumentatively to the pastor. Fanaticism is no stranger to religious belief, but from a psychiatric perspective, fanaticism of any kind can serve as an index of underlying paranoid pathology.

It should be added that religion has no prior claim on paranoia, but that paranoid dispositions and attitudes may focus in almost any field of human endeavor. However, religion and politics seem to be selective areas in which the kinds of issues that paranoid patients struggle with come to a particular focus. But these, after all, are areas in human experience in which beliefs and convictions carry much greater weight than factual evidence. It is not surprising, then, that they should become the privileged testing ground for paranoid issues.

Good pastors need to keep in mind that the paranoid potential is relatively widespread. Frank paranoid manifestations may seem to arise suddenly and unexpectedly, as if there were no prior context or backdrop out of which they had arisen. But frequently enough, on further examination, one finds some combination of paranoid characteristics either in the affected individual or in members of the family. The paranoid individual can go through many years of life with an attitude of isolated self-sufficiency, suspiciousness, and lack of trust, without this ever impairing the capacity to function effectively.

Often such characteristics, depending on one's position in life and work, can be relatively adaptive. If one thinks of the life circumstances of an FBI agent, or the average police, and even of a good lawyer, a touch of paranoia in the mix does not seem entirely uncalled for. An appropriate amount of lack of trust and suspiciousness about the motives and behaviors of others might serve very adaptive uses in certain areas of legal practice. Such characteristics or attitudes may persist for years sub rosa, only to erupt under a series of circumstances in which these characteristics no longer are adaptive but become maladaptive. The lawyer who begins to become increasingly mistrustful and suspicious of friends and family would have crossed the line from adaptive use of such characteristics to a use which becomes less than adaptive.

It is rare for individuals with paranoid dispositions to present themselves for treatment. In fact, insofar as the paranoia is operating effectively they do not need treatment, that is, the paranoia is effective in keeping any underlying anxiety or depression at bay and allowing individuals to convince themselves that external circumstances or other individuals are the cause of difficulties rather than themselves. More often than not, the vehicle by which paranoid difficulties come to attention is the complaints of others around these individuals. This may frequently be the situation in family contexts in which one or other member of the family has become increasingly paranoid and causes considerable distress, difficulty, or inconvenience to other family members. It may also be a difficulty in marital relationships where one of the partners becomes increasingly paranoid with disruptive effects on the marital relationship. In this context, it is not at all uncommon for married couples or the non-paranoid spouse to seek counsel and help from a religious minister.

A special word should be said about paranoia in elderly people. The onset of paranoid symptoms is generally a phenomenon of adult life, rather than early in life. In the early age group paranoid symptomatology is more frequently associated with schizophrenic illness. But in the elderly population, the inroads of paranoia are often widespread and marked. What passes for senile withdrawal or isolation may often have a paranoid component. This is not difficult to understand in view of what we know about the vicissitudes of growing old in our society. Elderly individuals suffer increasing degrees of debility and physical illness; they frequently suffer from the loss of sensory capacity, both visual and auditory; they are often socially isolated and economically deprived; the very process of growing old deprives them of the resources of family and friends and puts them at the mercy of strangers and social agencies whose intentions may or may not be benign, but whose practices are often inconsiderate and unfeeling, if not heartless and cruel. It is little wonder that older individuals would feel themselves victimized and might, in consequence, develop paranoid feelings. There is no parish or congregation that does not have its fair share of such elderly individuals, and it is the part of the good pastor to be attuned to and sensitive to their plight.

The role of pastor and pastoral counselors

I have undertaken this discussion of aspects of paranoid pathology and related forms of paranoid-like expression with a practical end in view. Perhaps the most important and most useful information that pastors or pastoral counselors can have is an awareness of when they are dealing with paranoid pathology and when not. If and when they have the sense that the difficulties being presented fall within the normal range, in other words, that these problems fall within the range of normal interactive behaviors in human affairs, there is good reason for them to feel that intervention in the form of support, advice, or counseling may have beneficial results. On the contrary, where they have the sense that they are dealing with a form of paranoid pathology, they are best advised not to try to deal with it alone, but to do what they can to facilitate getting the individual into proper medical and psychiatric treatment.

Consequently, referral and consultation must be regarded as matters of primary importance. To begin with, pastors or ministers should know the mental health resources of their area. They should not only know what and where these resources are and how one can mobilize them for assistance, but they should also have some sense of the quality and range of such services. Often where multiple such entities exist, in the form of hospitals or clinics, for example, the range and variety of services can vary considerably, and one such agency may be better equipped to deal with certain kinds of difficulties and another others.

Moreover, it is extremely helpful if pastors are known to such agencies, particularly to the administrative personnel. It is best when such relationships are personal and long-standing, so that when pastors refer someone to such an outlet, professional personnel know from whom the referral is coming and have a sense of what to expect. Good pastors should also know and have some familiarity with the mental health personnel in their parish or congregation. They should be able to call on these individuals for advice and consultation and should be able to make appropriate referrals to them when needed.

As indicated here, the treatment of paranoid psychopathology is a matter for fairly sophisticated psychiatric competence. Pastors or pastoral counselors should never try to deal with it on their own. The primary objective is always appropriate referral. Closely related to the question of referral, however, is the ever-present need for consultation. Wise pastors have at their disposal consultants who can be called upon for advice and support in dealing with the difficult questions and issues that almost inevitably arise with paranoid patients. Optimally, such consultation is carried on with an experienced mental health professional. Such an individual is by preference a psychiatrist, but not necessarily so. Experience and training are the key elements. The preference for psychiatrists rests on the relative depth of experience they may have had in the treatment of disturbed individuals and the medical background and training, which enable them to render a more professional judgment as to the advisability and extent of medical intervention where it is indicated.

It is also most advisable for the consultation to be carried on in the context of a long-term relationship, rather than to take place on an episodic basis dealing with particular cases that may arise. Psychiatric consultants work most effectively when they know their consultee, know their degree of knowledge, skills, and limitations, and also know the context in which pastors carry on their work, the nature of the population in the parish, and the sorts of problems and issues that arise in that context. None of this can be effectively known or integrated on a one-shot basis. Any pastor who has a large or busy parish, in which the likelihood of dealing with various forms of mental illness is significant, should have a psychiatric consultant to work with; the relationship should be professional, and the services of the psychiatrist paid for on a fee-for-service basis.

Given the kind of background and professional supports that have been suggested here, what can pastors do when confronted with paranoid parishioners? Whatever course of action pastors seek to follow, there are certain rules of thumb that they must constantly keep in mind. These rules of thumb are based on the inherent suspiciousness, lack of trust, vulnerability, and fragile autonomy of the paranoid individual. These rules of thumb can be listed as follows:

1. Openness and honesty are a primary requisite in dealing with paranoid individuals. There should be nothing hidden; everything should be above

board. Any concealment or deception will become meat for paranoid individuals' suspiciousness and will make them think that pastoral intentions are malicious rather than benign. In dealing clinically with paranoid patients, there is no transaction, no communication or dealing concerning patients of which they are not fully informed. There are no letters, telephone calls, insurance forms, or anything else regarding the patient about which they are not fully informed and over which they can exercise complete jurisdiction.

2. Related to the first rule is the essential respect for these individuals' confidentiality. No communications are to be made about them to anyone, whether family, friends, social agencies, insurance companies, doctors, lawyers, or anyone else, without their full knowledge and approval. Any violations of this principle will provide an opportunity and a stimulus for these patients' feelings of suspiciousness and persecution.

3. It is important in dealing with paranoid individuals to maintain an appropriate distance and objectivity. If pastors attempt to be too kind, too friendly, too helpful, too reassuring, this will serve only to activate paranoid patients' suspicions; they will suspect behind the overly friendly facade some more malicious intent, or they may experience the degree of closeness and involvement as itself threatening, a kind of impingement and influence that they will find it necessary to fend off. By the same token, if pastors are too cold, too distant, too dispassionate and uninvolved, they may be felt to be hostile or rejecting by the paranoid persons. This increases the liability that pastors will be seen as a persecutor or foe.

Perhaps the best attitude can be described as one of benign objectivity. Pastors must keep in mind that they can be most useful to paranoid individuals if the former can present themselves as persons who can be trusted and relied on. In dealing with paranoid individuals, the ground of trust is constantly being probed and tested. Essentially, paranoid individuals must be allowed to seek and find that degree of relationship and involvement with which they can be most comfortable. It is only within such context that the capacity for trust, however minimal, can be mobilized.

4. One of the great mistakes one can make in dealing with paranoid individuals is to get engaged in an argument about their delusions or to try to use logical arguments to dissuade them from irrational beliefs or suspicions. It never works, and pastors who make the attempt will only reinforce these individuals' suspicions and place themselves among such individuals' foes rather than their friends.

At times paranoid individuals will make an effort to convince pastors of the rightness of their (the patients') views and try to extort from them an acceptance or endorsement. Pastors do best to hold firmly to a position of benign objectivity or neutrality, neither arguing with nor rejecting patients' delusions on the one hand, nor giving them any support or credence on the other. An attitude of nonthreatening and interested concern is perhaps most useful. An attitude of empathy with patients' fright, sense of vulnerability or weakness, disappointment, disillusionment, or even resentment and rage can be very helpful. If paranoid persons try to force the issue, the best one can do is to express one's sympathy and understanding for their plight, but to firmly and nonthreateningly and nonargumentatively maintain one's own view of the reality. When it becomes clear to paranoid individuals that pastors are not going to threaten or counterattack or try to argue them out of their beliefs, the defensive need diminishes and they can more readily accept the pastors' insistence on maintaining an independent view.

5. Pastors should resist all attempts to gain allegiance on the part of others, who may be involved with the patient. The pastor's position must be one of consistent and absolute neutrality. If the paranoid individual gets the idea that pastors are taking sides with those "others," pastors thereby become the foe. This may be a difficult line to hew, particularly when the anxieties and distress created in others by the paranoid individuals' behavior may be rather intense.

6. Respect for the fragile autonomy of paranoid individuals plays a central role. Nothing should be forced on the paranoid individuals, but, insofar as possible, their sense of autonomy and free decision should be maintained intact. Whatever suggestions or interventions or courses of action might be recommended should be presented to the paranoid individual for consideration and approval, and any implication that they might be forced upon the patient should be assiduously avoided. In the treatment of such individuals, for example, the issue of medications often comes up. Paranoid patients do not like to take medications, particularly because such medications may diminish the state of hypervigilant scanning that these patients feel necessary for their survival. Doctors may suggest medications as useful and helpful for the patient's condition, but if they are wise they will not force them on the patient. Nonetheless, the issues related to the taking of medication, the exploration of patients' fears and motives, remains a focus of the therapy so that in time the patients themselves may see the wisdom of taking medication and accept it in a context of a trusting relationship with their physician and as a matter of their own determination.

There are times, however, when paranoid patients force the issue so that therapists must intervene and take decisive action that does in fact violate the patients' autonomy. Such is the case when the paranoia has reached psychotic proportions, as is often the case when it is linked with schizophrenic illness, or when patients have become a high risk for injury either to themselves or others. If, at such a point, the decision is reached to hospitalize the patient, the action is taken decisively and firmly, without equivocation or second thoughts or guilt, and is presented to the patient as necessitated by his or her condition. Fortunately, pastors are never in the position of making such a decision, or, at most, will only be tangentially involved in implementing or facilitating a decision that has been reached on medical or psychiatric grounds. In any case wise pastors do not take any course of action or do not suggest any intervention without previous consultation.

In the face of paranoid psychopathology, the difficulties are immense, and the line between what may be helpful and productive and what may be misguided and counterproductive is extremely narrow. Wise pastors will avail themselves of appropriate consultation in such a context and will work out an approach to this particular disturbed individual that is consistent with the role of pastor and makes good psychiatric sense.

Pastors who have a sense of their own limitations, who can approach their paranoid parishioners with an appropriate sense of humility and prudence, who can be both respectful and firm, tactful and objective, will be in the best position to do what is helpful. That optimal course is never the same in each case and must be tailored to the needs and vulnerability of each paranoid individual. Pastors who try to do it on their own risk not only not helping their parishioner, but may also put themselves at risk of paranoid hostility and even attack. Pastors who can enlist the aid of those who know best how to help gain strength and security and, more certainly, provide the assistance that the troubled parishioner needs.

REFERENCE

Meissner, William W. *The Paranoid Process.* New York: J. Aronson, 1978.

6

Adolescent Drug Abuse

CHARLES MCCAFFERTY

Would that we could forego the age between four and ten and one and twenty when youth do nothing but fight, drink, and get wench with child.

— *Shakespeare*

Since the late 1960s the use of non-medical drugs has become a common adolescent experience. A 1973 survey of illicit drug use indicated that 40.9 percent of adolescents used mind-altering drugs whereas recent surveys have suggested that more than 80 percent of adolescents of high school age have experimented at least once with marijuana. Drug experimentation in itself need not be considered evidence of psychopathology. Some have defined it as a self-administration of a drug to discover its psychological, physical, and social effects. However, in some adolescents, even with experimentation, the drug response may be unpredictable, and may, even in extreme cases, give rise to psychotic decompensation.

Enormous public concern over drug abuse among our young has brought about the appointment of presidential committees and the passage of legislation to cope with the problem. In spite of this the dynamics and the causes of drug abuse among adolescents have not been well delineated. The concept of identity provides a framework for understanding many aspects of both normal and pathological adolescent behavior. Adolescence is a period of flux with active psychobiological growth where personality and identity are forming — not formed. The problem with drug abuse is therefore much more complex in adolescents than in adults.

Alcoholism and drug abuse in adults traditionally have been looked on as either character disorders or evidences of an inebriate life-style. The traditional Alcoholics Anonymous philosophy sees alcoholism as primary, and once diagnosed, requiring life-long abstinence. These concepts are often extrapolated to adolescents. Labeling a thirteen-year-old as an alcoholic may create problems by providing the youngster with a pseudoidentity; it may interfere with vocational plans and create legal difficulties in adulthood which were not anticipated at the time of the diagnosis. It runs counter to adolescent psychiatry's concept of the adolescent as being amenable and accessible to psychiatric intervention, a person with a potential for cure rather than mere control.

The use of drugs by a depressed adolescent may be no more than the equivalent to other self-destructive behavior by such an individual, such as promiscuity or suicidal gestures. The diagnosis of substance abuse or chemical dependency should not be made merely because of the presence of substance abuse as a symptom. Such diagnoses are often made on the basis of "soft" data derived from questionnaires. The term *chemical dependency,* that originated in Minnesota, has no hard-and-fast definition that fits into the scientific framework. Strictly speaking, a diabetic or hypothyroid adolescent is chemically dependent on insulin and thyroid.

The diagnosis of alcoholism in some cases is most difficult in adults, but liver function tests, delirium tremens, and the physical stigmata of chronic, excessive alcohol use are often helpful diagnostic indicators. None of these, however, are useful in the adolescent. Diagnosis in adolescents differs not only psychologically but also physiologically from diagnosis in adults.

For a variety of reasons there is a tendency to overdiagnose substance abuse in the adolescent. In the past ten years it has become a more socially acceptable diagnosis than depression or schizophrenia, and insurance coverage is more readily available and payable for this diagnosis.

Many of the signs of abnormal behavior which suggest chemical dependency in an adult do not necessarily indicate behavior that is abnormal in an adolescent. The history of uncontrollable and destructive use is hard to document in the adolescent when the user's patterns are relatively short and possibly erratic. It has been suggested that most adolescent chemical use problems are episodic behavioral situations rather than actual dependency.

Case 1

A seventeen-year-old girl was brought in panic by her mother to the hospital emergency room after the mother had been awakened about

2:00 A.M. by a loud noise in the girl's bedroom. Upon investigation the mother found her daughter to be quite intoxicated with giddy behavior and unsteadiness on her feet to the point where she had tripped over some books on the floor and knocked her bedside table over, causing that commotion. The mother was particularly shocked because the girl was on the honor roll at school, was active in sports, and had been commended by her teachers for her creative talents in art and short story writing. There was no history of any serious behavioral problems or abuse of drugs or alcohol.

At the emergency room the girl's vital signs were stable, although there was some flushing of the face and a full, somewhat rapid pulse. Her breath smelled of beer. Urinalysis showed the presence of a moderate amount of alcohol but was otherwise normal. The alcohol blood level was well below the legal intoxication level.

The girl had admitted to the emergency room physician that she had been drinking beer. A beer party had been arranged by a victorious school football team in a park within walking distance of the girl's home. She and her girlfriend had arranged to go and with premeditation drank six cans of beer "just to see what it was like to get drunk." She admitted to getting sick prior to attempting to sneak quietly back into her bedroom.

The girl returned home with her mother, and a subsequent interview confirmed the above history and the parents were reassured. The girl continued to do well at school and eighteen months later graduated summa cum laude with subsequently a successful undergraduate career, finally being accepted into medical school.

The labeling of the adolescent as "chemically dependent" may distract from the recognition of more real adolescent psychopathology and may involve the "scienceless" oversimplification of the problem. The label of chemical dependency is often a more acceptable pseudodiagnosis to the adolescent's parents and may reflect unconscious resistance to exploration of the dynamic issues in the family or even to the genetic history of mental illness.

Case 2

A seventeen-year-old boy from a fashionable suburb was arrested by the police in a bank, where he was behaving bizarrely and had attempted to assault a woman customer. The police recognized that he was acutely psychotic, brought him directly for admission to the psychiatric unit. He was markedly regressed, in an agitated catatonic state, and needed to be restrained because of his behavior. He appeared to be actively hallucinating, and, at one point, without any provocation broke a staff member's arm. Because of the acuteness of the psychosis and the danger to himself and others, an emergency dose of an antipsychotic agent was administered.

When his parents arrived, having been contacted by the police, they were immediately incensed, pointing out that their son was chemically dependent and should not have been given a mood-altering medication. Subsequent history from them indicated that he had become gradually withdrawn over a period of six months with bizarre behavior, loosely associated conversation, impulsive assaultive behavior toward his pregnant mother, and had mentioned hearing voices and had felt himself to be influenced by electronic rays from the family's television. He had been admitted by the parents to several drug treatment programs in the previous three months, but had dropped out almost immediately before any assessment could be undertaken. The parents remained convinced that his behavior was secondary to the use of street hallucinogens, although they had never seen him in possession of drugs, and they reported he did not associate with drug-using peers at school.

What motivates the adolescent to take drugs? Or is the drug use merely a currently popular mode of finding new experiences that differs from and defies the establishment? Does the increased popularity of drugs among adolescents reflect serious psychopathology? There is certainly evidence that drug abuse in adolescents, in the majority of cases, appears to be a transient phenomenon resulting from the particular developmental stresses of that period. It may represent rebellious acting out and defiance toward parents, and in some cases, it may be a conscious decision to use the drug, not to relax or transcend a crisis situation, as might be the case in adult use, but rather to discover what kind of new sensation it produces and to see whether the individual can measure up and somehow master this dangerous new adventure.

In an attempt to explore the psychological reasons why young people, many of whom place a high premium on intellectual functioning, took drugs that were potentially dangerous to the mind, some college students who had taken LSD were investigated. Findings included the following: the initial experience with LSD usually resulted from the information from a peer who reported pleasurable reactions to the use of the drug; the influence of a roommate or friend carried more weight than newspaper articles and reports concerning the dangers of the drugs or rumors about psychotic breakdowns. In the minds of the students, the promises about what the drug could do for them far outweighed the risk. The expectation was that the drug could make them overcome a sense of loneliness, help them feel love for others, and be more socially and sexually effective, as well as more productive and creative. Many also felt the drug might fill a moral and spiritual void. When college students finally discovered the drug's failure to meet these expectations, the use of LSD on college campuses rapidly declined, and today marijuana and alcohol, and to a lesser extent cocaine, are more widely used.

There are more and more data being compiled on the relationship between drug abuse in adolescents and the dysfunctional family. The parents may unconsciously foster drug abuse to resolve their own conflicts over the adolescent's impending separation from the family. Drugs hold out the promise of magical solutions, and their use is clearly related to the ambivalence of both the child and the parents about separation. The youngster's symptomatology may validate the parents' fantasy that the child is helpless, dependent, socially incompetent, and not yet ready to matriculate into adulthood. In some cases the parents may simply derive vicarious gratification from the adolescent's drug abuse. The parents' role in placing the youngster in an institutional program may represent an unconscious need for control. As mentioned earlier, the youngster may take a shortcut in the path of adolescence by settling for a pseudoidentity—for example, as an "alcoholic"—while other adolescents may embrace drug abuse as a diversionary tactic for holding the parents together in their crumbling marriage. The antisocial behavior of the child may preserve psychological homeostasis for the parents and an interpersonal balance for the family. With the above in mind, it is crucial that the developmental history and current family dynamics be explored in attempting to understand the basis for the youngster's drug-abuse symptomatology. Commonly the feeling of rejection by the family may bring about a reactive depression, and the lack of an affectionate, trusting relationship may cause the adolescent to attempt to compensate with a purely counterfeit closeness and acceptance in a drug-using peer group.

Many psychiatrists feel that drug abuse in adolescence always is a symptom of underlying emotional turmoil or ego deficit. Drugs may be used in a variety of ways as a transient, occasional, recurrent, or chronic phenomenon. Their use may be concealed from the parents or they may be flaunted in a provocative manner. Borderline and prepsychotic adolescents may rely on drugs to shore up and supply controls and gratifications. Drugs may be used as a "structural prosthesis" or a crutch for the vulnerable ego. During adolescence there is a regressive resurgence of archaic childhood fears and wishes that may temporarily raise the threat of loss of social adaptation, rationality, and maturity. Drugs may be seen to hold out the magic panacea for this distress.

Conflicts in certain stages of early personality development, "fixations" in Freudian terminology, may come to the surface again in adolescence. It has been suggested that the blissful satiation of marijuana may symbolize a narcissistic regressive phenomenon of the earlier symbiotic maternal relationship while amphetamine abuse may be an attempt to recreate the experience of the second year of life where the toddler who discovers walking is elated with his seemingly magical omnipotence.

Drugs produce pharmacologically for the adolescent the reduction of distress that the individual cannot achieve by his or her own psychic efforts. The adolescent is not interested in the drug itself but in the experience it produces. The concept is worth considering that adolescent drug abuse is a transitional experience to deal with the turmoil of adolescence. During early childhood the still incomplete personality structure, in the early stages of separation from the nurturing mother, may use a transitional object to relieve anxiety. A teddy bear or special blanket may suffice as a maternal substitute to bolster the still incomplete personality structure and maintain psychic stability. This transitional object compensates for the immaturity of the ego until its functions have developed. During adolescence drugs may be used as the transitional experience in the transitional phenomenon that is adolescence.

During the Viet Nam conflict there was well-documented use of hard narcotics, including heroin and opium, among American servicemen. As in any war in any culture, usually the majority of the fighting force are late adolescents. Following the rundown of that conflict, our government was concerned with the possible epidemic of the use of hard narcotics among returning veterans. Previous studies had shown that individuals who had become dependent on narcotics had an extremely low success rate in rehabilitation programs even with the most intensive treatment efforts. Millions of dollars were set aside in the federal budget to cope with the expected return of these seriously physically dependent youths. Happily, the threat never materialized, and the vast majority of these young men were able to be received back into a culture without any continuing narcotic abuse. Again, it would appear that the drug abuse was merely a transitional phenomenon occurring as a result of unusual transient, psychosocial stress in a battle situation in an alien culture and environment.

The distinction between psychotic episodes produced by hallucinogenic drugs and functional psychoses derived from schizophrenic illness often produces particular diagnostic difficulties during adolescence. The incidence of schizophrenia tends to peak in adolescents in the same age framework where adolescent drug abuse is also common. In fact, the old terminology for schizophrenia, *dementia praecox* or adolescent dementia, reflects this observation. As noted in the previous case example, a genuine schizophrenic illness can be labeled as a drug abuse phenomenon because it meets the psychological needs of the family to see it as such. However, there are situations where toxic psychosis, specifically amphetamine psychosis, may exactly mimic paranoid schizophrenia. The clinical picture of amphetamine abuse may include paranoid delusions, auditory hallucinations, assaultive behavior, and extreme anxiety. In particular, amphetamines may be dangerous in uncovering underlying aggressive impulses which may be acted out in the period of intoxication with the drug, sometimes with fatal results.

Case 3

A youth thrown out of his home a week earlier because of repeated drug abuse decided to celebrate his seventeenth birthday by "really getting stoned." He began by drinking beer, continued with several joints of marijuana, then, by his report, consumed six tablets of an amphetamine type drug. He invited a fifteen-year-old girl back to his newfound apartment, and on impulse without any premeditation whatsoever, picked up a knife from a nearby table and stabbed her to death.

The chronically depressed adolescent may also go unrecognized because of overly repeated drug abuse.

Case 4

An eighteen-year-old male with a four-year history of drug abuse had been referred by his divorced mother to a series of drug treatment programs, but returned to drugs shortly after discharge. As a result of several suicidal gestures, including attempting to throw himself in front of a car, jump off a bridge, and cut his wrists, he had been admitted to several adolescent psychiatric units. Invariably his divorced mother, who was pathologically overprotective of him, would sabotage any attempts to develop an alliance with him in individual psychotherapy and would sign him out of the psychiatric unit against medical advice. Following such a withdrawal from a hospital setting, he was found dead of carbon monoxide poisoning in his mother's car on Mother's Day. The mother later unsuccessfully sued the hospital for malpractice.

We must keep in mind the differences between drug abuse in teenagers and that in adults. The causes of drug abuse in adolescents range from the search for new experiences to a response to the pressures and uncertainties of adolescence. Adolescents respond more readily to individual psychotherapy, which usually needs to be directed at something other than the drug problem per se. Helping the youngster recognize areas of unconscious conflict, particularly in the parent-child relationship, together with an empathic approach in helping the adolescent bring anger and depression to the surface, may yield dramatic results.

Appealing to the adolescent's sense of idealism and offering a set of alternative activities to drug abuse may also be useful. Introducing the youngster to other experiences which can contribute to self-reliance and which offer physical, mental, or emotional satisfaction may also be needed. These experiences would include such things as specific recreational activities, esthetic appreciation, learning, spiritual exercises, as well as social and political activities.

Treatment Considerations

In the adolescent where the presenting problem appears to be alcohol or substance abuse, obviously a detailed history from the young person is required, including details about the dose and frequency of use of the primary drug of abuse. Alcohol and marijuana seem to be more common among older adolescents including college students, the latter occasionally also using cocaine. In earlier adolescence, in the twelve and thirteen age group, one will occasionally see youngsters using inhalants such as glue or gasoline, but this is rare in older adolescents. One should attempt to get a picture of whether the youngster feels he or she does indeed have a problem with drug or alcohol use and at what age drug use began. The frequency of use and the conscious rationale for using the drug should also be explored. Are the drugs used at school or on the job, and is the use the result of pressure from peers or because of an association with a particular friend? One should also inquire as to whether the young person has been in trouble with the legal system because of drug abuse, including citations for driving while under the influence of intoxicants. It is important also to get some feeling as to whether the adolescent is using the drug as a form of self-medication. Schizoid, withdrawn youngsters may find that marijuana or even amphetamines appear to help them socialize. One should inquire whether the drugs are used only in company or when the individual is alone. Occasionally an adolescent will claim to have used a multitude of street drugs and present a list with an air of provocativeness and bravado. Asking about the subjective effects of the various intoxicants may give some help in deciding whether the youngster in fact has used drugs or is exaggerating in an attention-seeking tactic. One often finds that a drug will be used only once, perhaps experimentally in a very small dose, although at first it is presented as if it is being used regularly.

As in any other interaction for therapeutic purposes with adolescents, it is important to gain the youngster's confidence and not to allow oneself to be provoked by the often defiant and limit-testing behavior that is common in the early stages of the first interview.

Having gotten as clearly as possible an idea of what, in reality, the adolescent is using and how often and in what context, one should then take a more complete history. It should include an early childhood history, relationships with family and peers, together with a past medical history, including any serious physical or mental conditions, and whether the individual has been hospitalized or is on any prescribed medication. In the family history, exploring the relationship with parents and siblings is important, as well as attempting to get some feel for any unusual tensions in the home, such as conflict between the parents or an impending breakup in the parents' marriage.

It is hoped that by the end of the first interview, one can have some idea of what lies behind the presenting problem. Later interviews will usually clarify dynamic considerations. If the youngster's drug abuse is chronic, repetitive, seriously interfering with functioning, including academic work at school, and he or she is unable to muster impulse controls to discontinue the drug, it may be necessary to have the youngster admitted preferably to a hospital setting such as an adolescent psychiatric unit. There external controls will provide a drug-free milieu and an opportunity for undertaking further diagnostic assessment. Immediately on admission it is often a good idea to have a sample of urine subjected to a chemical screen so that one can have some actual objective evidence of what, in fact, the youngster has been taking. Later on, psychological testing including the MMPI and other projective tests such as the Rorschach may be useful. A detailed history from an interview with both parents is often necessary in understanding the family dynamics that may be contributing to the substance-abuse disorder.

More and more evidence is surfacing to point to the ineffectiveness of using, for teenagers, programs designed primarily for adult alcoholism. Many such programs, while working well for adults, use chemical dependency counselors who vary in their knowledge of adolescent developmental processes and psychopathology. It is important that youngsters not be shortchanged by being placed in programs that, at best, they do not need and which, at worst, are not equipped to recognize serious adolescent psychopathology, such as suicidal depression and schizophrenia.

In many cases a short period of individual psychotherapy, perhaps with adjunctive family therapy on an outpatient basis, is all that is needed. Adolescents generally do not respond to a rigid authoritarian approach and coercive treatment, sometimes under the threat of being expelled from school unless the youngster satisfactorily completes a drug treatment program. One often comes across adolescents who have been through a series of programs, having been summarily discharged because of their failure to comply with a philosophy of treatment that is essentially one of behavior-modification orientation.

In summary, the successful counseling of drug-abusing adolescents and their families must rest in a detailed exploration of family dynamics with an attempt at some form of psychotherapy to resolve the underlying conflict resulting in the drug abuse. The old medical dictum *primum non nocere*, "first do no harm," should always guide us in judging the risk-benefit factors in deciding on the indications or contraindications for any form of coercive treatment for adolescents with a history of drug abuse. Above all, we must remain flexible in designing a treatment plan, resisting any rigid, dogmatic approach and remembering the words of H. L. Mencken: "For any complex problem there is always a simple solution, which is always wrong."

REFERENCES

Egan, Katherine. *Youth Experience "Drug/Alcohol Rehabilitation": An Interactionist Perspective.* Dissertation, Syracuse University, June 1978.

Hartmann, Dora. *A Study of Drug-Taking Adolescents.* Topeka: Bulletin of the Menninger Clinic, 1969, 384–97.

McCafferty, C., Cline D., & Jordan, J. Issues in the psychiatric approach to substance abuse in adolescents, *Psychiatric Annals* II (8), August 1981.

McCafferty, Charles. Adolescent murder, *Adolescent Health Care, Clinical Issues,* Robert M. Blum, ed. New York: Academic Press, 1982, chapter 27.

Meeks, John E. *Psychiatric Treatment of the Adolescent: Comprehensive Textbook of Psychiatry II,* vol. 2, 2nd ed., 2262–69.

Nicholi, Armand M., Jr., ed. *The Harvard Guide to Modern Psychiatry.* Cambridge: Harvard University Press, 1978.

Sederberg, Rick. *Adolescent Drug Use—Epidemic or Epicurean?* Minneapolis: Minnesota Behavioral Institute.

Setle, Peter, & Sherman, Charles L. Adult alcoholism regimen said useless for teenagers, *Psychiatric News,* March 5, 1982.

Wieder, Herbert, & Kaplan, Eugene H. *Drug Use in Adolescents.* Topeka: Bulletin of the Menninger Clinic, 1969, 399–430.

7

Alcoholism

JOSEPH CIARROCCHI

No area of pastoral care better validates the emerging identity of pastoral counseling than alcoholism. No field provides more opportunity to demonstrate the usefulness of a pastoral counseling model that goes beyond the role of a "mental health affiliate" and accepts its place within a multimodal approach to an enormously complex illness. Indeed, the points of convergence for this model, as outlined by Estadt (cf. chapter 2), with the modern understanding of the illness are many and varied.

Alcoholism is one public health problem that is interdisciplinary in fact as well as concept. Although widely accepted as a major health problem, this illness permits specialists from many different disciplines, medical and nonmedical, to contribute their expertise, thereby augmenting everyone's understanding of this illness. Although it is normal for tensions to occur, professionals collaborate increasingly in alcoholism research and treatment. Pastoral counselors are as easily drawn into this effort as any other professional discipline. Further, the unabashedly spiritual nature of the most influential self-help group, Alcoholics Anonymous, provides a hospitable environ for the transpersonal dimension central to the task of pastoral ministry. Finally, an interdisciplinary effort permits the pastoral counselor to appreciate alcoholism in the context of a systems model because it is a devastating societal illness. The pastoral counselor, because he or she is involved in the system at points inaccessible to even the most creative mental health professional, may ultimately be the most influential resource in terms of system intervention.

Effective pastoral ministry, however, will depend upon knowledge and skill, and the pastoral care functions of guiding, healing, reconciling, and sustaining (cited by Estadt, chapter 2) certainly describe well the pastoral counselor's role with regard to alcoholism counseling.

The present chapter can only highlight some of the more important concepts regarding alcoholism. Detailed descriptions of the pastoral counseling process itself with the alcoholic are described elsewhere (Ciarrocchi, 1983; Clinebell, 1978).

Scope of the problem

The economic and human toll of alcohol-related problems generates statistical data that, like the national debt, defy the mind's ability to interpret. One study estimates that in a single year, the economic effects of alcohol-related problems cost United States society $42 billion (*Alcohol and Health,* 1981). The breakdown occurs along the following lines: $19 billion in lost production, $12.5 billion in health and medical costs, $5 billion in motor vehicle accident costs, $2.5 billion in violent crime costs, and $2 billion in other costs such as fire losses. The toll in terms of human suffering is not calculable by empirical methods.

Public health specialists measure the medical impact of the disease in two ways: mortality and morbidity. Mortality refers to the disease's impact on loss of life. From this perspective, alcoholism ranks third in the United States as the leading cause of death, behind cancer and cardiovascular conditions. However, in terms of morbidity, that is, a disease's ability to produce symptoms severe enough for medical treatment, alcoholism ranks as the number one health problem in the United States (Selzer, 1980). Recent investigations have also triggered a new wave of concern by linking maternal alcohol consumption during pregnancy to a variety of birth defects in the newborn. These studies have generated widespread publicity in the media. While the more dramatic consequences of heavy drinking, for example, growth retardation, facial abnormalities, and deficient cognitive development, are better known as fetal alcohol syndrome (FAS), more modest alcohol consumption in mothers is related to other significant, if less striking, fetal anomalies. These lesser irregularities are termed fetal alcohol effects (FAE) and include effects such as behavior and learning problems despite normal intelligence, milder facial irregularities, and other organ damage (Little, Graham, & Samson, 1982). Also disturbing are recent reports that cite the increased risk of spontaneous abortion for women drinking as little as one to two drinks daily to be double that of non-drinking mothers (Harlap & Shiomo, 1980). As these latter authors note, the medical profession has been remiss in reminding expectant mothers that alcohol is, after all is said and done, a toxin.

Alcohol-related problems also have societal impact beyond health issues. Alcohol is related to the whole spectrum of violent behavior and accidents. High level of alcohol intake is related to one-fourth of all suicides, half of all homicides, half of all traffic fatalities, 45 percent of all rapes, 40 percent of fatal industrial accidents, nearly 70 percent of drownings, plus strong associations with child and spouse abuse. The domestic impact, of course, is also considerable. The rate of divorce where alcoholism is present in at least one partner is considerably higher than for the general population, with estimates as high as 40 percent. Conversely, separated and divorced persons are likely to have higher rates of alcoholism (Nace, 1982).

Common misconceptions

Misconceptions about alcoholism are likely to impede treatment efforts, and pastoral counselors are as susceptible to these misconceptions as any member of the helping profession.

ALCOHOLISM IS A SYMPTOM

A belief natural to a psychodynamic model of human behavior holds that alcoholism is the symptomatic expression of a severe personality conflict or problem. Such a model is more interested in the supposed underlying causes of behavior rather than the mere symptom, i.e., the drinking. While such a model has widespread acceptance for many disorders, it has not demonstrated much utility in treating alcoholics. The model ignores the powerful reinforcing properties, both psychological and physiological, of the chemical. While many alcoholics suffer from a host of difficulties, few such problems can be seriously addressed as long as the alcoholic is actively drinking. Furthermore, treatment strategies based on a psychodynamic model have had little success in solving either the maladaptive drinking or its related problems.

RECOVERY IS THE ABSENCE OF DRINKING

For many years alcoholism treatment has been evaluated in terms of one dimension only: sobriety. Treatment success has been judged by the length of sobriety. More complex evaluation methods, however, now suggest that recovery is multidimensional—that a variety of criteria constitute recovery in addition to merely not drinking. For example, these methods can discriminate between groups of sober alcoholics who are employed at full capacity, maintain varied social and recreational activities, function adequately in their families and relationships, and achieve a reasonable measure of good physical health, from those groups of sober alcoholics who do not meet these performance levels (Pattison, Sobell, & Sobell, 1977). Treatment programs have adjusted their goals and strategies accordingly to attain the multiplicity of goals noted here, in addition to the traditional one of sobriety.

A RIGID SEQUENCE OF SYMPTOMS

"She can't be an alcoholic; she hasn't sold her body yet." This statement was made by a husband in defense of his wife's drinking patterns to her concerned friends. The implication here is that there are rigid diagnostic criteria for alcoholism and no intervention is required until they are met. In one sense such a stance arises from the denial mechanism that is characteristic of the illness. For example, in the above case, the friends were too discreet to remind the husband that when intoxicated his wife gave her body away and that selling her body was therefore unlikely. At another level many view alcoholism as a discrete entity, characterized by a rigid sequence of symptoms. If the behavior patterns have not emerged, neither has the illness.

An emerging concept, however, suggests that alcohol-related problems involve a continuum of difficulties concerning health issues, social and occupational functioning, legal/normative behavior, and psychological well-being. This emerging concept suggests that intervention and treatment may be appropriate at any point, as long as alcohol is related to significant life problems.

MOTIVATION FOR TREATMENT

"No one can be helped unless he wants to be." This adage is a truism among counselors and therapists and has reached the status of an inviolable precept. Alcoholism is one human problem that violates this maxim. Since denial is the underlying characteristic of the illness, many alcoholics lack the necessary "motivation" to enter treatment. Consequently, many alcoholics die without treatment, since they refuse to seek help on their own initiative. Many years ago industry learned that excellent recovery rates were obtained for alcoholics who were "forced" into treatment through threat of loss of employment. Rather than hire new employees, thus requiring expensive retraining programs, industry found that their alcoholic employees could return to their jobs with significantly improved productivity after recovery. Since industrial managers were not trained as mental health professionals, they did not know their approach violated basic counseling wisdom.

This experience has led to carefully conceived intervention strategies toward treatment for alcoholics, which will be described below. The pastoral minister can be most helpful in assisting families and colleagues of alcoholics in putting significant "pressure" on alcoholics to enter treatment, without being harsh or violating the alcoholic's personal freedom.

Basic concepts and diagnosis

Traditionally addiction to any kind of drug has been defined as substance use resulting in dependence and/or tolerance. Dependence may be physiological or psychological. Physiological dependence refers to the characteristic withdrawal effects that come with cessation of intake of a drug. In the case of alcohol, these effects range from mild to severe reactions: tremors, vomiting, nausea, sweating, anxiety, increased heart rate, elevated blood pressure, delirium, hallucinations, etc. Psychological dependence involves a felt need for the drug, despite its many untoward complications. This dependence is not necessarily generated by the chemical properties of the substance. Rather the expectancy or psychological set generates this dependence, which influences the person to attribute special properties to the substance. In other words, some individuals resonate to the mood-altering properties of alcohol and find its effects powerfully rewarding, while others, experiencing the same effects, do not develop this craving.

Tolerance refers to the necessity of increasing the amount of drug consumed over time in order to achieve the same mood-altering effects. Depending upon the particular drug, tolerance may develop rapidly or slowly. A related phenomenon is cross-tolerance, the ability to substitute one drug in a class for another in the same class, and so prevent withdrawal. For example, heroin addicts turn to inexpensive alcoholic beverages during periods of decreased drug supply to prevent heroin withdrawal. In this instance, alcohol, a central nervous system depressant, prevents withdrawal from heroin, which is also a central nervous system depressant. Many alcoholics in our society are cross-addicted, for example, employing an early morning Valium pill to overcome the inevitable withdrawal effects. This gives them a socially acceptable means of preventing morning shakes, rather than resorting to the taboo morning drink, which even the least enlightened drinker realizes reflects alcoholic behavior. This pattern also characterizes women drinkers in the

United States to a greater extent than men, possibly because there is less social stigma attached to using pills and/or decreased tolerance to alcohol (Gomberg, 1979). This "balance" of alcohol and pills allows the chemically dependent person to maintain a state of mood equilibrium while avoiding the socially disapproved consequences of heavy alcohol intake.

DIAGNOSIS

Several systems have established criteria for the diagnosis of alcoholism, including the World Health Organization (WHO), the National Council on Alcoholism (NCA), and the *Diagnostic and Statistical Manual* (3rd ed.) of the American Psychiatric Association (DSM-III, 1980). DSM-III recognizes two classes of alcoholic disorders, which are labeled substance use disorders: alcohol abuse and alcohol dependence. The advantage of DSM-III is that it presents straightforward criteria and recognizes that some patterns of alcohol use, while not technically speaking dependent patterns, are nevertheless severe disorders warranting treatment.

Alcohol abuse is defined as a pattern of pathological use of alcohol, lasting at least a month, and causing impairment in social or occupational functioning. The following represent the criteria for a pattern of pathological use of alcohol:

1. Need for daily use of alcohol for adequate functioning
2. Inability to cut down or stop drinking
3. Repeated efforts to control or reduce excessive drinking by "going on the wagon" (periods of temporary abstinence) or restricting drinking to certain times of the day
4. Binges (remaining intoxicated throughout the day for at least two days)
5. Occasional consumption of a fifth of spirits (or its equivalent in wine or beer)
6. Amnesia for events occurring while intoxicated (blackouts)
7. Continuation of drinking despite a serious physical disorder that the individual knows is exacerbated by alcohol use
8. Drinking of non-beverage alcohol

Similarly, impairment in social or occupational functioning due to alcohol use includes the following:

1. Violence while intoxicated
2. Absence from work
3. Loss of job
4. Legal difficulties (for example, arrests for intoxicated behavior, traffic accidents while intoxicated)
5. Arguments or difficulties with family or friends because of alcohol use

Alcohol dependence (alcoholism) is defined as either a pattern of pathological use or *impairment in social or occupational functioning plus either tolerance or withdrawal.* Some researchers are criticizing these formulations on technical, empirical grounds, saying that, by definition, the system tends to diagnose alcohol dependence more frequently than abuse, which appears to lack face validity. Nonetheless, the definitions are useful in describing more than one pattern of alcohol misuse requiring treatment. No counselor should be locked into any one set of symptoms or any rigid "progression" of the disease, since research demonstrates many patterns (Pattison, Sobell, & Sobell, 1977).

The hidden nature of the illness, as well as the drinker's own denial system, complicate the diagnostic process. The pastoral counselor, in a similar vein, faces the necessity of making practical decisions concerning intervention. Traditional diagnostic systems generally focus on symptoms related to advanced alcohol tolerance and are not as useful for decisions concerning early intervention or alcohol problems where loss of control is not an issue. While never easy to intervene, the counselor at least has greater confidence when faced with a drinker who clearly meets the DSM-III criteria or some other similar diagnostic system. Great problems arise, for example, when the person "has never lost a day of work," is physically healthy, but whose drinking is associated with severe marital and family crises.

A more current approach is to see alcohol problems associated with use, misuse, and abuse (Pattison & Kaufman, 1982). In this model alcoholism is seen as a syndrome, a cluster of signs and symptoms constituting a disease, rather than a single, clearly-defined entity. In this regard problems associated with a wide variety of drinking patterns may require intervention by the pastoral counselor.

Alcohol *use,* distinct from dependent patterns, may result in physical abuse, psychological deterioration, legal difficulties, or social ostracism. For example, an elderly parishioner might enjoy his dinner wine, but cerebral deterioration will maximize motor coordination problems, creating risk of injury from falling. The concerned family might enlist the minister's aid, but to approach this gentleman as an "alcoholic" is neither clinically helpful nor scientifically precise.

Through the *misuse* of alcohol, drinkers justify socially unacceptable behavior. For example, a married man has an adulterous affair or abuses his wife or child only "when under the influence." Once again, alcohol dependency may not be an issue, but its adverse consequences are; certainly the minister must address the person's alcohol misuse directly if he or she is to deal effectively with the problem. Labeling the behavior "alcoholism" would not be the best approach here either.

Finally, the *abuse* pattern involves true dependence along with severe consequences. This pattern most closely reflects the traditional definition of alcoholism and its attendant symptoms—morning drinks, denial, gulping drinks, sneaking drinks, blackouts, protecting the supply—and may include adverse physical consequences.

CAUSES OF ALCOHOLISM

The mechanisms of addiction are not at all understood. About 50 percent of people who experiment with drugs other than alcohol never repeat the experiment. Ten percent of those who drink develop alcoholism, yet 30 percent of tobacco users become dependent, an addiction rate higher than heroin.

Investigators focus on several influences in the etiology of alcoholism. Constitutional factors have long been suspected, but their exact relationship is still not clear. Alcoholism is well known to run in families, but only in the last few years has research indicated inheritance as a factor. This has been elucidated through adoption studies which demonstrate that children whose biological parents are alcoholic, when adopted by nonalcoholic parents, develop alcoholism three to four times more than adopted children whose biological parents are nonalcoholic (Goodwin, 1981).

If alcoholism is inherited, what factor is transmitted that accounts for its development? Many have been investigated, in particular certain groups' "intolerance" of alcohol (for example, Orientals), which is physiologically measurable and documented in the newborn. This intolerance appears related to a low incidence of alcoholism in such groups. Some would speculate further that groups with high rates of alcoholism inherit a lack of this intolerance for alcoholism and hence can consume large quantities without feeling the effects, thus laying the groundwork for alcohol dependence.

Sociocultural and environmental factors are also implicated in the etiology of alcoholism and associated drinking problems. For example, ethnic groups that encourage daily drinking may have high rates of liver disease and other medical problems, but fewer alcohol-related accidents, violence, or crime. Groups that encourage binge drinking are more likely to have higher accident and crime rates, but fewer medical conditions (Heath, 1982). Ethnic groups that associate alcohol consumption solely with religious ritual would also show different patterns from groups that use it for times of conviviality or initiation into adulthood.

Finally, investigators have expended much energy trying to identify the "alcoholic personality" in the search for causes of alcoholism. It is now fairly clear that no such personality exists, that earlier studies are flawed in not distinguishing between the causes and effects of alcoholism in relationship to one's personality. Individual differences that have emerged relate to less global, but perhaps ultimately more meaningful characteristics. Nonalcoholics, for example, differ from alcoholics in their ability to discriminate blood alcohol levels without training. Further, nonalcoholics used both internal and external cues to discriminate blood alcohol levels, while alcoholics utilize only external cues (Lipscomb and Nathan, 1980). Ability or inability to tell "when one has had enough" may be useful diagnostically as a marker of high tolerance.

Other laboratory investigations demonstrate that persons will drink more alcohol when provoked to anger and under frustration, even when the alcoholic beverage is so disguised as to be imperceptible (Marlatt, Kosturn, & Long, 1975). Identifying such antecedents to problem-drinking behavior is no doubt more useful to the counselor in helping recovering alcoholics than lists of alcoholic "traits" of dubious validity. For example, altering an alcoholic's "desire to control" is a vague therapeutic task, whereas training the alcoholic to be more assertive in anger-provoking situations permits greater specificity of therapeutic goals.

Treatment

SETTING

Alcoholics are treated in a variety of settings, the most popular of which for middle class patients is residential, intermediate care. These programs may be attached to a general or psychiatric hospital or be independent (free-standing), and residents generally stay twenty-eight days. The length of stay is largely dictated by the limits placed on reimbursement for alcoholism treatment by health insurance carriers. Programs differ in philosophy, but most have common features. After detoxification has occurred, the patient typically participates in a highly structured schedule, including group sessions, lectures, and films related to alcohol or chemical dependency, individual counseling, and participation in Alcoholics Anonymous meetings. Most programs emphasize family participation and arrange for counseling sessions and education with the patient and his or her family. Medical evaluation and care are provided according to staff resources and specialized mental health personnel; for example, psychiatrists or psychologists may be available as consultants.

Halfway houses provide less in the way of structured programming, but offer recovering alcoholics temporary residence as they are reintegrated with family or job. Sobriety is one criterion for continued residence, along with active A.A. participation.

Alcoholics are also treated in nonresidential outpatient settings. Innovative methods have developed due to some insurance carriers' dropping residential alcoholism treatment from their coverage. Some programs offer day treatment, a special convenience for homemakers or not fully employed persons. These programs have schedules similar to residential treatment schedules. An alternative approach provides a full therapeutic program every evening for the employed person, so that no occupational break is necessary while receiving treatment. Once again, treatment is intense, comprising four to five hours nightly, and including the traditional therapeutic component. Aside from the reduced cost of such programs, other positive features include intensive treatment while the alcoholic deals with day-to-day problems as they occur in their real-life setting, plus greater opportunity to involve families in treatment. The disadvantage is that some alcoholics' problems may be related to harsh environmental stress and require respite from these factors. While many may consider such programs "diluted" in contrast to residential treatment, research to date is not definitive. Some data suggest outpatient treatment is effective for many (Schuckit, 1979). What remains unclear is which treatment works for which population.

If the pastoral minister plays a significant role in the life of an alcoholic or the alcoholic's family, most programs will welcome the minister's participation in the treatment process as part of the alcoholic's extended family. Since most programs provide after-care components for a number of weeks following the intensive treatment phase, the knowledgeable minister can easily be incorporated as a resource person for the long-term support of the recovering alcoholic.

METHODS

Probably every known approach in the behavioral and medical sciences has been used at one time or another in alcoholism treatment. Individual alcoholism counselors employ a variety of models, and some popular approaches have evolved based on Gestalt or transactional analysis methods (Silverstein, 1977). These approaches are also popular in pastoral counseling training programs and would not seem foreign to pastoral ministers. Ministers may be less acquainted with pharmacological or behavioral treatment methods, however.

Pharmacological treatment, for the most part, involves the daily administration of the drug disulfiram (Antabuse), which blocks alcohol metabolism resulting in accumulation of acetaldehyde in the body—in turn causing a toxic reaction. If a person drinks alcohol after taking the drug, a most unpleasant physical reaction occurs, for example, nausea and vomiting. Disulfiram is often used by family physicians or internists to treat their alcoholic patients, by some programs where the patients have a measure of freedom to come and go (for example, halfway houses), and by psychiatrists who treat alcoholics on an outpatient basis. Some drawbacks to this treatment include the need for high motivation in the alcoholic to take the drug daily, rather high noncompliance rates, and if used alone, disregard for developing new coping skills, as well as medical contraindications for some of the very conditions endemic to alcoholics: cirrhosis, diabetes mellitus, or organic brain disorders.

Behavior therapy is an umbrella term for a host of strategies ranging from electrical aversion therapies to social skills training. To further complicate matters, behavior therapists who treat alcoholism strongly disagree among themselves on the relative merits of each strategy. A consensus appears imminent, however, that electrical aversion therapies are not specifically related to positive outcome for alcoholics (Nathan, 1976). Chemical aversion therapies are another matter. The procedure involves injecting the alcoholic with emetine, an emetic drug, whereupon the alcoholic sees, smells, and tastes a favorite alcoholic beverage. The administration of the drug is so timed that nausea and vomiting follow the alcohol presentation. Conditioning theory predicts that repeating this experience several times results in the unpleasant association to alcohol, thereby facilitating abstinence. Several hospital groups treating alcoholics have used this method as their primary treatment mode. Descriptions of the treatment method frequently generate negative reactions among some alcoholism professionals, but nevertheless there exists an impressive array of empirical data documenting its effectiveness (Bandura, 1969).

More recent behavioral strategies in alcoholism treatment focus on treatment "packages," that is, combining various behavioral techniques to combat the human problems associated with excessive alcohol consumption. Young drinkers or drinkers in the earliest stages of problem drinking may be taught to assess their alcohol intake through blood alcohol level discrimination training. Alcoholics themselves may be taught self-monitoring techniques to assess the different emotions that trigger the craving for alcohol. Specific strategies based on this assessment are then taught. For example, if excessive anxiety is related to alcohol consumption, the patient will be taught relaxation methods either through self-regulated means or assisted through biofeedback. Depression may be treated through cognitive behavioral methods or establishing reinforcing events (Beck, Rush, & Shaw, 1979; Lewinsohn, 1981). Since research has established that interpersonal anxiety is related to relapse, social skills and/or assertiveness training may be emphasized (Cummings, Gordon, & Marlatt, 1980). If marital difficulties or unemployment appear to be associated with excessive drinking, specific behavioral marriage counseling is employed or structured groups such as the "job-finding club" may be utilized (Azrin, Naster, & Jones, 1973; Azrin, Flores, & Kaplan, 1975). Behavioral approaches, therefore, rely on very highly individualized assessment of the antecedents to drinking behavior followed by specific treatment strategies to cope with these negative events.

Role of the pastoral counselor

From a practical standpoint most pastoral counselors, unless they choose a specialty in alcoholism counseling, will not be involved in the acute treatment phase of the alcoholic. Their more common involvement will center on the family issues, in particular preintervention, intervention, and recovery phases.

PREINTERVENTION

Initially the minister becomes involved with either the alcoholic or some family member. At times alcohol will be identified quickly as the major problem, but often the minister begins helping the family and only gradually uncovers alcoholism as the difficulty. The minister's role is to clarify for the family the part alcohol plays in the family dysfunction. This task is quite difficult in that not only does the alcoholic defend him- or herself through denial but so do the family members. Once this task is accomplished, the family is left with three choices: to continue as is, to keep the family together and learn to distance themselves emotionally from the devastation of the illness, or to separate themselves physically and emotionally from the alcoholic (Pattison & Kaufman, 1982). The choice belongs to the family members and the minister's role is to support them as they clarify the task for themselves. The minister will rapidly experience his or her own powerlessness over the disease of alcoholism in that families will make blatantly maladaptive choices and not be receptive to guidance. In such circumstances the minister may find it helpful to follow his or her own advice and attend Al-Anon meetings, which can assist the minister in coming to terms with powerlessness over the disease.

The minister can educate the family in the dynamics of alcoholism as a family disease. The role of the family as enablers of the disease can be illustrated in an objective, non-guilt-provoking manner, which may help the members develop the strength to confront the alcoholic and recommend treatment (Kellermann, 1978). Further, the minister can educate members about the roles children frequently play and act out in alcoholic families, thereby perhaps forestalling some of the more self-defeating aspects of these roles.

INTERVENTION

Intervention involves significant family members, employers, and/or friends confronting the alcoholic with his or her alcoholic behavior with the goal of having the alcoholic accept treatment for the disease. The intervention process is well formulated and consists of three steps (Johnson, 1980). First, concerned individuals share their observations with the alcoholic despite the potential denial and anger such communication may generate. Each participant is instructed to write detailed accounts including specific behavioral observations of the alcoholic's drinking, the drinking-related behaviors, and the emotional impact these behaviors have on the participants. Preparation usually includes discussion and rehearsal of the data to be presented.

Second, members deliver their observations in a nonjudgmental manner, expressing a spirit of concern for the alcoholic's health. Presentations with a moralistic tone will only intensify the alcoholic's shame and guilt, ultimately increasing denial and rendering effective intervention less likely.

Third, since the goal of intervention is for the alcoholic to accept treatment, specific treatment options should be outlined and encouraged. Optimally a trained alcoholism counselor will be present to facilitate the intervention process. Depending on the level of denial and/or the difficulty level in motivating for treatment, the presence of the employer may be necessary to ease the alcoholic's acceptance of treatment. Many employers are quite adept at intervention based on data obtained from the work setting alone. Frequently it will be possible for a family to set up the intervention collaboratively with the employer.

The minister can fit quite naturally into the intervention process, first as a participant supporting both the alcoholic and the family, and gradually with experience and further training as facilitator of the intervention process. An excellent resource that the minister may recommend to the family at this phase, particularly to the spouse, is T. R. Drew's *Getting Them Sober*. This popularly written book provides practical advice on living with an alcoholic and in preparing oneself psychologically for the confrontation.

RECOVERY

With the alcoholic's acceptance of treatment, the minister's role may be just beginning. Certainly the minister may become involved subsequent to formal treatment in long-term pastoral counseling of the recovering alcoholic. This process may be conceptualized in developmental stages quite intricate in themselves; these are spelled out in detail elsewhere (Ciarrocchi, 1983).

Beyond helping the individual alcoholic, however, the minister may have much work left in assisting the family through the stage that has been termed "the family's recovery and reorganization" (Jackson, 1954). Now that the alcoholic is sober, family roles must be readjusted and revamped, a process which does not occur automatically or without pain and stress. Despite the dysfunctional nature of families with actively drinking alcoholics, these family units are systems nonetheless and are as resistant to change as any organization. Even dysfunctional roles are not easily surrendered, and the minister's support may be more essential during this phase than any other. The minister may be inclined to "take a breather" and leave the family alone; but in reality since the family system is so fluid at this stage, it will require delicate renegotiation of roles. Conversely, due to the stress of the years of dysfunction, the morale of family members may be at its lowest ebb, and members may have a diminished capacity to carry out this renegotiation. In such a situation there is great need for the minister's supportive role.

Conclusion

This chapter provides little more than an outline of the salient characteristics of the illness and suggests points of entry in the healing process for the pastoral counselor. Technically speaking, the pastoral counselor's role and the natural flow of recovery from alcoholism are closely allied. Once appropriately trained and supervised, therefore, the pastoral counselor will feel confident in his or her place in the process without endless scrutiny over one's identity. While sometimes ambivalent about the role of organized religion in their recovery, alcoholics themselves are often quite sophisticated in their spiritual thirst and thus open to the transpersonal "message" of the pastoral counselor. Official Churchdom's support of A.A. is also a well established tradition leading to a common saying in A.A. that alcoholism is an Irish Catholic disease, which is cured in the basements of Protestant churches.

The care of alcoholics and their families also fits well the everexpanding ministry of the pastoral counselor as outlined in this volume and elsewhere (Estadt, Blanchette, & Comptom, 1983). As pastoral counselors and ministers seek to understand their roles in the contemporary Church, alcoholism counseling and supporting the families of alcoholics permit maximum extension of these roles. The involvement of pastoral counselors with alcoholics and their families also leads to further reflection on the very nature of the pastoral counseling experience, thereby providing guideposts for the profession's future development.

REFERENCES

Alcohol and Health. Fourth special report to the United States Congress, January 1981. U.S. Department of Health and Human Services, publication no. ADM 81-1080.

Azrin, N.; Flores, T.; & Kaplan, S. Job-finding club: A group-assisted program for obtaining employment. *Behaviour Research and Therapy* 13, 17–27, 1975.

Azrin, N.; Naster, B.; & Jones, R. Reciprocity counseling: a rapid learning-based procedure for marital counseling. *Behaviour Research and Therapy* 11, 365–82, 1973.

Bandura, A. *Principles of Behavior Modification.* New York: Holt, Rinehart & Winston, 1969.

Beck, A.; Rush, A.; Shaw, B.; & Emery, G. *Cognitive Therapy of Depression.* New York: Guilford, 1979.

Ciarrocchi, J. Counseling with the recovering alcoholic. In B. Estadt; M. Blanchette; & J. Compton, eds. *The Ministry of Pastoral Counseling.* Englewood Cliffs, N.J.: Prentice-Hall, 1983.

Clinebell, H. *Understanding and Counseling the Alcoholic.* Nashville: Abingdon, 1978.

Cummings, C. J.; Gordon, J. R.; & Marlatt, A. Relapse: Prevention and predition. In W. Miller, ed., *The Addictive Behaviors: Treatment of Alcoholism, Drug Abuse, Smoking, and Obesity.* Oxford: Pergamon Press, 1980.

Diagnostic and Statistical Manual of Mental Disorders, 3rd ed. Washington: American Psychiatric Association, 1980.

Drews, T. R. *Getting Them Sober.* Plainfield, N.J.: Haven Books, 1980.

Estadt, B.; Blanchette, M.; & Compton, J. *The Ministry of Pastoral Counseling.* Englewood Cliffs, N.J.: Prentice-Hall, 1983.

Gomberg, E. Problems with alcohol and other drugs. In E. Gomberg & V. Franks, eds. *Gender and Disordered Behavior.* New York: Brunner/Mazel, 1979.

Goodwin, D. Alcoholism and Heredity. *Journal of the National Association of Private Psychiatric Hospitals* 12, 94–96, 1981.

Harlap, R., & Shiomo, P. Alcohol, smoking, and incidence of spontaneous abortions in the first and second trimester. *Lancet* 2, 173–76, 1980.

Heath, D. B. Sociocultural variants in alcoholism. In E. Pattison & E. Kaufman, eds. *Encyclopedic Handbook of Alcoholism.* New York: Gardner Press, 1982.

Jackson, J. The adjustment of the family to the crisis of alcoholism. *Quarterly Journal of the Studies of Alcohol* 15, 562–86, 1954.

Johnson, V. *I'll Quit Tomorrow.* New York: Harper & Row, 1980.

Kellermann, J. *Alcoholism: A Merry-go-round Named Denial.* Center City, Minn.: Hazelden Press, 1978.

Lewinsohn, P. Behavior treatment of depression: a social learning approach. In J. Clarkson & N. Glazer, eds. *Depression: Behavioral and Directive Intervention Strategies.* New York: Garland STPM Press, 1981.

Lipscomb, T. R., & Nathan, P. E. Effect of family history of alcoholism, drinking pattern, and tolerance on blood alcohol discrimination. *Archives of General Psychiatry* 37, 571–76, 1980.

Little, R.; Grahan, J.; & Samson, H. Fetal alcohol effects in humans and animals. *Advances in Alcohol and Substance Abuse* 1 (3): 103–25, 1982.

Marlatt, A.; Kosturn, F.; & Long, R. Provocation to anger and opportunity for retaliation as determinants of alcohol consumption in social drinkers. *Journal of Abnormal Psychology* 84, 652–59, 1975.

Nace, E. Therapeutic approaches to the alcoholic marriage. *Psychiatric Clinics of North America* 5 (3): 543–64, 1982.

Nathan, P. Alcoholism. In H. Leitenberg, ed. *Handbook of Behavior Modification.* New York: Appleton-Century-Crofts, 1976.

Pattison, E., & Kaufman, E. The alcoholism syndrome: definitions and models. In E. Pattison & E. Kaufman, eds. *Encyclopedic Handbook of Alcoholism.* New York: Gardner Press, 1982.

Pattison, E.; Sobell, M.; & Sobell, L. *Emerging Concepts of Alcohol Abuse.* New York: Springer, 1977.

Schuckit, M. Treatment of alcoholism in office and outpatient setting, and inpatient and residential approaches to the treatment of alcoholism. In J. Mendelson & N. Mello, eds. *The Diagnosis and Treatment of Alcoholism.* New York: McGraw-Hill, 1979.

Selzer, M. Alcoholism and alcoholic psychoses. In H. Kaplan; A. Freedman; & B. Sadock, eds. *Comprehensive Textbook of Psychiatry,* 3rd ed. Baltimore: Williams & Wilkins, 1980.

Silverstein, L. *Consider the Alternative.* Minneapolis: CompCare Publications, 1977.

Index